psychiatric
liaison nursing

authors

Anita Lewis, RN, MS
Psychiatric Nurse Consultant,
New England Medical Center,
Boston, Massachusetts
Assistant Clinical Professor in Psychiatry,
Tufts University School of Medicine
Assistant Clinical Professor,
Boston University Graduate School of Nursing

Joyce Levy, RN, MS
Psychiatric Liaison Nurse,
Associate Director, Consultation–Liaison Service
The Cambridge Hospital,
Cambridge, Massachusetts
Lecturer on Psychiatry,
Harvard Medical School
Assistant Clinical Professor,
Boston University Graduate School of Nursing
Adjunct Instructor,
Boston College Graduate School of Nursing

contributing authors

A Peer Group of Liaison Nurses/Greater Boston Area
Jane Barbiasz, Kathleen Blandford, Karin Byrne, Kathy Horvath,
Joyce Levy, Anita Lewis, Susan Pell Matarazzo,
Kathleen O'Meara, Linda Palmateer, and Marilyn Rossier

Kathleen Blandford, RN, MS
Clinical Director-Psychiatric Nursing,
    Mount Auburn Hospital,
    Cambridge, Massachusetts
Adjunct Instructor,
    Boston College Graduate School of Nursing
Clinical Supervisor,
    Boston University Graduate School of Nursing

Nancy Neble, RN, MS
Psychiatric Liaison Nurse,
    Beth Israel Hospital,
    Boston, Massachusetts

Janice Runzheimer, RN, MS
Psychiatric Liaison Nurse,
    Parkland Memorial Hospital,
    Dallas, Texas

Kathleen O'Meara, RN, MS
Mental Health Nurse Consultant,
    Childrens Hospital Medical Center,
    Boston, Massachusetts
Assistant Clinical Professor,
    Boston University Graduate School of Nursing

Marilyn Rossier, RN, MS
Psychiatric-Mental Health Nurse Specialist,
    Department of Psychiatry,
    The Cambridge Hospital
    Charlton Memorial Hospital,
    Fall River, Massachusetts

psychiatric liaison nursing:
the theory and clinical practice

Anita Lewis RN, MS
Joyce Levy RN, MS

Reston Publishing Company, Inc.
A Prentice-Hall Company
Reston, Virginia

Library of Congress Cataloging in Publication Data

Lewis, Anita, (date)
   Psychiatric liaison nursing.

   Includes index.
   1. Psychiatric consultation. 2. Sick—
Psychology. 3. Psychiatric nursing.
I. Levy, Joyce, (date). II. Title.
[DNLM: 1. Psychiatric nursing. WY 160 L673p]
RC455.2.C65L48   610.73'68   81-15366
ISBN 0-8359-5706-3   AACR2

Portions of Tables 2–3 and 2–4 were designed by
Nursing Staff Development at The Cambridge
Hospital.

The term *Kardex* is used with permission of
Victor Systems and Equipment, division
of Kardex Systems, Inc., Marietta, Ohio.

Editorial/production supervision and interior
   design by Norma M. Karlin
Manufacturing buyer: Ron Chapman

To Philip and Michael,
who shared in common their first experience
with sibling rivalry

contents

contents

foreword

This book demonstrates dramatically the revolution in the nursing profession which has taken place in recent decades. Moving beyond their role as providers of bedside care, in which they have worked largely as helpmates to physicians, nurses have, as Anita Lewis and Joyce Levy describe, taken responsibility for "the delivery of psychological health care in the general hospital."

Perhaps it is natural that this evolution in the functioning of nurses should eventually have taken place. Involved intimately with the physical care of patients, nurses have always needed to confront on a daily basis the emotional stresses which accompany physical illness. Thus strategically situated to experience the meaning and impact of illness as "a personal and social crisis" in the lives of patients and their families, it may have been inevitable that nurses would emerge as leaders among health care professionals in addressing the affective dimensions of medical and surgical illness and in developing new and creative approaches to the core issues of life and death that are encountered on hospital wards and intensive care units. Working in collaboration with psychiatrists and other mental health professionals, nurses have a unique opportunity to reduce for patients the emotional stress associated with physical illness. They are also ideally situated to take part in research that will add to our understanding of psychosomatic illness and of the impact of the care system itself on the course of a variety of medical and surgical conditions. It is possible that the evolving status of women in recent decades has had a liberating effect here too and has accelerated the emergence of nurses as increasingly sophisticated and skilled health care professionals. Certainly the expanded education of nurses in colleges and universities has contributed to this evolution.

Nowhere are the increased knowledge and capabilities of nurses more clearly in evidence than in the consultation and liaison field. Here the psychiatric nurse works as an autonomous professional, employed by the department of nursing, strongly supported by the department of psychiatry, and functioning in close collaboration with hospital nurses, psychiatrists, and other physicians and health professionals. This book is a larger effort than its title would suggest. For in addition to their thorough exposition of the field of psychiatric liaison nursing, Lewis and Levy provide an ideal model for the functioning of a psychiatric nurse in the multidisciplinary context of the general hospital.

The model which the authors provide is "holistic" or "systemic." By these terms it is meant that clinical assessment, consultation, and care are provided within the context of the total health system, with as full knowledge as is possible of the parts played by all the actors in the drama of the patient's life and illness, inside and outside of the hospital. Latent meanings, or unexpressed communications, in requests for consultation are carefully assessed so that interventions can be selected that will be appropriate and useful in the actual clinical context. Ideas and experience derived from psychoanalysis, clinical psychiatry, systems theory, and many other disciplines are brought together with previous work in nursing itself to provide a comprehensive theory of psychiatric liaison nursing. Innovative methods of teaching and supervision are carefully described, and creative use is made of nurses' groups as an effective consultation modality. Working independently, or as part of a multidisciplinary team, the liaison nurse can be highly effective in introducing mental health concepts into the everyday functioning of a variety of hospital personnel. The authors have provided a rich supply of detailed clinical illustrations that document comprehensively their major points. In addition to its value for nurses, this book has much to teach psychiatrists and other mental health professionals about the psychological aspects of physical illness and the strategies for reducing its human cost.

JOHN E. MACK, MD
Professor of Psychiatry
Harvard Medical School at
The Cambridge Hospital

preface

In the vanguard of a nursing trend that is gaining high visibility, *Psychiatric Liaison Nursing: The Theory and Clinical Practice* is a timely and intellectually provocative book that is on the leading edge of expanding the dimensions of nursing practice in a variety of settings. Anita Lewis and Joyce Levy have brought theoretical coherence to a field known for its diversity. In an exemplary way, this book captures the depth and breadth of liaison nursing.

Due to nursing's historical commitment to and responsibility for improving the quality of life, liaison nurses give particular attention to the psychological component of health care. Patients *need* nursing care when they come to the hospital. Liaison nursing recognizes the mind–body relationship and emphasizes the techniques for delivering psychological care within a holistic approach to patient care. Of particular note is the application of developmental theory and crisis intervention in working with the hospitalized patient.

The chapters in this book come alive with the rich clinical vignettes that provide a vivid sense of the translation of theory into practice. A strong theme throughout the book is that liaison nursing is a complex activity requiring the identification of patients' needs and the utilization of a broad range of interventions and skills.

The authors call our attention to the research potential in liaison nursing to validate nursing practice. Research is needed to specify and operationalize the principle concepts of liaison nursing and to develop and test the linkages between patient care and patient outcomes. A major direction will be to interconnect the differential use of techniques, resources, and methodologies with nursing diagnosis. These steps, according to the authors, include the development of well designed nursing research projects.

The authors provide many insights into the patient's experience in the hospital and the role of the liaison nurse in the health care delivery system. They show the way to develop the consultation program and how to achieve the objectives within the realities of the practice setting. This book is a major contribution to practitioners, both in explicating a basic practice model and in applying it to different nursing situations. It serves a twofold purpose: (1) as a textbook for graduate nursing students learning the liaison-consultative model, and (2) as a guide to nurses who wish to establish a liaison program within their practice setting.

Clearly, this book does more than fill an important gap in the clinical literature. It illustrates a growing trend in nursing of the collaborative relationship between nursing service and nursing education. Anita Lewis and Joyce Levy have clinical appointments to Boston University School of Nursing and are actively involved in teaching a graduate nursing consultation seminar. Thus this book exemplifies the breaking of new ground in psychiatric-mental health nursing that has high hopes of being translated into many areas of nursing.

ANN WOLBERT BURGESS, RN, DN Sc
Professor and Dean ad interim
Director of Nursing Research
Boston University School of Nursing

acknowledgments

Although an academic endeavor, writing a book is an uniquely intense, highly gratifying experience. The creation of this text holds a very special significance for the authors. The relationship between coauthors assumes a life of its own as the initial anxieties of working together are mastered. Sharing clinical experiences, successes, errors, philosophy, conceptualizing theoretical models, and editing each other's contributions comprise a small part of the relationship.

Friends and colleagues consistently expressed curiously, "How was it going for us? What was it like working together?" It has been extraordinary. Our relationship is best described as a marriage, of sorts, the initial and sole purpose of which was the creation of an object. What has been difficult to describe, and what does not appear on these pages, is the separate world that was also created and shared by the authors: broken fingers that went unrecognized, the restructuring of two households, ignored and disgruntled husbands, flat tires, endless weekends at the library or at the office, ongoing adolescent issues, frustration, exhaustion, humor, and exhilaration. Also experienced was the enormous sense of satisfaction as each milestone was reached.

On an airplane trip to Philadelphia, we discovered, quite by chance, that the roots of our relationship existed prior to the writing of this text. Although years apart, we had both attended the Sarah J. Rawson School in Hartford, Connecticut. Furthermore, our parents knew each other within the parameters of a close family/friend relationship characterized by a warmth and depth that supercedes blood relationships. The names of Lewis, Apter, Sasson, and Saffir are our common heritage.

During the crisis of physical illness, the constriction of interest and egocentricity are adaptive. Our families, friends, and colleagues would probably agree that for us this phenomenon also applied to the writing of this book. We are grateful not only for their belief in us, but also for their patience and endurance as we arduously completed this awesome task.

The support and interest of the departments of nursing at the New England Medical Center and The Cambridge Hospital, as well as the departments of psychiatry at Tufts University School of Medicine and Harvard Medical School, have been sources of intellectual stimulation and encouragement. Our fifteen years of clinical work with students, members of the nursing staff, medical-surgical colleagues, and patients established the essence of this text. As we have attempted to provide them with consultation-liaison services, they have, in turn, provided us with innumerable opportunities for learning, personal and professional growth, and reflection. Graduate students in psychiatric nursing have motivated us to define and refine our teaching. The contribution in the text by graduate students regarding their experience has been especially rewarding. A Peer Group of Liaison Nurses/Greater Boston Area, has been a major professional support to which we are indebted. The total group, as well as individual members, has made valuable contributions to this text. It was through this Peer Group that we met.

Also included in this text is the influence of our teachers. Over time, their ideas and knowledge have begun to feel like our own. We leave the distinction to our revered and respected teachers. The influence of Herbert Brown, Myrna Weiss, Philip Gottlieb, Bennett Simon, Jerald Grobman, Norman Zinberg, Carol Nadelson, George Vaillant, Vickie Roemele, and Henry Grunebaum are present throughout the text. We are appreciative of their hours of reviewing manuscripts, analyzing cases, and offering constructive criticism. Their greatest contribution, however, was their honesty, availability, confidence, and encouragement. We would also like to thank Paul Myerson, Richard Shader, Myron Belfer, Ann Wolbert Burgess, Ruth Borofsky, Suzanne O'Connor, Alan Marks, Peter Reich, Stephen Kemble, James Harburger, Marion Garey, John Mack, Marta Frank, Dianne Schilke Davis, Martha Sacci, Sandra Twyon, and Kathleen Bower, who have supported and influenced us. Lee Macht died tragically as the manuscript was being completed. His vision, creativity, and commitment to mental health care was an inspiration. Lee consistently expressed personal interest and encouragement regarding this text.

Behind the scenes were Carol Kassabian, Rheta Stanton, Kay Shanahan, and Mary Lynch, who were patient with our impatience. Our final typist, Alice Powers, never faltered while maintaining a sense of humor against the greatest of odds. While introducing us to the computer word processor, she helped to make the intolerable tolerable.

Adam left home to attend Haverford College. Josh pursued academics and athletics at Wayland High and Belmont Hill and maintained his sense of humor as the book became a part of the family. Gregg became a Bar Mitzvah. Scott wrote supportive and funny letters. Our husbands, Philip and Michael, experienced a different family lifestyle. Humor, reality testing, roses, brandy, briefcases, gourmet dinners, elegant manuscript containers, fancy red editing pens, and electric pencil sharpeners sustained us.

As we created this book, we have learned professionally and personally from each other within a relationship that cannot be duplicated.

A.L.G.
J.S.L.

introduction

During our first years as professional nurses, mastery of the technical elements of general nursing care practice were of high priority. Over time, we found ourselves becoming more interested in the relationship of the psyche to the soma, the stress of illness, and the psychologically therapeutic role of a nurse. As we developed skills in the technical aspects of clinical nursing, we continued to experience as problematic the provision of therapeutic psychological care and subsequent patient management. Although we had acquired reasonable understanding of the psychodynamics of illness and were aware of some supportive nursing interventions, we recognized that significant gaps in our knowledge remained.

As staff nurses, these gaps evidenced themselves in personally painful ways. We remained puzzled in fully understanding how our patients and their families were dealing with illness and hospitalization. We experienced both helplessness and frustration in identifying when patients and/or families were receptive to learning about their illness, assessing the level of autonomy of patients, planning therapeutic nursing interventions, and so on. It was not difficult to recognize the depressed patient, the angry patient, or the resistant family. However, obtaining useful help or consultation from colleagues was either unavailable or inconsistent.

Perhaps the most painful issue involved in the care of our patients was how the patient and/or family made us feel. The next step, tinged with confusion, was in examining the possible influence that our reactions and feelings were having on the tone, style, and effectiveness of our interactions. How were personal feelings inhibiting the formulation and accomplishment of nursing care goals? Would our growing competence in handling complex and technical situations leave room for empathic professionalism? Would we find desensitization to the emotional concerns of our patients our only option?

Where can the nurse take personal, sometimes unacceptable feelings, about patients and/or their families? What can nurses do with feelings about the patient in terrible physical pain, the dying patient, the hostile patient, the mistrusting family member, pediatric or adult patients crying for their mothers or begging the nurse not to hurt them again? What options are available to nurses for dealing with or containing their feelings of anger and their frustration when faced with the hallucinating and combative medical patient? What about the guilt-ridden discomfort of sadistic tendencies, which frequently become stimulated by outrageous or unmanageable patient behavior? How could nurses develop self-assurance that would aid them with feelings of helplessness? With experience some nurses are able to deal comfortably with these situations. However, a common response is a blend of confusion, avoidance, anger, depression, and fatigue.

Sensitivity to the complex facets of illness and hospitalization for the nurse and the patient/family must be combined with a solid foundation in psychiatric principles. Although we maintain a professional interest in psychiatry, the application of mental health principles to common life experiences and stresses has been our overriding interest. As a result of this aim, our clinical direction has developed.

A psychiatric nurse educated in the principles of consultation-liaison is the appropriate professional to assist nurses in providing psychological care to patients. Psychiatric nursing consultation resources are often not available. In some instances, the role has been neither well understood, well formulated, nor used appropriately.

The goals of this text, based on our fifteen years as practicing psychiatric liaison nurses, are to describe the theory and clinical practice of psychiatric liaison nursing in a general hospital and to validate that practice by illustrating the impact on patients and on other members of the health care team. Part One, with a description of the history, presentation of a theoretical model, and discussion of the creation and development of the role, will set the stage for the clinical practice of the liaison nurse described in Part Two. Part Three includes contributions of other liaison nurses. This text is enriched by presentations based on their clinical practice, which also further illustrate many of the basic concepts described earlier.

Our theoretical model is based on an holistic approach to clinical practice. It combines pertinent concepts in understanding the patient, the medical illness, the nurse, the milieu, and their relationships to the psychiatric liaison nurse. These are integrated within the framework of consultation theory. Various consultation modalities are discussed, which illustrate the core of our clinical work, that is, "diagnosing the total consultation."

This text is geared primarily for graduate students in psychiatric nursing who are interested in learning and practicing liaison nursing. There is a paucity of literature in this area, with the exception of specific consultation cases, articles of limited scope, and texts on the psychosocial or psychological needs of patients. This text encompasses a comprehensive appraisal of the illness experience based on the views of the nurse, the patient/family, and the psychiatric liaison nurse. It may also prove valuable to graduate nursing students studying nonpsychiatric specialties. The specific psychodynamics and needs of nursing staff, the identification of patient problems, and the implementation of nursing interventions would certainly be applicable to the masters level nurse. The concepts and consultation techniques used by the psychiatric liaison nurse in the hospital can be applied to other health settings. Finally, it is our hope that our colleagues and other mental health professionals will be able to increase their knowledge regarding the role of psychiatric liaison nurses, psychologically based nursing care, its impact on the patient, and ultimately its impact on the professional nurse.

ANITA LEWIS–GOTTLIEB

JOYCE SASSON LEVY

psychiatric
liaison nursing

part one
psychiatric liaison nursing in a general hospital

1

origin of nursing consultation

The history of science is science itself;
the history of the individual, the individual.

GOETHE

section 1   historical perspective

Psychiatric liaison nursing has its origins in both nursing and psychiatry. Historical developments in both professions have directly influenced the emergence and growth of the role of the psychiatric liaison nurse.

At the end of the nineteenth century, the care provided by nurses to the mentally ill was mainly custodial. The nurse's responsibility was to meet the physical needs of patients. Psychological care consisted merely of expectations that the nurse be kind and tolerant. The training of nurses at that time was divided between general hospitals and psychiatric hospitals, which in itself reflected the lack of an holistic approach to nursing practice. The fact that the formal preparation for nurses was referred to as "training," as opposed to "education," symbolized the task-oriented approach to nursing. Psychiatric nurses received their education/training at psychiatric institutions with the emphasis on the physical and custodial care of the mentally ill. General nurses received no training in psychiatric nursing. Johns Hopkins School of Nursing first included a course in psychiatric nursing in the general training of nurses in 1913. Not until 1930 was the importance of psychiatric knowledge recognized in general nursing care.

After World War II the Veterans Administration was faced with the care of many patients suffering from psychiatric illnesses. Nurses, although they were not sufficiently trained/educated in the principles of psychiatric care, were faced with a patient population requiring immediate psychological care. The necessity of educating nurses became apparent. Although there were few graduate nursing programs by the early 1940s, psychiatric nursing had become part of nursing curriculums. This was the beginning of the trend to combine all basic nursing knowledge into one general program. By 1950 the National League for Nursing required psychiatric clinical experience for accreditation of nursing programs.

In 1946 the National Mental Health Act was passed by Congress, and new opportunities for psychiatric nursing became available. This Act meant the beginning of federal funding for nursing education. At the same time, the nursing profession was beginning to recognize the necessity for graduate programs that emphasized clinical practice. Eight graduate programs in psychiatric nursing were in existence by 1947.* By 1981 graduate progams numbered over ninety. Concurrent with this development, a major text, published in 1952 by Peplau and titled *Interpersonal Relations in Nursing*, was viewed as the theoretical framework for psychiatric nursing. By 1962 psychiatric nursing was based on interpersonal techniques and on nursing process. Counseling was recognized as a primary function of psychiatric nursing while debates began about nurses as psychotherapists.

The National Working Conference on Graduate Education in Psychiatric Nursing, held in Williamsburg, Virginia in 1956, was a milestone in the development of psychiatric nursing. The results of the conference were described in the report called "The Education of the Clinical Specialist in Psychiatric Nursing." Thus the title of "clinical specialist" was established, although not generally recognized.

The Community Mental Health Centers Act, passed as federal legislation in 1963, made money available for the development of comprehensive mental health services in the community. This Act influenced the involvement of psychiatric nursing as a component of a multidisciplinary treatment team which was needed to provide care in the community. The emphasis on the prevention of mental illness, as well as its treatment, was noteworthy. During the next ten years psychiatric nursing continued to develop and expand. The Standards of Psychiatric–Mental Health Nursing Practice were identified by the American Nurses' Association in 1973 (see Appendix F). Formulated on the nursing process, these standards were a prescription for quality nursing care.

-----

*Programs included were at Columbia University, Yale University, University of Pittsburgh, Boston University, University of Minnesota, Catholic University, and the University of Washington.

section 2   *consultation-liaison psychiatry*

The development of psychiatric units in the general hospital has influenced the growth of consultation-liaison psychiatry. Albany Hospital in 1902 was the first general hospital in the United States with a psychiatric in-patient unit. As units continued to open in general hospitals, psychiatric consultation became more readily available.

In 1934 the Rockefeller Foundation provided the funds for the establishment of five psychiatric liaison departments in general hospitals. These departments provided the framework for bridging the gap between psychiatry and medicine. During World War II the medical profession was, for practical reasons, required to recognize and treat psychiatric problems on a short-term basis. As psychiatrists returned to civilian life, some incorporated these clinical experiences into their practice.

Psychosomatic medicine, which represents the view of man as a body-mind complex, emerged in the 1920s and influenced the development of consultation-liaison psychiatry:

> ... liaison is derivative from consultation psychiatry and may be viewed as the process through which the interrelationships sought by psychosomatic medicine are identified, formulated, clinically tested, and transmitted to our colleagues in other areas of medicine [1].

The increase in technology in medicine during the 1950s and 1960s resulted in less of an holistic approach to patient care. As medicine became more specialized, a greater emphasis was placed on the disease entity than on the individual patient. As more mechanical devices were utilized in the care of patients and as more complicated treatments and procedures were made available, intensive care units multiplied. Patients were living longer, yet they were subject to a new kind of psychological stress. The return of the generalist, in medicine described as the "primary care physician," indicated a recognition of the impact not only of the illness but also of the health care delivery system on the individual patient. Primary nursing may be viewed as paralleling this development.

The expansion of the psychopharmacology field in the 1950s had an impact on psychiatry in general. It also provided the psychiatric consultant with a useful and effective tool to aid the medically ill, when indicated, as well as offering expert advice and guidance about

psychotropic medications to the medical doctor. Psychopharmacology provided a bridge between psychiatry and medicine, and it
strengthened the consultation alliance.

Consultation, not an unfamiliar method of practice for psychiatrists, refers to the provision of expert diagnostic opinion and advice
on management regarding a patient's mental state and behavior at
the request of another health professional [2]. Therefore, initially at
least, psychiatrists have been able to make the transition to the role
in consultation–liaison psychiatry due to their familiarity with both
medicine and the concept of consultation. In contrast, nurse-to-nurse
consultation has been much less common.

section 3   nursing consultation

Psychiatric liaison nursing is a model for nursing practice that has
developed from the consultative process and psychiatric nursing. In
1963, cross-service consultation was first reported by Betty Sue
Johnson at Duke University. Although the concept of consultation
was well accepted within the medical field, nurses were not accustomed to utilizing each other's skills. In the program at Duke, nurses
in all nursing specialties acted as resources to each other. As psychiatric units in general hospitals became more prevalent, psychiatric
nurses became more visible and available in the general hospital.
Medical-surgical nurses logically sought assistance from psychiatric
nurses to help them provide more comprehensive psychological care
to patients. Within this framework, psychiatric nurses, based on the
general hospital psychiatric unit, began consulting to general medical
units. The medical-surgical staffs and the psychiatric nurses understood that the psychiatric nurses would assist the nursing staff in
problem solving and increase their sensitivity not only to the emotional concerns of patients, but also to the impact these concerns had
on the patient's illness and recovery [3]. The complexity of the emotional problems of the medically ill, the time commitment for effective consultation, the need for follow-up—all contributed to limiting
the success of nursing consultation in this model. The recognition of
the need for more extensive and multifaceted involvement by the
psychiatric nurse as consultant paved the way for the development of
the specialty of psychiatric liaison nursing. Adhering to the basic
principles of consultation, as described by Caplan, the psychiatric

liaison nurse's role evolved more in response to the needs of individual institutions than as a theoretical model.

In attempts to provide consultation to medical-surgical nurses,
various models were used. Jackson worked with the nursing staff, at
their request, to help those patients whom they identified as being
"disturbed," "problems," or "troubled" [4]. Holstein and Schwab
described a coordinated consultation program as an outgrowth of an
inefficient noncoordinated psychiatrist and nurse consultation approach. In this program the nurse was recognized as a consultation
team member. As a participant observer in the general hospital
milieu, the "consultation team nurse" was able to aid ward nurses in
facilitating patients' psychological adaptations by reinforcing the
therapeutic relationship and by intervening in situations where anti-
therapeutic emotional responses to patients had developed [5].

The need for theoretical and clinical guidelines for effectively
functioning as a liaison nurse became evident through the experiences
of psychiatric nurses attempting to provide consultation without formal education. The lack of a clinical framework allowed for a personalized, gut-level, "trial-by-fire" approach to what were complicated and involved patient management and consultation-liaison
problems. The concept and process involved in considering all
aspects of consultation were not formally integrated into practice.
However, the enthusiasm, disappointments, and frustrations of the
early liaison nurses validated the need for education in psychiatric
consultation liaison nursing. Graduate schools began to respond by
offering specialized programs in liaison nursing. The University of
Maryland and Yale University were the first two graduate programs
to provide a special program or "track" for liaison nursing [6,7].

Additional factors have influenced the practice of psychiatric
nurses as consultants in the general hospital. In conjunction with
deinstitutionalization of the mentally ill, the psychiatric patient has
returned to the community and, in some instances, to the general
hospital. The visibility of psychiatry in the local community has
helped the medical community and private citizens to become more
familiar and aware of emotional or mental problems.

Within this framework, the psychiatric liaison nurse in the
general hospital has evolved to become a vital mental health team
member, who provides not only consultation to medical-surgical
nurses but also an opportunity to incorporate mental health and psychiatric principles into the total care of the patient. The psychiatric
liaison nurse crosses the boundaries between medical-surgical and
psychiatric nursing.

section 4   philosophy of clinical practice

With the preceding historical perspective as a foundation, a philosophy of psychiatric liaison nursing is proposed. This specialty area of clinical practice within psychiatric nursing is based on the synthesis and application of theoretical models in nursing, psychiatry, systems theory, crisis intervention, and adult learning theory. Psychological care has been acknowledged as an integral part of comprehensive nursing care [8]. Approaches have been considered for meeting the psychological needs of the hospitalized patient [9]. The basis of this philosophy is founded in a strong belief in the integration of mental health concepts into general nursing practice. The interaction of medical illness and of its psychological effects on the hospitalized patient are so complex that understanding, availability, reassurance, anxiety reduction, empathy, and support prove in many instances inadequate. Every individual who is hospitalized brings in with him or her an emotional, as well as a physical, life. The challenge is to psychologically assess each individual to provide therapeutic interaction and intervention. Psychiatric liaison nurses are faced with the responsibility not only of confronting this challenge, but also of encouraging, educating, and supporting the nurse consultees to do the same.

Experienced psychiatric liaison nurses are presently practicing effectively in a variety of hospital settings. As the role itself has evolved, expectations of additional formal education have increased. The climate within nursing fosters a trend towards a combination of advanced education and clinical experience. If the historical perspective is to be acknowledged, along with the present issues of practice and the future arenas for professional expansion, then the need for standardization in preparation is obvious. Based on these factors, we support the following suggestions and criteria for optimal role practice.

Psychiatric liaison nurses are specialists within psychiatric nursing and generalists within nursing. Preferably they should be masters-prepared clinicians who not only possess a strong clinical base in psychiatric nursing, but who also have practiced as registered nurses in some area(s) of medical-surgical nursing. Clinical experience has demonstrated that this educational and clinical preparation proves valuable. This rich foundation can help to demystify the role, to assist in its development within the general hospital, and to provide the role occupant with an increased sense of professional gratification. Clinical experience as a registered, medical-surgical nurse serves to augment the liaison nurse's credibility as a nurse and role model. The quality rather than the quantity of this clinical experience is of importance. Obviously, extensive practice in specific areas of medical-surgical nursing can provide the liaison nurse with a greater reservoir of information from which to draw when engaging in clinical work. Some administrative experience as a head nurse or as a nurse manager also proves helpful as an adjunct to understanding the consultee and the system. Professional development is an evolving process that occurs in identifiable steps. Omitting any of these steps may result in limitations in competence, effectiveness, gratification, and success.

Liaison nurses are in a staff position within the nursing department. Although individual relationships may vary, they are not usually peers in relation to the consultees. In fact, an easily identifiable peer group does not always exist for them, which can become a problem. Liaison nurses are neither supervisors nor omnipotent experts. They are consultants, providing psychiatric nursing consultation relevant to the particular slice of the patient/family's life presented to them. They are not mandated with any evaluative responsibilities. Since a great deal of the actual work is based on the liaison nurse's ability to establish consultation alliances, these responsibilities would prove counterproductive to clinical practice.

Liaison nurses are nursing colleagues who are "invited in" to provide psychiatric nursing consultation. Although remaining available to other members of the health care team and working within a collaborative model, they provide consultation primarily to members of the nursing staff. As knowledgeable resources, they are specifically concerned with psychological issues that relate to nursing care and to nursing management. Their clinical work is focused on the promotion of quality nursing care practice and of professional self-esteem within nursing.

Psychiatric liaison nurses are valuable members of a nursing department. When based within this department, they are more clearly regarded as nursing colleagues. When the consultees identify them as such, the clinical effectiveness of psychiatric liaison nurses is enhanced. This is not to say that psychiatric nursing consultation cannot be provided if the role is based in another department, such as psychiatry. Yet both nursing identity and role validity are augmented when the psychiatric liaison nursing role is based in and funded through a department of nursing. In this area of clinical practice, which demands flexibility, each hospital system is assessed to ensure the most feasible administrative organization.

Confidentiality is another hallmark of clinical practice. Liaison

nurses assume a respectful, confidential stance in terms of the information shared with or gathered by them. Unless such information
indicates grossly inappropriate nursing care actions and/or a potential danger to patients, confidentiality is maintained. In the rare situation in which confidentiality is threatened, the liaison nurse initially
discusses the problem with the nursing colleague in both a professional and responsible manner. She encourages the consultee to
actively participate in the necessary problem solving process and in
the notification of the appropriate nursing managers. The liaison
nurse may accompany the consultee, if doing so is appropriate. If the
consultee is unable or unwilling, then the liaison nurse is compelled
to break their confidentiality agreement. Although this option has
never been exercised in our practice, it is a prudent alternative.

The psychiatric liaison nurse is clinically competent and possesses the ability to diagnose situations and to set appropriate limits.
Recognition of internal as well as external pressure to react, to do
something, is apparent. The art of therapeutic listening [10] must be
coupled with the art of therapeutic nonlistening—that is, the conscious process in which the listener refrains from actively responding
(to gossip, for example). Appreciation of the value of listening, both
as a diagnostic tool and as a supportive intervention, is paramount.
Preservation of consultation alliances within the context of realistic
goals of practice cannot be ignored. The documentation of clinical
work, the evaluation by appropriate nursing and psychiatric supervisors, along with self-evaluation and feedback from consultees are
all segments of professional practice.

Liaison nurses are responsible for their clinical practice, that is,
for their nursing actions and the content of their consultation. Clinical supervision, preferably by an experienced liaison nurse, is both
appropriate and essential for effective practice. Psychiatric back-up
from a psychiatrist in the context of a collaborative relationship is a
crucial dimension to effective practice. When either of these elements
is weakened, the role and clinical practice of the liaison nurse becomes
threatened.

To be sincere, rather than viewing the general hospital as a laboratory for applying mental health concepts, liaison nurses must have
a passion for medicine. The light in which they regard their past
medical-surgical nursing experiences is inevitably communicated to
the consultee. If they view their own medical-surgical experience as
exciting and challenging rather than as dreaded and burdensome,
then their role satisfaction and professional credibility as liaison
nurses are enhanced. Liaison nurses have made a choice in their spe-

cialty, but not due to a revulsion to medicine. Their effective role practice is based on an appreciation of medicine, along with a desire to enrich their understanding of the impact of the psyche on the soma and of the illness experience for the patient, the family, and for the health care providers.

Professional and personal maturity is a necessary attribute for successful clinical practice. Professional maturity is demonstrated in the liaison nurse's ability to take carefully thought-out, clinically sound risks, to assess a situation, and to develop a formulation and a nursing diagnosis. A critical element is the liaison nurse's ability to accept the reality and anxiety of not always having sufficient data or the privilege of obtaining it. Reasonable nursing interventions are still developed if at all possible. Personal maturity is demonstrated through tolerance of the humbling experience of being personally and professionally visible, vulnerable, sometimes rejected, and often alone. Other indicators are the capacity and willingness to tolerate the intolerable, to be able to maintain professionalism and self-control when under extreme stress, to be flexible, to work respectfully and helpfully with patients and with health care providers who are also very stressed.

As the role of the liaison nurse becomes integrated within the hospital, two problematic areas evolve. Although the liaison nurse emphasizes mental health concepts, staff members may at times be unwilling or unable to accept this emphasis and therefore reject the liaison nurse. At other times, staff members may feel unable to integrate these concepts into their practice and expect the liaison nurse to assume responsibility for the psychological care of the patient. On some level the problem of dependency may be appealing to the liaison nurse who consistently works towards acceptance as a colleague. In certain crises or complicated situations, temporary dependency may be therapeutically sound for the patient and the consultee. However, in an ongoing relationship, dependency interferes with the consultation process and alliance. The goal with consultees is to aid their professional development so that they are less dependent on the liaison nurse and are able to be more proficient and confident in integrating mental health concepts into their own clinical practice.

The issue of psychotherapy is the second problem area. When the liaison nurse is working directly with patients, the clinical approach is individualized and based on a thorough assessment. It is best to begin with the least complicated intervention, and then to evaluate, reassess, and modify the approach as necessary. An intervention may be as simple as the recommendation that a patient's room be changed, or it may consist of crisis intervention or brief psychotherapy. When working with consultees, alliances and collegiality are crucial so that negotiation for and provision of psychotherapy to nursing colleagues are always inappropriate. Although tempting at times, psychotherapy of consultees is contrary to our philosophy of psychiatric liaison nursing, and we believe it may even prove disastrous. However, if a consultee is directly or indirectly requesting psychotherapy, this request should not be ignored. The liaison nurse can discreetly provide the consultee with an appropriate psychiatric referral.

The psychiatrist represents the resource in psychopathology, psychosomatic medicine, pharmacology, and differential diagnosis. The social worker represents the resource in family dynamics, as well as in the social and family-related aspects of patient care. Together with the liaison nurse, the psychiatrist and social worker are resources in psychodynamics, psychotherapy, crisis intervention, and other areas. The authors fully support an interdisciplinary approach to care delivery, but we emphasize the necessity of recognizing each clinician's individual base of operation. The psychiatric liaison nurse represents the resource in the psychological nursing care and subsequent management of patients. Through the process of "diagnosing the total consultation," the liaison nurse expands the traditional model of singular consultation into a liaison model of clinical practice. *Consultation* is defined as the provision of clinical expertise regarding the delivery of psychological care in response to a request from a health care provider(s). *Liaison* is the process of facilitation of the relationship that exists among the patient, the adjustment to the illness, the consultee(s), and the hospital/ward milieu. Consultations may as well be done in a closet if the consultant does not recognize, accept, and include milieu-related issues. The psychiatric liaison nurse holds special membership within the medical milieu. In the liaison model consultation is ongoing, while follow-up and reassessment become a non-negotiable responsibility of the psychiatric liaison nurse.

The theoretical framework for effective practice can be clinically illustrated and taught. In conjunction with the philosophical beliefs presented, an awareness of self is emphasized as a necessary tenet of all clinical practice.

references

1. Chase Kimball, "Liaison Psychiatry of Approaches and Ways of Thinking about Behavior," *Psychiatric Clinics of North America* 2:2 (August 1979): 201–210.

2. Z. J. Lipowski, "Consultation Liaison Psychiatry: An Overview," *American Journal of Psychiatry* 131 (1974): 623–630.

3. Jill Nelson and Dianne Schilke, "The Evolution of Psychiatric Liaison Nursing," *Perspectives in Psychiatric Care* 14:9 (1976): 61–65.

4. Harriet Jackson, "The Psychiatric Nurse as a Mental Health Consultant in a General Hospital," *The Nursing Clinics of North America* 4 (1969): 327–340.

5. David Barton and Margaret Kelso, "The Nurse as a Psychiatric Consultation Team Member," *International Journal of Psychiatry in Medicine* 2 (1971): 108–115.

6. Lisa Robinson, "A Psychiatric Nursing Liaison Program," *Nursing Outlook* 20:7 (1972): 454–457.

7. Jill Nelson and Dianne Schilke Davis, "Educating the Psychiatric Liaison Nurse," *Journal of Nursing Education* 18:8 (1979): 14–20.

8. Florence Nightingale, *Notes on Nursing* (Philadelphia: J. B. Lippincott Co., 1946), p. 34.

9. Lisa Robinson, *Psychological Aspects of the Care of Hospitalized Patients* (Philadelphia: F. A. Davis Company, 1972).

10. Hildegard Peplau, "Professional Closeness," *Nursing Forum* 8:4 (1969): 343–360.

bibliography

books

CAPLAN, GERALD. *The Theory and Practice of Mental Health Consultation.* New York: Basic Books, Inc., Publishers, 1970.

HACKETT, THOMAS and CASSEM, NED, eds., *Massachusetts General Hospital Handbook of General Hospital Psychiatry.* St. Louis: The C. V. Mosby Company, 1978, pp. 1–14.

KALISCH, PHILIP and KALISCH, BEATRICE. *The Advance of American Nursing.* Boston: Little, Brown & Co., 1978.

MERENESS, DOROTHY and TAYLOR, CECILIA. *Essentials of Psychiatric Nursing.* St. Louis: The C. V. Mosby Company, 1978.

PEPLAU, HILDEGARD. *Interpersonal Relations in Nursing.* New York: G. P. Putnam's Sons, 1952.

ROBINSON, LISA. *Liaison Nursing: Psychological Approach to Patient Care.* Philadelphia: F. A. Davis Company, 1974.

STRAIN, JAMES and GROSSMAN, STANLEY. *Psychological Care of the Medically Ill: A Primer in Liaison Psychiatry.* New York: Appleton-Century-Crofts, 1975.

STUART, GAIL and SUNDEEN, SANDRA. *Principles and Practices of Psychiatric Nursing.* St. Louis: The C. V. Mosby Company, 1979.

articles

BARTON, DAVID and KELSO, MARGARET. "The Nurse as a Psychiatric Consultation Team Member," *International Journal of Psychiatry in Medicine* 2 (1971): 108–115.

GRACE, MARY JO. "The Psychiatric Nurse Specialist and Medical/Surgical Patients," *American Journal of Nursing* (1974): 481–483.

HOLSTEIN, SHIRLEY and SCHWAB, JOHN. "A Coordinated Consultation Program for Nurses and Psychiatrists," *Journal of the American Medical Association* 194:5 (1965): 491–493.

JOHNSON, BETTY. "Psychiatric Nurse Consultant in a General Hospital," *Nursing Outlook* 11 (1963): 728–729.

KUNTZ, SANDRA; STEHLE, JOAN; and MARSHALL, RUTH. "The Psychiatric Clinical Specialist: The Progression of a Specialty," *Perspectives in Psychiatric Care* 18:2 (March–April 1980): 90–92.

LEGO, SUZANNE. "The One-to-One Nurse Patient Relationship," *Perspectives in Psychiatric Care* 13:2 (March–April 1980): 67–89.

2
definition and application of the psychiatric liaison nursing role

Clear and distinct ideas are terms which,
though familiar and frequent in men's mouths,
I have reason to think everyone who uses
does not perfectly understand.

JOHN LOCKE [1]

section 1   *a theoretical model*

The clinical practice of psychiatric liaison nursing is multifaceted. As will be illustrated, areas of practice include a wide variety of consultations, liaison work, and educational responsibilities. The content of the work, as well as the strategies used, vary in response to each request and situation. A synthesis of theoretical models in nursing, psychiatry, systems theory, consultation theory, crisis intervention, and adult learning theory blend to create the proposed theoretical model. This holistic model is comprised of principles that form a comprehensive foundation for psychiatric nursing consultation and liaison work. This model, applicable to all areas of clinical practice, is in concert with the goals of psychiatric liaison nursing. The goals in turn remain consistent, irrespective of the consultation-liaison modality utilized, and serve as guidelines to practice.

goals of psychiatric liaison nursing

1. To demonstrate and to teach mental health concepts and their application to clinical nursing practice.
2. To effect appropriate psychiatric and nursing intervention.
3. To support nurses in continuing to provide quality nursing care.
4. To promote and to develop the professional and personal self-esteem of the nurse.
5. To encourage among the members of the nursing staff tolerance of situations in which immediate and/or effective intervention or resolution is unattainable.

A theoretical model—a type of staging apparatus from which to

17

build and develop guidelines for clinical practice—is founded in our philosophy of nursing, clinical knowledge, and clinical practice. The theoretical model is an holistic approach to consultation with the following five basic principles, each of which deals with specific elements of professional practice and therefore represents an important delineation. Each of these principles is of equal significance and blends with the others.

- *Principle one: Consultation-liaison model*
  The clinical practice of psychiatric liaison nursing is firmly based on principles inherent in consultation-liaison theory.
- *Principle two: The patient*
  An assessment of the patient's psychological status includes history, personality style, defensive structure, and present level of functioning.
- *Principle three: The medical illness*
  The patient's psychological response to illness and hospitalization is assessed in conjunction with the medical illness, its symptomatology, and the patient's physical status.
- *Principle four: The nurse and the system*
  The elements of the medical milieu and its subsystems are components necessitating incorporation.
- *Principle five: Preventative management*
  Therapeutic prophylactic psychological care is accomplished through the recognition of predictable responses to specific illnesses, along with the application of adult learning theory and crisis theory.

The specific content of each theoretical principle will be discussed at length. This holistic model, however, becomes cohesive and clinically applicable only through the process of "diagnosing the total consultation." This is the process of comprehensively assessing and evaluating aspects of the consultation that are beyond the consultant–patient interaction. Data obtained as a result of this process provides a foundation upon which to formulate interventions. In Chapter 4, "The Consultation Process," areas that are reflected in the "total" consultation and these five theoretical principles are further identified, examined, and diagnosed.

The knowledge and skill of the psychiatric liaison nurse enable her to apply this theoretical model in accurately "diagnosing the total consultation," within the guidelines of the goals of practice. In addition to basic psychiatric and nursing education, clinical expertise is based on an awareness of the reactions to receiving and giving care, on the knowledge of responses to stress and illness, and on the knowledge of predictable and normal responses to medical illness.

principle one: consultation-liaison model

Clinical responsibilities are fulfilled within the boundaries of a consultation-liaison model, which is characterized by:

1. an educative, collaborative alliance with medical and nursing colleagues;
2. a consciousness-raising approach to recognizing the psychological care needs of patients and families, as well as the emotional and professional self-esteem needs of the consultee(s); and
3. a definition of the consultant's responsibilities, as they are limited to the context of the recommendations submitted and the interventions effected. The primary responsibility for the patient remains within the jurisdiction of the consultee, who may accept or reject the offerings of the liaison nurse. Administratively, the liaison nurse has neither power over nor supervisory responsibility for the consultee.

Consultation has been defined as the process in which one person, termed an expert, undertakes to advise another [2]. Psychiatric consultation has been defined as the "provision of expert advice in the diagnosis, management and prevention of mental disorders by specially trained mental health professionals at the request of other health professionals and within the constraints of available knowledge and techniques [3]." The necessity of solid psychiatric knowledge for a complete evaluation of the patient is without question. At the core of every consultation is the "psychiatric ear." At times the impact or presence of psychiatric illness demands full attention and assessment. The concepts inherent in consultation-liaison are integrated and viewed in perspective. Therefore, consultation, an interactional process, is defined as the provision of clinical expertise regarding the delivery of psychological care in response to a request from a health care provider(s).

The diagnostic process inherent in psychiatric nursing consultation is the formulation of a "nursing diagnosis [4]." A theoretical framework for psychiatric consultation incorporates the complexities of the social world in which consultant, patient, and consultee participate [5]. The liaison nurse may assume the position of the patient's therapist, the consultee's advisor, the educator, or the role model—whichever is relevant to the diagnosed needs manifested in the consultation and the goals of consultation. There is no absolute "distinction between case-centered and consultee-centered consultation.... A consultation request results from both the needs of the patient and the needs of the consultee [6]."

Hackett describes consultation as the process of responding to a request for help with a particular problem, while intervention is left in the domain of the consultee. Liaison work includes preventative management, teaching, and active participation in ward rounds [7]. The liaison component of this theoretical principle recognizes that a mutually complementary relationship exists between consultation and liaison work [8]. Liaison is the process of facilitation of the relationship that exists among the patient, the adjustment to the illness, the consultee(s), and the hospital/ward milieu. Taking this viewpoint one step further, consultation and liaison clearly become inseparable areas of clinical practice. If the liaison nurse is to work toward the achievement of clinical goals, then the expansion of a purely consultative model to include a liaison model becomes paramount. After diagnosing the consultation regarding a medical patient, whose behavior is maladaptive in dealing with a physical illness, short-term psychotherapy may prove beneficial. Educating health care providers in terms of the psychological needs of this patient and of therapeutically enhancing their intervention in such a case is of equal benefit and importance. A supportive, collaborative, and consultative alliance with the consultee(s) enables the liaison nurse to clarify the quality of communication among patients, families, and health care providers. Mediation by the liaison nurse can occur if necessary, while both patient and consultee(s) presumably gain greater psychological understanding of their mutual and individual experience within the hospital.

principle two: the patient

A thorough psychiatric assessment of the patient is a fundamental component of client-centered consultation. It can provide data that not only elucidates the etiology of the patient's psychological responses and defensive strategies, but that may also further clarify the client-focused problem originally defined by the consultee. Either direct or indirect assessment of the "identified" patient may, under specific circumstances, be an appropriate approach to providing psychiatric nursing consultation. Accurately "diagnosing the total consultation" aids in clarifying whether or not the patient should be interviewed. Obviously, there is the risk of misdiagnosis of the consultation, which may lead to serious consequences when a decision is made not to interview the patient. A misdiagnosis may include:

1. underestimating the patient's psychopathology or degree of stress,

2. overestimating the consultee's ability to intervene independently,
3. underestimating the consultee's anxiety or fear in working with the patient, and
4. jeopardizing the consultation alliance.

In 1961, Orlando described the nursing process as the relationship of three elements:

1. the behavior of the patient,
2. the reaction of the nurse, and
3. the nursing actions that are designed for the patient's benefit [9].

This definition has been expanded to include identifiable steps. The nursing process begins with the objective assessment of the patient. Subjective views are noted and labeled as such. Areas of health are noted, while problems and care needs are identified. These needs are prioritized as short- and long-term goals.

Section 3 of Chapter 5 is devoted to a detailed description of the assessment of the patient. This principle of the theoretical model is based on psychiatric interviewing skills, combined with the steps of the nursing process and nursing diagnosis.

A well integrated psychoanalytic-developmental approach is used in formulating patients' personality styles and character structures. In an attempt to understand patients, their ego strengths, their capacity for adaptation and learning, and their potential for mental health are all considered.

Anxiety and fear represent one segment of the etiology of the patient's reactions [10–12]. Freud distinguished anxiety from fear and fright.

> "Anxiety" describes a particular state of expecting the danger or preparing for it, even though it may be an unknown one. "Fear" requires a definite object of which to be afraid. "Fright," however, is the name we give to the state a person gets into when he has run into danger without being prepared for it [13].

It is useful, in conceptualizing the patient's experience, to differentiate anxiety from fear and fright. This formulation is the basis for empathic interaction and effective intervention. When engaging in direct patient assessment, this differentiation in concepts proves helpful in identifying id, ego, and superego influences in presenting behavior.

An equally important concept is regression. In most instances, regression, as manifested by the hospitalized patient, is in the service of adaptation. Kris refers to this phenomenon as a "primary process in the service of the ego [14]." In other words, when faced with a perceived threat or conflict, the ego responds with any one of a variety of defensive strategies, the goals of which are comfort and self-preservation. The most commonly observed response of the hospitalized patient is regression. Either the unwillingness to regress (and the accompanying fear) or, on the other end of the spectrum, the proclivity for regression may be a serious impediment for the patient. Erikson's discussion of the "eight stages of man" [15] provides a theoretical framework from which to conceptualize the development of the ego and the key issues to be negotiated at each developmental stage. This model is recommended, because it enhances recognition of the use of regression by both the patient and the consultee(s). It also crystallizes the source and intrapsychic level of the perceived threat or conflict. Because "the ego is first and foremost a body ego" [16], a developmental approach to diagnosing psychiatric symptomatology also heightens the liaison nurse's awareness of the significance of body image and of body integrity in the life of the patient.

principle three: the medical illness

The disease or illness itself demands close scrutiny. An appreciation of the etiology of the illness, its anticipated course, the resultant symptomatology, and the prescribed treatment is necessary in understanding the impact of the illness on the patient. The prospect or reality of medical illness precipitates both a generalized and individualized emotional response, which constitutes the psychological significance of illness and the patient's response to it.

When entering a situation, each individual brings certain values, beliefs, and behavioral expectations. When confronted with actual or fantasized stressors, any or all of these elements may be affected. Three major categories of causes of psychological stress have been identified: "(1) loss or threats of loss of psychic objects, (2) injury or threat of injury, and (3) frustration of drives and drive derivatives or threats thereof." Every stressor has some specific effects and does not always elicit exactly the same response, since the same stressor acts differently on different individuals, whose responses depend on both internal and external factors [17]. Selye's physiologic view identifies stress irrespective of the stressor that causes wear and tear to the body [18]. Illness and hospitalization certainly create a situation characterized by stress and disequilibrium. The individual patient's cognitive and psychological appraisal of this situation, coupled with his or her assessment of the degree and quality of the personal threat posed, will color the patient's responses. These responses may be adaptive or maladaptive in nature, and the patient may be viewed as existing somewhere on an illness–wellness continuum. Chapter 5, "Experience of Illness and Hospitalization," elaborates on the special meaning of illness and hospitalization to the individual patient.

The task for medically ill patients is to accurately identify their stressful states and to mobilize intrapsychic energies to initiate adaptive behavior. Sometimes, these objectives are not attainable. Erikson's developmental stages are described as crises that must be mastered to achieve psychological growth. The manner in which each developmental crisis has been negotiated can influence the patient's ability to successfully adapt to medical illness.

principle four: the nurse and the system

Life on the ward, the quality of relationships, and the subsystems in operation are significant factors affecting the consultee's motivation for requesting psychiatric liaison nursing services. The social matrix of the ward has a direct influence on the behaviors, emotional responses, and attitudes of its patients and its health care staff. The exact content of a consultation request cannot be examined in a vacuum. Doing so would prove self-defeating in terms of the goals of psychiatric liaison nursing. Meyer and Mendelson describe an "operational group model" [19], which is useful in understanding the process of requesting consultation. This model emphasizes the identified patient, a crisis within the patient–health care provider relationship, and the provision of therapeutic care. This is akin to our model of "diagnosing the total consultation." Weisman and Hackett have identified a "therapeutic consultation model" [20] in which the major orientation is the patient. The focus of this model is the development of a psychodynamic formulation of the patient's problems/behavior, strengthening the alliance with the patient and offering psychotherapy. Sandt and Leifer discuss a "communication model" [21] wherein the language utilized in requesting consultation is regarded as significant. The language serves as a source in understanding the problem presented for consultation.

Our holistic theoretical model combines these elements with an emphasis on a comprehensive appraisal of the entire medical milieu. It clarifies the complex dynamics of the consultation question.

Bertalanffy (1956), Boulding (1951), Rapoport (1966), and

many others have defined and described general system theory [22]. Bertalanffy regards a system as a set of elements standing in interaction [23]. Hall and Fagan define a system as the relationships between objects and their attributes [24]. Power, control, responsibility, accountability, stress, identification issues, performance expectations, and the individual psychology of each member of the medical milieu comprise elements of subsystems warranting consideration. The response and behaviors of health care providers in relation to the patient's illness and in relation to the liaison nurse are also examined.

principle five: preventative management

The intent of the liaison nurses is to utilize data, derived from their assessment of the total consultation, to create a treatment matrix through which patients may best employ their adaptive capacities. In conjunction with the principles of this theoretical model, liaison nurses draw on their knowledge of personality development and medical psychology for their formulations. There is no simple equation for minimizing psychological trauma, that is, for achieving preventative management. An additional aspect of preventative management is to promote flexibility and adaptation of the hospital system to the needs of patients.

As previously stated, psychological responses to illness and hospitalization are, in some measure, predictable [25]. Medical-surgical nurses are in a unique position to diagnose sources of psychological stress for the patient and family, as well as to identify maladaptive responses to stress. An increased awareness of predictable psychological problems of the patient and family may result in the promotion of adaptive strategies and the creation of an increasingly psychotherapeutic environment within the medical milieu.

Utilizing andragogical assumptions regarding the adult learner, the liaison nurse can identify a potential crisis or danger for patients as they experience illness and hospitalization. Knowledge of the process by which patients learn is a prerequisite to prophylactic psychological nursing care. The following tenets of adult learning theory are pertinent:

As a person matures, (1) his self-concept moves from one of being a dependent personality toward one of being a self-directing human being; (2) he accumulates a growing reservoir of experience that becomes an increasing resource from learning; (3) his readiness to learn becomes oriented increasingly to the developmental tasks of his social roles; and, (4) his time perspective changes from one of postponed application of knowledge to immediacy of application and accordingly his orientation toward learning shifts from one of subject-centeredness to one of problem-centeredness [26].

Liaison nurses educate the consultee in regard to the possible psychological reactions of hospitalized patients, their needs, and the interplay of these andragogical beliefs. The diagnostic and therapeutic care-giving role of the consultees proves effective only in light of their ability to be knowledgeable and competent in adult learning theory. "As an open system constantly exchanging matter, energy and information with the environment, man is capable of maintaining pattern and organization and proceeding toward increased growth [27]."

An understanding of crisis theory and of illness/hospitalization as a crisis is a crucial element in terms of the principle of prevention in this theoretical model [28]. *Crisis* has been defined as an obstacle to life goals that is temporarily insurmountable through the usual problem-solving methods and that is followed by a period of disorganization [29]. The minimum goal of crisis intervention is to aid individuals in regaining the level of functioning they experienced before the crisis. With appropriate intervention, a crisis may be resolved in such a way as to promote the growth and achievement of a higher level of functioning. During the crisis of illness, a patient may be afforded a singular opportunity to achieve emotional growth. When the crisis has passed, often so has the motivation and energy of the individual. Crisis, although most commonly viewed as negative, is applied to common positive occurrences such as marriage or parenthood.

Some of the techniques of crisis intervention are similar to, if not the same as, the steps in the nursing process and in the process of psychiatric consultation. A comprehensive assessment of the problem and of the individual, in tandem with the formulation of individualized therapeutic interventions that capitalize on the individual's strengths, is geared toward the restoration of cognitive, emotional, and physical control over the identified stress. Psychological pain may be minimized for the patient when the liaison nurse and the consultee(s) are attuned to appropriate interventions based on the probable responses to the crisis of the illness/hospitalization. The least complex interventions are employed first and may become more complex as necessary. Identifying and building on ego strengths, clarifying conflicting areas and areas of need with the patient, recognizing that the stressful situation itself is usually time-limited, and establishing realistic short- and long-term goals apply to each intervention. "Man must come to be more effective and able to perceive himself as the determiner of his fate if he is to live comfortably with himself [30]."

Consultees, responsible for the patient's care, may improve the delivery of their psychological care through interaction with the liaison nurse. Combining the basic elements of the nursing process with a diagnosis of the total consultation, which incorporates the principles previously identified, the liaison nurse is able to make a thoughtful, scientific, and clinical contribution to the psychological care of the hospitalized patient. This contribution is evidenced in:

1. increasingly therapeutic psychological care for the patient,
2. increasing professional growth and sophistication of the consultee(s), and
3. the enhancement of professional self-esteem in the consultee(s) as an adjunct to recognizing the fruits of one's efforts.

With a well defined theoretical model, liaison nurses are prepared to begin the work of creating, negotiating, and implementing their role.

section 2   creating and negotiating the role*

Psychiatric nurses have been involved in consultation and liaison activities in general hospitals since the early 1960s. Reports of these activities in the literature have consisted primarily of descriptions of individual experiences in implementing this role within a specific institution [31–35]. In this section general considerations in creating the role of the psychiatric liaison nurse will be explored.

As a group of experienced psychiatric liaison nurses, our belief is that, prior to role implementation, the necessary first steps of role creation and system entry need to be addressed. The process of role creation is clarified, and recommendations for specific steps for entry into the system proposed. This view is based on a composite of ten liaison nurses' experiences in ten different institutions. Our recommendations constitute areas for consideration rather than a prescription for action. The format in which the information is presented is sequential in nature. In practice, there is a blending and overlapping of the outlined steps.

---

*This section has been contributed by A Peer Group of Liaison Nurses/Greater Boston Area.

The following terms are defined to aid in the clarity of creating and negotiating this nursing position:

- "A role is a set of expectations about how a person in a given position in a particular social system should act [36]."
- Role creation refers to the process of establishing the need for, as well as the broad parameters of, the position within the system.
- System entry refers to strategies that introduce and integrate a position into the system with the appropriate administrative sanctions.
- Role implementation refers to specific behaviors that allow the person within that position to fulfill the system's expectations.

The rationale for the creation of the role of the psychiatric liaison nurse is inherent in the philosophy previously discussed in Chapter 1, Section 4. The following brief encapsulation may prove helpful in validating the role to those unfamiliar with it.

Illness is often viewed as a life crisis or as a stressful situation that has the potential to disrupt psychological equilibrium. The patient progresses through certain describable stages of psychological adaptation. The nurse's interaction with the patient during these stages plays a significant part in the patient's healing. This philosophical orientation emphasizes wellness rather than illness. It is assumed that any nursing department needs a psychiatric liaison nurse with the educational and clinical experience to function within a collaborative-consultative model to assist nurses in meeting the psychosocial needs of patients.

Psychiatric liaison nurses implement this role by serving as resource persons who consult with nursing staff in assessing, planning, implementing, and evaluating the psychosocial needs of patients. They are concerned with facilitating communication between nurses and other members of the health care team. As strong advocates of preventative care, their goal is to increase staff awareness of potential stress and to make appropriate interventions in situations that may eventually develop into an emotional crisis for the patient.

The ability to implement this role successfully depends on broad clinical expertise, as well as on a working knowledge of the descriptive liaison nursing literature. Even the most clinically competent nurse, however, may have difficulty implementing the role without careful attention to the following stages of role creation and system entry.

The process of role creation begins with the recognition of the needs of nurses in providing for the psychosocial care of patients.

The inherent difficulties in providing this care may be identified in a variety of ways, that is, by staff nurses, a head nurse, a nursing administrator, a psychiatric consultant, or a psychiatric nurse interested in liaison work. More specifically, a nursing service, in the process of ongoing evaluation of the quality of nursing care, may become aware of the nurses' needs in meeting the psychosocial needs of patients. Or a nursing administrator may possess the necessary knowledge and sophistication to develop a role for the liaison nurse. Perhaps a psychiatrist within a consultation liaison service may become aware of the need to develop a closer liaison with nursing to address issues of patient management. In recognizing the uniqueness of nurse-to-nurse consultation, the psychiatrist begins to seek ways for the institution to develop a role for the liaison nurse. Finally, the psychiatric nurse who is interested in liaison work might point out the need to a nursing administrator and/or to a consulting psychiatrist, offering the liaison nurse role as a solution.

With the need for the role established, the next phase of role creation is negotiation. During this phase, the system and the candidate for the position of psychiatric liaison nurse assess each other as part of the decision-making process leading to a contractual agreement for employment. Even at this early phase, the style and content of candidates' communication with various people within the system can set the tone and blueprint for how they intend to implement their role. It is therefore important for candidates to quickly clarify their expectations to avoid irreversible or tenacious myths about their role and functions.

This phase of negotiation is of equal importance to nursing administrators. The role is sanctioned by its relationship to positions of authority and power. Therefore, its viability within the system requires active support by nursing administrators. In order to provide this support without interdepartmental or intradepartmental conflict, it is useful for nursing administrators to also clarify expectations during this early phase of negotiation.

Thus it is crucial to the process of role creation for the candidate and the nursing administrators to discuss the following questions:

- Which department will hire the liaison nurse? Where is the position relative to others in the organization? To whom will the new employee be accountable? (Refer to Table 2–1.)
- Who are the key people within the system to interview the candidate?
- Is this a system within which the candidate would want to work?
- Are there adequate supports and supervision within the system? Or is

it necessary to develop them outside the system? Are outside supports and supervision sanctioned and funded?

- Who will evaluate the performance and functioning of the psychiatric liaison nurse? Have adequate criteria for evaluation been developed? By whom were the criteria developed, and are they open for discussion? Does the evaluator understand the role adequately and possess the necessary expertise to evaluate the work of the liaison nurse?
- What is the philosophy and model that underlies the delivery of nursing services? What is the philosophy, modality, and method of evaluating the quality of nursing care within this system?
- What are the expectations on the psychiatric liaison nurse in terms of administrative meetings and responsibilities, teaching responsibilities, and committee work? Do these expectations interfere with the development of the consultative relationship? That is, do they pose a threat to confidentiality? Does the liaison nurse have the flexibility to participate in the activities of his or her choice?
- Will the salary be competitive with similar positions at other hospitals and comparable with the salaries of other positions within the hospital of similar responsibility and independent functioning?
- What is the philosophy and scope of clinical practice of the department of psychiatry? What is the psychiatrist's understanding of the role of a psychiatric liaison nurse? How will the liaison nurse interface with this department? Is there any history of liaison nursing within this system?
- What is the availability of consultation with members of the department of psychiatry? Is there a psychiatrist available if the clinical situation warrants?
- How will the liaison nurse interface with the other major clinical services within the hospital, such as social service, pastoral counseling, occupational and physical therapy, and the like?

After considering these questions, candidates must determine if their professional interests and goals coincide with the needs of the system. Likewise, the nursing administration must determine how suitable a particular candidate is for the position of psychiatric liaison nurse. Further, both the candidate and the system must determine how flexible they will be in this process of role creation.

Sometime during this process of negotiation, the content of the job description is considered. Although a general agreement of the scope of clinical practice must exist, a written description is crucial to clarify expectations. Each institution has individual needs, interests, assets, and problems that will be reflected in the requirements for the job. (Refer to Table 2-2, which serves as a guide [37].)

Once the parameters of the role and contract for employment

TABLE 2–1   ORGANIZATIONAL CHART

Title and Hospital	Employed by:	Administratively Responsible to:	Clinical Supervision
1. Clinical Specialist for Psychiatric Nursing* Beth Israel Hospital Boston, Mass.	Dept. of Nursing	Associate Director of Nursing for Education and Research	Private Nurse Consultation
2. Psychiatric Liaison Nurse The Cambridge Hospital Cambridge, Mass.	Dept. of Nursing	Psychiatric Nursing Supervisor	Dept. of Psychiatry Consultation Liaison Service
3. Mental Health Clinical Spec. Children's Hospital Boston, Mass.	Dept. of Nursing	Associate Director of Staff Development	Dept. of Nursing
4. Psychiatric Nurse Clinical Specialist Massachusetts Rehabilitation Hospital, Boston, Mass.	Dept. of Nursing	Director of Nursing	Dept. of Nursing Dept. of Psychiatry Liaison Service
5. Psychiatric Liaison Nurse The Miriam Hospital Providence, Rhode Island	Dept. of Psychiatry	Dept. of Psychiatry Chief, Liaison Service	Dept. of Psychiatry Chief, Liaison Service

	Column 1	Column 2	Column 3
6. Clinical Director of Psychiatric Nursing Mount Auburn Hospital Cambridge, Mass.	Dept. of Nursing	Director of Nursing	Dept. of Psychiatry Liaison Service
7. Psychiatric Liaison Nurse Mount Auburn Hospital Cambridge, Mass.	Dept. of Nursing	Psychiatric Clinical Director of Psychiatric Nursing	Dept. of Psychiatry Clinical Director— Psychiatric Nursing
8. Psychiatric Nurse Consultant New England Medical Center Boston, Mass.	Dept. of Nursing	Assistant Director of Nursing	Dept. of Psychiatry Consultation/Liaison Service Dept. of Nursing
9. Psychiatric Nurse Clinician Peter Bent Brigham Hospital A Division of the Affiliated Hospitals Center	Dept. of Nursing	Associate Director of Staff Education	Dept. of Psychiatry
10. Psychiatric/Mental Health Nurse, Somerville Hospital Somerville, Mass.	Independent Contractor	Director of Nursing	Dept. of Psychiatry
11. Psychiatric/Mental Health Nurse, Youville Hospital Cambridge, Mass.	Dept. of Psychiatry The Cambridge Hospital	Dept. of Psychiatry The Cambridge Hospital	Psychiatric Liaison Nurse

*During the course of preparing this manuscript, this position was retitled as "Psychiatric Liaison Nurse," accountable to the Coordinator for Psychiatric Nursing Services.

have been agreed on, the psychiatric liaison nurse begins planning an entry into the hospital system. He or she develops strategies for implementing this role and requests administrative support as necessary. The following section discusses various factors that the psychiatric liaison nurse addresses to become successfully integrated into the hospital. As in role creation, many of these activities overlap and are not necessarily sequential.

An initial step in entering the system involves a continuing assessment of the system's formal and informal power structures. A key factor in this continuing assessment is a knowledge of the history of nursing in general, as well as of psychiatric liaison nursing within the system. This step is so important to the process of system entry that it cannot be sacrificed to the impulse to begin "functioning." Just as one might assume that a nursing intervention would be inappropriate without exercising the assessment steps of the nursing process, one may also assume that to begin "functioning" as a liaison nurse

---

TABLE 2–2 A MODEL JOB DESCRIPTION

PSYCHIATRIC LIAISON NURSE

Definition

The psychiatric liaison nurse is a registered professional nurse, with a master of science degree in psychiatric nursing, who practices predominantly in the general hospital. Functioning in accordance with the philosophy, objectives, and standards of nursing care within this institution, the focus of the clinical practice is the psychosocial and psychological aspects of the patient's illness.

Qualifications

1. Master's degree in psychiatric nursing.
2. Clinical experience in general nursing practice.
3. Demonstrated competence in psychiatric nursing.
4. Expert interpersonal skills with colleagues and patients.
5. Teaching ability.

Characteristics

1. Self-directed and able to function autonomously.
2. Committed to quality patient care.
3. Skilled in multidisciplinary approach to patient care.
4. Able to initiate and support change for the improvement of patient care.
5. Demonstrated ability in problem solving.

TABLE 2–2 (*continued*)

Responsibilities

1. To serve as a resource person by consulting with nursing staff regarding the management of patients with behavioral problems, patients who are experiencing difficulty with their medical illness, and milieu issues.
2. To serve as a liaison between nursing and psychiatry.
3. To participate with other disciplines in problem solving, education, and other patient-related issues.
4. To function as a role model in demonstrating therapeutic nursing relationships either directly or indirectly with patients and/or families.
5. To assess and meet the educational needs of nursing personnel by teaching on the unit level and by functioning closely with staff development in formal education programs and their evaluation.
6. To participate as needed and appropriate in meetings, seminars, and the clinical practice of the department of psychiatry.
7. To maintain professional competence through continuing education courses and other relevant learning experiences.

Responsible to:

Director of Nursing. Maintains a close working relationship with and clinical supervision from the Director of the Consultation-Liaison Service.

without acquiring an adequate history of the system may result in a disastrous first consultation encounter.

Questions to consider during this history-gathering phase include:

- How much impact has the nursing department had within the system in terms of improving and assuring quality patient care? What are the current attitudes toward and the present understanding of emotional care needs, not only within nursing but throughout the system?
- Which departments within the system are united by mutual goals and approaches to administrative and clinical problems?
- Are there any traditions of territoriality within the system? Might some members of the system block the implementation of the psychiatric liaison nurse role? Is there acceptance of the philosophy of nurse-to-nurse consultation, not only with the nursing department but throughout the system?
- Have there been any previous attempts to implement the role? Successful? Unsuccessful? Why? Might any remaining myths or expectations from these previous attempts hinder the present attempt to implement the role?

To understand these questions, the psychiatric liaison nurse should meet not only with nursing administrators, but also with department heads in areas such as psychiatry, social service, medicine, and pastoral care. These meetings should be legitimized by the director of nursing, and they should also be formal sessions rather than casual chats over a cup of coffee.

In addition to this overall system assessment and history gathering, the liaison nurse recognizes that each patient care unit is a subsystem with distinct strengths and needs that warrant identification. It is important to become cognizant of the uniqueness of each unit. The psychiatric liaison nurse meets with the head nurse of each unit to gain an understanding of the head nurse's philosophy and approach to managing the unit. The type of care and patient diagnosis is assessed to assist in understanding the type of patient care problems that each staff encounters within the realm of its unit. Meetings with the key nursing administrators involved in each unit are arranged, as it is important that nursing coordinators, supervisors, or area directors sanction the validity of the unit staff utilizing the psychiatric liaison nurse as a consultant. Finally, at this point in system entry, formal meetings with the staff of each unit are scheduled, and introductions take place. During these introductory meetings, liaison nurses elicit staff expectations and articulate their role.

In conjunction with assessing the system and beginning introductions, the process of establishing relationships and working alliances begins to emerge. The success of these initial discussions contributes to the eventual use of the liaison nurse in the consultation-liaison role. During system entry the liaison nurse develops lines of communication within the nursing department and with other departments. These lines are rarely static and, once established, are kept open and functioning; they are then used for the necessary task of continually defining and redefining what the psychiatric liaison nurse is there to do.

As the liaison nurse gathers data, assesses individual nursing units, and begins to establish relationships and alliances, the informal power structure of the system begins to unfold. As described, "...the influence of the informal system is not an exception or an aberration but a continuing element in the organizational process [38]." Liaison nurses remain cognizant of the fact that they will initially be presented with the formal power structure, such as policies and job descriptions, rather than the "...informal system of relationships and information sharing, ties of loyalty and of dependence, of favors granted and owed, of mutual benefit, of protection..." that constitutes the informal power structure [39].

In planning for entry into the system, liaison nurses are aware that establishing credibility is their ultimate goal and may well be the key factor in successful role implementation. They are aware that system entry may not proceed in the outlined orderly fashion. They may receive requests for service prior to any meetings on a particular unit and be forced to define their role by means of "trial by fire." Answering a call for help when a patient's behavior suddenly becomes unmanageable, even when the request comes before the liaison nurse has been fully oriented to the system, can sometimes establish the position's usefulness in a dramatic and effective way. It is important that the psychiatric liaison nurse maintain flexibility in response to these requests for service that occur during the initial stages of system entry. A helpful guiding principle in determining an appropriate response should be: "How can I best establish my credibility as a useful consultant?"

Credibility is also enhanced by liaison nurses' personal and professional presentations. Based on their assessment of the system and the system's perception of psychiatric nurses, they consider what style of dress is appropriate. In addition, they identify ways of communicating theoretical knowledge in a manner that fosters comprehension by nonpsychiatric personnel. Thus their written and verbal statements are clear, concise, and devoid of psychiatric jargon.

A final factor in establishing credibility is the initial investment of time on units that are most receptive, with the hope of developing a reputation for being useful and of transmitting it to units whose staff appear less ready to seek consultation. It is helpful, however, for the psychiatric liaison nurse to maintain visibility on those units that are less receptive. The act of maintaining visibility and availability initially may include attending many long meetings that may appear irrelevant to the liaison nurse's role, such as a change-of-shift report or supervisors' conferences. Since out of sight is sometimes out of mind, the nursing staff may need many reminders that the liaison nurse is available.

Each hospital system is unique and the importance of addressing specifics when creating the psychiatric liaison nurse role cannot be overemphasized. Equally important is adhering to the philosophy and goals of psychiatric nursing consultation and the overall responsibilities of the agreed-upon job description. When the role is created and the initial negotiations completed, attention is then directed toward concrete, pragmatic, and effective ways to carry out the clinical work of the psychiatric liaison nurse.

section 3 implementing and developing the role

The effectiveness of nursing consultation is correlated with a clear understanding by liaison nurses of their job. "When the nurse is not certain of what her role is and what expectations others hold for her, then confusion and conflict may result [40]." In their eagerness to develop alliances and to begin clinical practice, they are tempted to gloss over the early phases of negotiating the role. The early weeks or months of any position are fraught with anxiety, insecurity, and an urgent need to feel like a part of the system. The inherent isolation of psychiatric liaison nursing, combined with its clinical infancy, magnifies the problem for the newly hired liaison nurse. This overall feeling results in liaison nurses using situations to implement their role that are not only inappropriate but damaging to the further development of the position.

Two causes of failure of the liaison process have been described: Either the staff has unrealistic expectations, or they distort the purpose of the consultation [41]. It behooves liaison nurses to remain aware of these tendencies as they seek to gain acceptance. There is no cookbook guide for the implementation of the role. Not only is each institution unique in structure and needs, but so are the clinical or administrative situations influencing implementation. A commitment to the development of a consultation relationship is imperative.

Jackson describes an errant consultation as a result of her initial eagerness. She negotiated her intervention with the supervisor and failed to inquire about the head nurse's thoughts and observations. "Basically it was part of my own need to prove myself in the new role, a need to be the 'rescuer' at once—without a sensitivity to the head nurse as a person, and without conforming to the appropriate channels of communication [42]."

Especially during the initial stages of implementation, liaison nurses should evaluate each request for involvement, opinion, action, or any kind of assistance, along with its relationship to their job description. Implementation, although it begins immediately, can vary from a request for consultation on the first day to a lapse of several weeks.

One liaison nurse, while driving to work the very first day of employment, heard on the news that a gun fight resulted in two deaths and the admission of three critical patients to her hospital. Upon arriving at work, the head nurse in the ICU contacted the liaison nurse and asked for help. In the midst of the tension and confusion in the ICU, the liaison nurse began the assessment process with two of the patients. In this situation, implementation was required immediately. One of the patients was paralyzed from the bullet and faced prolonged hospitalization. The liaison nurse was involved, both directly and indirectly, for three months in the psychological care of the patient.

Most initial involvements are not as dramatic and urgent as this illustration. More commonly, the first case is the more difficult, demanding, and intractable patient. The covert message from the consultee may be, "Show us your stuff." Your message back might be, "I'm no magician, but I'll try." Attempts should continue thoughtfully and impartially to evaluate each opportunity to begin the work. Supervision, discussed in more detail in Chapter 3, Section 4, is a critical element during the early phases of the job.

There are multiple appropriate areas for liaison nurses to begin to clinically define their role in the hospital. The possibilities are of varying interest, and some may prove less exciting than others. They are, however, the nuts and bolts. In the long run, these openings are the building blocks to strong alliances, to increased utilization, and to the germination of the sought-after reputation that the liaison nurse is competent, available, helpful, and effective. A legacy develops and alliances with new staff occur in a manner similar to any accepted aspect of nursing care within the institution with increased rapidity each year. The result is that psychiatric nursing consultation becomes a valuable part of professional nursing care that is available to patients and nurses.

As a guide for the liaison nurse, each request for involvement and/or consultation that permits implementation of the role can be quickly evaluated by the who, what, where, when, and how approach. This is a *beginning step* toward engaging in the more complex process of "diagnosing the total consultation."

- **Who** is requesting the consultation? Does the identity of the consultee itself indicate another agenda? Another health professional, such as a physical therapist, may present a reasonable and viable reason for nursing consultation. An important consideration for the liaison nurse is the nursing staff's view of the patient. Checking with the nurses strengthens alliances, aids in avoiding traps, and fosters a nursing identity.

Example: The nursing supervisor may ask the liaison nurse to speak with a patient who is refusing her medications. Some questions to be considered are: Why is the supervisor telling the liaison nurse and not the staff nurses? Is there a conflict between the supervisor and the nurses? Is the patient creating an unidentified problem for the supervisor, but she prefers to phrase it in the context of a "patient problem"?

- **What** are they asking of you? Is the request for consultation about a patient who is belligerent in the evening an attempt to expose the problems of the 3-to-11-o'clock staff? Does the nursing staff see the liaison nurse as an outside resource to solve staff problems? Are they asking you to do nothing because they are afraid and threatened? Is a staff member seeking individual counseling? Is the request for your services a set-up for your intervention in a political struggle? What is the liaison nurse's previous experience on this ward?
- **Where** is the request made? Is it written? Do you receive a phone call? Is it casual? Does the consultee ask you to talk in a private place? Is the request made in the nurses' station in the presence of other staff members? Consideration of these factors is important for an appropriate response by the liaison nurse.
- **When** is the request for psychiatric nursing consultation made? Is this the first time consultation has been requested? Has the patient just been admitted? Has the patient been hospitalized for three months? Is this the first time in many months that the ward has requested assistance? Have they tried other interventions and are regarding psychiatric nursing consultation as a last resort? Are the nurses feeling overwhelmed and frustrated, and do they just want the liaison nurse to stand by for validation of their feelings? Is the liaison nurse being requested to do an in-service program that would be inadequate without sufficient time for preparation?
- **How** can the role be implemented in this situation? Is this the time to make a direct intervention? Should the liaison nurse carefully avoid becoming involved because it might conflict with the role and its implementation? Is this a situation that necessitates an interdisciplinary approach? Should the liaison nurse give an impromptu ward conference on the drug-abusing patient to demonstrate flexibility? How will involvement strengthen consultation alliances?

Using this set of questions—who, what, where, when, and how —as a guideline, liaison nurses can conceptualize quickly whether the situation is an appropriate one for the implementation of their role. There are multiple avenues for increasing visibility, availability, and "showing your wares." The careful identification of appropriate arenas for clinical practice, combined with some risk avoidance, results in effective implementation. The willingness to recognize an effective and/or dangerous place for role implementation is crucial.

A liaison nurse who had prior pediatric experience negotiated attending patient care rounds on a very small pediatric unit with the hope of becoming actively involved with the psychological nursing management of the patients. After two years, the liaison nurse recognized that the low patient census, skilled nursing staff, extensive psychiatric input from child psychiatrists, and the consistent availability of social workers who focused on the multiple social problems of the families, resulted in diminished necessity for liaison nursing. Although the liaison nurse maintained contact and remained available, full implementation of the role at this time was not attempted. Psychiatric nursing consultation certainly had a place on this unit, but the need was a low priority. The amount of energy required to implement the role was not justifiable.

The following examples are of activities that have been effective in beginning the job. The list, though not exhaustive, illustrates possibilities and encourages creative adaptations.

daily rounds

Visibility is a precursor to implementation. The sight of the liaison nurse serves as a concrete reminder of the psychological care of the patient. Experience has proven that issues are presented to liaison nurses when they are seen on the unit. Consultations are less likely to occur if they require seeking out the liaison nurse. Initially, making the daily rounds can be very difficult because the new liaison nurse is unfamiliar with the staff. However, it is essential to lay the groundwork of availability, consistency, and concern.

in-service programs

Exposure and publicity are provided to liaison nurses through their participation in hospital education programs. Especially in the initial stages of implementation, their involvement in such programs provides identity, purpose, and direction for their efforts. When programs are integrated into general educational presentations, they portray the liaison nurse as an integral and coordinated part of patient care rather than as a separate entity. For example, the psychological care of the oncology patient may be more effectively communicated when it is part of an overall program concerning the medical-surgical care of oncology patients. Alliances can be built with the staff development/in-service department, as well as with the general nursing staff. Tables 2–3 and 2–4 are brief outlines illustrating this type of educational presentation.

As the ongoing assessment of the system continues and as implementation progresses, the involvement in educational programs can become increasingly creative, sophisticated, and stimulating for both the liaison nurses and the staff. Timing, again, is crucial. Even though the liaison nurse may have a special interest in the manage-

---

TABLE 2–3 TEACHING THE DIABETIC PATIENT—
THE STATE OF THE ART

Content

1. Nature and Causes of Diabetes
2. Medical Management and Complications
3. Research in the Field of Diabetes
4. Dietary Considerations
5. **Psychosocial Aspects of Diabetes**

   The role of a psychological assessment for the diabetic will be discussed as a prerequisite to the learning process. Consideration will be given to the grief process as related to the patient's adjustment to the disease.

   The effect of diabetes on the patient's life will be stressed, with emphasis on his pre-morbid personality and social and family strengths. The relationship of exacerbations of the disease, as they are related to events in the broad psychosocial environment, will be included.

6. Teaching the Diabetic—One Nurse's Perspective
7. Teaching the Nurse to Teach the Diabetic
8. The Diabetic Teaching Clinic

Bibliography

Isenberg, P. L. and Barnett, D. M. "The Psychological Problems in Diabetes Mellitis," *Medical Clinics of North America* 49:1 (1979): 123.

Kahana, R. and Bibring, G. B. "Personality Types in Medical Management," in *Psychiatry and Medical Practice in General Hospitals*, edited by N. Zinberg. New York: International Universities Press, Inc., 1964.

Kimball, C. P. "Emotional and Psychosocial Aspects of Diabetes Mellitis," *Medical Clinics of North America* 55:7 (1971): 160.

Lipowski, Z. J. "Physical Illness, the Individual, and the Coping Process," *International Journal of Psychiatry in Medicine* 1:2 (April 1970): 91–102.

———. "Psychosocial Aspects of Disease," *Annals Internal Medicine* 7 (1969): 1197.

TABLE 2–4 YOU HAD AN MI—TEACHING THE PATIENT

Content

1. Review of Cardiovascular Anatomy and Physiology
2. Complications of Acute Myocardial Infarction
3. The MI Teaching Protocol—How To Use It
4. Rehabilitation of the Coronary Patient
5. **Psychological Assessment of the MI Patient**

   Through case-centered discussions, the elements of a psychological assessment will be illustrated. Attention will be given to various personality types, as well as to the importance of recognizing the meaning of the illness to the patient. The emphasis will be on how to listen for and to explore with the patient reactions to his or her MI.

6. Problems in Convalescence

Bibliography

Cassem, Ned and Hackett, Thomas. "Psychological Aspects of Myocardial Infarction," *Medical Clinics of North America* 61:1 (July 1977): 711–721.
————. "Psychological Rehabilitation of Myocardial Infarction in the Acute Phase," *Heart and Lung* 2 (May–June 1973): 382–388.
Skelton, M. and Dominian, J. "Psychological Stress in Wives of Patients with Myocardial Infarction," *British Medical Journal* (April 1973): 101–103.
Snyder, Joyce and Wilson, Margo. "Elements of a Psychological Assessment," *American Journal of Nursing* (February 1977): 235–239.
Soloff, Paul. "Denial and Rehabilitation of the Post-Infarction Patient," *International Journal of Psychiatry in Medicine* 8:2 (1977–78): 125–132.
Storlie, Frances. "Learning as a Life Experience: The Case of the Cardiac Patient," *Supervisor Nurse* (July 1977): 64–67.
Wishnie, Howard et al. "Psychological Hazards of Convalescence Following Myocardial Infarction," *Journal of the American Medical Association* 215:8 (1971): 1292–1296.

ment and assessment of terminally ill patients, right now may not be the "right time" to do a program on this subject. What is the history within the institution concerning programs on death and dying? Who taught these programs? How were they received? Is there a need for another program? What resources within the system concern the care of the terminally ill patient? Will the liaison nurse become identified as the "death and dying" nurse? Is there a hidden issue in the milieu regarding management of terminal patients? That is, have nurses been criticized for their work in this aspect of patient care? Will they be threatened? Is the liaison nurse being encouraged to present this topic because there has been a flood of complaints from patients and families regarding this issue?

Even more critical than the possible bad timing is the negative effect it has on the acceptance of liaison nurses as providers of helpful patient care. Their role is implemented through in-service programs by presenting themselves and the programs as timely, realistic, and appropriate adjuncts to the care of patients.

Some possible programs that may be presented are:

1. interviewing patients,
2. suicidal patients,
3. psychotropic medications,
4. psychosis,
5. human sexuality,
6. angry or hostile patients,
7. agitated or combative patients,
8. drug-abusing patients,
9. alcoholism,
10. death and dying,
11. hospitalization as a crisis, and
12. the over-compliant patient.

TABLE 2–5 PAIN MANAGEMENT IN CHILDREN AND ADOLESCENTS

Content

Psychosocial variables in pain perception from the patient's, the family's, and the staff's points of view. The meaning of pain to children at different developmental levels.

   I. The Reality of Pain
     A. A socially unacceptable phenomenon
     B. The symbolic meaning and experience of pain
     C. Defining pain

  II. A Developmental Approach to Assessment and Intervention

 III. The Parental Position
     A. Coping strategies and character style
     B. Experience with and expectations of pain
     C. Perceptions of the parental role

 IV. Nursing Intervention
     A. "Painful" experiences and memories
     B. Symbolic meanings and definitions

TABLE 2–5 (*continued*)

C. Developmental considerations
D. Family/social/cultural components

V. Implications for Nurses
  A. The nurse's experience
  B. The pain-fear-stress cycle
  C. Interventions for nurses

Bibliography

ARONOFF, GERALD M. and WILSON, R. REED. "How to Teach Your Patients to Control Chronic Pain," *Behavioral Medicine* (July 1978): 29–35.

BOND, M. R. "Psychological and Psychiatric Aspects of Pain," *Anesthesia* 33:4 335–61 (April 1978): 489–520.

COPP, L. "Pain and Suffering"–special supplement, *American Journal of Nursing* 7:3 (March 1974): 489–520.

ELAND, J. "Chronic Intractable Pain—Living with Pain," *Nursing Outlook* (July 1978): 430.

ENGEL, GEORGE. "Psychogenic Pain and the Pain-Prone Patient," *American Journal of Medicine* (June 1959): 899–918.

EPSTEIN, MEL H. and HARRIS, JAMES. "Children with Chronic Pain, Can They Be Helped?" *Pediatric Nursing* (January–February 1978): 42–44.

FAGERHAUGH, SHIZUKO Y. and STRAUSS, ANSELM. "How to Manage Your Patient's Pain and How Not To," *Nursing '80* (February 1980): 44–47.

GILDEA, JOAN and QUIRK, TINA. "Assessing the Pain Experience in Children," *The Nursing Clinics of North America* 12:4 (December 1977): 631–637.

JACOX, ADA, ed. *Pain: A Source Book for Nurses and Other Health Professionals.* Boston: Little, Brown & Company, 1977.

JACOX, A. and STEWART, M. L. *Psychosocial Contingencies of the Pain Experience.* College of Nursing, The University of Iowa, 1973.

JOHNSON, MARION. "Pain—How Do You Know It's There?" *Nursing '76* (September 1976): 48–50.

LARKINS, FABIENNE R. "The Influence of One Patient's Culture on Pain Response," *The Nursing Clinics of North America* 12:4 (December 1977): 663–668.

McCAFFREY, MARGO and HART, LINDA L. "Undertreatment of Acute Pain with Narcotics," *American Journal of Nursing* (October 1976): 1586–1591.

McMAHON, MARGARET A. and MILLER, PATRICIA. "Pain Response: The Influence of Psycho-Social-Cultural Factors," *Nursing Forum* 17:1 (1978): 58–71.

SCHMITT, MARY. "The Nature of Pain," *The Nursing Clinics of North America* 12:4 (December 1977): 621–629.

STORILE, FRANCES. "Pointers for Assessing Pain," *Nursing '78* (May 1978): 37–39.

WOLF, BARBARA. *Living with Pain.* New York: The Seabury Press, 1977.

WOLF, ZANE ROBINSON. *Topics in Clinical Nursing: Pain Management.* Germantown, Md.: Aspen Systems Corporation, 11:1, April 1980.

ZBOROWSKI, M. "Cultural Components in Responses to Pain," *Journal of Social Issues* 8 (1952): 16–30.

TABLE 2–6 COPING WITH EVERYDAY DEPRESSION

Content

I. Defining Depression
  A. Psychoanalytic view
  B. Behavioral view
  C. Interpersonal theory
  D. Organic theory

II. A Description of Affect
  A. Signs and symptoms
  B. Use of defense mechanisms

III. Intervention for staff and patients

Bibliography

Books

ANTHONY, E. J. and BANEDEK, T., eds. *Depression and Human Existence*. New York: Little, Brown & Co., 1975.

ENGEL, G. L. *Psychological Development in Health and Disease*. New York: W. G. Saunders Co., 1962.

SELYE, H. *The Stress of Life*. New York: McGraw-Hill Book Company, 1956.

Articles

BOWLBY, J. "Grief and Mourning in Infancy and Early Childhood," *Psychoanalytic Study of the Child* 15 (1960): 9–52.

ENGEL, G. L. "Grief and Grieving," *American Journal of Nursing* (September 1964): 93–98.

FISDEN, H. K. "Faces and Masks of Depression: The Psychodynamic Side," *Psychosomatics* 20:4 (April 1979): 254–268.

HALL, R. C. et al. "The Professional Burnout Syndrome," *Psychiatric Opinion* (April 1979): 12–17.

IVANCEVICH, J. M. and MATTESON, M. T. "Nurses and Stress: Time to Examine the Potential Problem," *Supervisor Nurse* (June 1980): 17–22.

MASLACH, C. "Burned-Out," *Human Behavior* (September 1976): 1–12.

MULLINS, A. C. and BARSTOW, A. E. "Care for the Caretakers," *American Journal of Nursing* (August 1979): 1425–1427.

POE, R. O.; LOWELL, F. M.; and FOX, H. M. "Depression—Study of 100 Cases in a General Hospital," *Journal of the American Medical Association* 195:5 (January 31, 1966): 345–350.

SHUBIN, S. "Rx for Stress—Your Stress," *Nursing '79* (January 1979): 53–55.

Tables 2–5, 2–6, and 2–7 are examples of educational programs that are primarily psychologically focused. The possibilities are endless, and involvement is ongoing.

TABLE 2–7 RENAL CONFERENCE—COPING WITH CHRONIC ILLNESS

Content

I. Illness as a Life Stress
    A. A personal definition
    B. Coping versus adaptation
    C. Defining "chronic"
    D. The sick role

II. The Crisis Is Experienced
    A. Grief and the capacity to bear it
    B. Dependency-interdependency conflicts
    C. Working through: the defensive structure
    D. Psychotropic medication—psychotherapy

III. Behavioral Predications
    A. Pre-morbid assessment
    B. Helplessness in service of the ego
    C. Denial in service of hope
    D. The role of motivation

IV. Nursing Intervention—A Psychological Approach

Bibliography

Articles

ANGER, DIANE. "The Psychologic Stress of Chronic Renal Failure and Long-Term Hemodialysis," *The Nursing Clinics of North America* 10:3 (September 1975): 449–458.

BASCH, S. H. "The Intrapsychic Integration of a New Organ," *The Psychoanalytic Quarterly* 42:3 (July 1973): 364–384.

BEARD, BRUCE H. "Fear of Death and Fear of Life: The Dilemma in Chronic Renal Failure, Hemodialysis and Kidney Transplantation," *Archives of General Psychiatry* 21 (1969): 373–380.

LIPOWSKI, Z. J. "Psychosocial Aspects of Disease," *Annals of Internal Medicine* 71:6 (December 1969): 1197–1206.

————. "Physical Illness, the Individual and the Coping Process," *International Journal of Psychiatry in Medicine* 1:2 (April 1970): 91–102.

MLOTT, S. A. and WHITING, S. M. "Superstition and the Renal Nurse," *JAANNT* 5:2 (1979): 92–99.

SAND, P.; LIVINGSTON, G.; and WRIGHT, R. "Psychological Assessment of Candidates for Hemodialysis Program," *Annals of Internal Medicine* 54:3 (March 1966): 602–610.

TUCKMANN, A. J. "Brief Psychotherapy and Hemodialysis," *Articles of General Psychiatry* 23 (July 1970): 55–59.

There are potential in-service programs that are wise to avoid. Topics involving supervision, evaluation, or job performance are inadvisable to discuss. As a nurse, involvement in teaching programs about psychiatric diagnosis or an in-depth description of psychoanalytic theories and therapeutic techniques may represent dangerous bridges to cross. As liaison nurses implement their role, silent observers may have a variety of reactions. The politics and administration of the institution with regard to any teaching program should be acknowledged and respected.

Teaching through in-service programs progresses in concert with the overall advancement, utilization, and integration of the role of liaison nurses. An assessment is recommended of the general impact, as well as of the possible hidden agendas, of all in-service programs in which the liaison nurse is involved.

nursing orientation

Through orientation programs required by nursing departments, liaison nurses have an opportunity to introduce and to promote their availability to the new nursing staff. The offer is both time-effective and welcomed by those required to acquaint new employees to hospital services. By open-ended discussions in orientation, liaison nurses can begin to assess the new employees' level of experience with psychological intervention. Since the effectiveness of liaison nurses' intervention is influenced by the staff's participation, it is helpful to acquire and encourage support early on in the nurses' careers in the institution.

Liaison nurses, recognizing the inherent stress and tension for staff beginning a new job, can utilize their initial contact with new nurse employees by offering support and understanding. Alliance building is slow and steady, based on genuine feelings of caring about both staff and their patients. Just as new liaison nurses hope for a warm response from hospital staff, so do any new employees hope to feel accepted and recognized as an integral part of the staff. As liaison nurses meet new employees in orientation they can, by fostering a warm welcome, lay the groundwork for appropriate utilization of their skills.

committees and meetings

Within the structure of the department of nursing are numerous opportunities for liaison nurses to become involved, to promote their role, and to build critical alliances. As each institution is unique, the responsibility of liaison nurses is to assess for themselves which path provides the best opportunity professionally. For example, a newly hired liaison nurse learned that a bright, energetic staff nurse, who had been informally responsible for ostomy teaching, wanted to coordinate the teaching program for in-patients and out-patients. Cognizant of the large psychological component in the teaching of ostomy patients, the liaison nurse joined the committee, which was comprised of the in-service director, the ostomy teaching nurse, the out-patient head nurse, and the nutritionist. The committee's work together ended with a day-long Staff Workshop on "Teaching the Ostomy Patient." The liaison nurse presented material on the psychological care of the ostomy patient and the meaning of the illness.

Some committee work can be endlessly time-consuming with little or no potential for the implementation of the psychiatric liaison role. The effects of the committee work on the role of the liaison nurse should be carefully weighed. Similar criteria can be applied to regularly scheduled meetings. Initially it is helpful for liaison nurses to assess the individual system to ascertain the most beneficial way to spend their time. The necessity to attend meetings varies with their length of employment in the system and the issues being addressed.

department of psychiatry

Whenever there is an acute psychiatric problem with a medical-surgical patient, the nursing staff will probably experience anxiety, tension, and stress. Even though the patient may be receiving psychiatric intervention from a member of the department of psychiatry, the liaison nurse can still assess the degree of comfort and ease that the nursing staff is experiencing in their care of the patient. The liaison nurse may be helpful by expressing interest in how the staff is managing with the patient. There may be questions about the procedure involved in committing a patient, how to care for a suicidal patient, how to talk to a psychotic patient, and so on. Interventions with staff and/or patients include collaboration with the psychiatrist, or with any other mental health professional involved, in order to provide optimal care. The willingness to stand by, to help, to teach where needed, and to be available is a concrete, effective, and essential way to implement the role. Even without a direct intervention one psychiatric patient on a medical ward may have the potential of exposing the liaison nurse to twenty staff members. Visibility, availability, flexibility, and involvement are the hallmarks of role implementation with the identified psychiatric patient on the medical-surgical ward.

nursing assessments

Accurate, comprehensive, and thorough health assessments have become a vital tool to hospital nurses. Some nurses experience difficulty in acquiring data about personal issues or those essential to a psychosocial history. When appropriate, liaison nurses can assist staff in gathering information required for a nursing assessment. This involvement is not only an aid to the staff, but it also gives added exposure to the liaison nurse.

interviewing patients

A psychosocial assessment of the patient is based on proficiency in interviewing the patient. Clearly the best way to learn how to interview a patient is to watch someone who is skilled in interviewing. It makes sense then to ask the consultee to join liaison nurses as they talk with a patient who is presenting a problem. Liaison nurses demonstrate data-gathering techniques and the integration of this information into plans for intervention. The consultee may then understand more clearly the way in which liaison nurses can make a valuable and helpful contribution to the care of the patient.

cardiac or respiratory arrest

When stress and tension are prevalent on a ward during an arrest, liaison nurses can implement their role by being available. Maybe a staff member, for a variety of reasons, is experiencing difficulty. If family is present, they may require assistance that is not, for the moment, available due to the medical crisis. Furthermore, the other patients in the ward may be stressed by the arrest and possible subsequent chaos. Responding to codes and their aftermath may provide numerous opportunities for intervention.

deceased patients

Death on a ward is met by staff with a variety of reactions, including relief, anger, sadness, guilt, or helplessness. Liaison nurses may provide support to the young nurse who has never done post mortem care. They may also just be there as a silent support for what, at that time, may be unspeakable. Liaison nurses, in their quest for implementation, can be role models not only during a crisis but during the aftermath. The opportunities are endless. What do you say to the family of the deceased patient whom you have never met before?

What happens if they become hysterical or angry? What do you tell other patients? More painful still, how do you cope with the way you feel as a nurse and human being?

The guidelines of who, what, when, where, and how—blended with a well thought-out professional stance and fortified with enthusiasm and energy—aid the process of role implementation. Creativity is essential, both initially and in the further development of the role, to realize the fullest potential of the work of liaison nurses.

section 4   potential problems of role practice

As the psychiatric liaison nursing role develops, there are opportunities for increased acceptance. As discussed previously, implementation is an ongoing process that continues as long as the role itself exists within the hospital. The goals of clinical practice remain constant, while the liaison nurse's consultation alliances are established and strengthened. In the course of working with consultees, liaison nurses are afforded the opportunity to increase their knowledge of the milieu and its members. Over time, they become increasingly proficient in their practice, and the result is a positive role legacy. The role becomes more established within the hospital and recognized as an important adjunct to comprehensive patient care.

The following developments are a sampling of our observations:

1. The number of appropriate consultation requests increases.
2. The nature of the consultations change from those that are solely crisis-oriented to those that are prophylactic.
3. Professional growth in the consultees is demonstrated through their ability to recognize more subtle psychological care issues and to carry out more sophisticated interventions, as well as by their comfort with increased clinical autonomy.
4. The clinical competence and reliability of the liaison nurse is acknowledged by other disciplines.

It has been documented that over time changes occur in the quality of nursing consultation referrals. Referrals become more patient-specific, patient-focused, psychological, and comprehensive [43].

Problems and/or rejection are also experienced in the implementation and development of the role. Gertrude Flynn describes the process of consultation "as a love affair of the French variety [44]."

She emphasizes the significance of time, the mode of entry into the system, the charisma to stimulate interest and trust, and the need for a contract that clearly specifies mutual expectations, responsibilities, and time-frames. Nevertheless, not every love affair, even those of the French variety, are satisfying. Liaison nurses may incorporate into their practices the elements that Flynn mentions, only to find that their consultations are not well received. Teaching the consultee about some aspect of psychological care does not guarantee a successful consultation. Quite often, liaison nurses learn that the information that they are so eager to provide is already in the consultee's knowledge base. Interviewing the identified patient and formulating psychotherapeutic interventions do not always guarantee success. Although it is essential that liaison nurses be supportive, available, and visible, these characteristics of practice do not ensure acceptance.

Role implementation and development are accompanied not only by increased opportunities for clinical practice, but also by temptations, inappropriate consultation requests, clinical risk taking, clinical errors, and the hearing of painful as well as of positive feedback. Confidence can sometimes breed carelessness. It would behoove liaison nurses to carefully consider the following professional tasks and personal issues, lest they fall prey to incorrectly viewing their clinical work as reasonable and therapeutic, while projecting their clinical mistakes onto the consultee(s).

Liaison nurses may experience a variety of baffling and upsetting situations. Increased visibility may strengthen their consultation alliances, but it may also make them targets for projection. Members of the health care team may incorrectly believe that the liaison nurses are providing psychotherapy for a patient whom they do not even know, or that they have consulted on issues outside the realm of their clinical practice. Liaison nurses may lose their invitation to consult on a ward or in regard to a specific situation and not be able to clarify the etiology. They may listen to the hospital grapevine, only to learn that disharmony exists between the manner in which they are perceived and the manner in which they thought they were perceived by their nursing colleagues. Contradictions may also exist in terms of their interactions with other departments. Liaison nurses may be devalued by anyone on the health care team. Unbeknownst to them, they may be tested, set up to fail, or caught in a clinical split. Their clinical recommendations may be misinterpreted by the consultee(s), which may result in recommendations not being followed, being only partially carried out, or being incorrectly carried out. Misinterpretation may also result in the inappropriate generalized application of clinical recommendations from one patient situation to another.

The intent of a consultation request may not always be clear. Sometimes the consultees cannot formulate consultation questions, or they formulate them inaccurately. It is not unusual for the consultee to merely state that the patient is "crazy" or that something about the patient "isn't right." The consultee may be acutely aware that a problematic situation exists, but also unclear as to what the liaison nurse should provide. If the consultee is confused in terms of clarifying the need for psychiatric nursing consultation, the liaison nurse may find clinical formulation just as baffling. As discussed in Chapter 4, "The Consultation Process," a request for consultation may prove vague or confusing in reference to the overt and covert agenda contained in it. The overt agenda is most usually expressed in terms of an appropriate request for consultation. The hidden agenda emerges as the consultation is diagnosed, or it may become evident while clinical recommendations and interventions regarding the overt problem are either in progress or completed. At this time, a hidden agenda may be directly or indirectly expressed by the consultee(s). Or it may be demonstrated behaviorally or affectually; for example, the consultee(s) may continue to be upset regarding the overt situation even though this situation is at some stage of resolution. Failing to correctly carry out clinical recommendations suggested by the liaison nurse may also be a symptom of a hidden agenda.

Expectations of the liaison nurse by the consultee(s) and/or by the hospital system itself may be realistic or unrealistic. They may reflect hidden agendas, a lack of understanding of the liaison role, or a lack of agreement with the theoretical definition. As a consequence of such expectations, liaison nurses may be called upon to become involved in areas of clinical work that are contrary to and/or outside the boundaries of their role. The temptation to comply with the request can be very great. The short- and long-term results of giving into this temptation are rarely benign. Rigid policies regarding clinical work on the part of liaison nurses are not the solution. A careful evaluation of all consultation requests, clinical temptations, and administrative/supervisory directives is combined with open discussion with the consultee(s) and/or the clinical supervisor.

Although the consultee's perception and opinion regarding consultation is important, other aspects of this issue also warrant prudent examination. Liaison nurses' expectations of themselves as clinicians, coupled with a personal and professional appraisal of their performance, always reflect realistic and unrealistic values, hopes, and ambitions. To objectively evaluate one's clinical work is difficult at best. Although not a completely impossible task, liaison nurses accomplish objective self-evaluation as a result of their ability to recognize subjective elements.

- Do they view their work as being clinically sound only if a patient's behavior or mood improves?
- If their consultation alliance is strengthened with a specific ward or consultee, does this indicate work well done?
- Does the number of consultation requests received validate clinical competence and clinical acceptance?
- Do liaison nurses need to be held in high esteem by all members of the health care team?
- If their clinical recommendations are not followed, is this evidence of poor performance in the liaison role?
- How bothered are liaison nurses when the social worker or the psychiatrist is called in by the nurses to assist in managing a nursing issue with a patient?
- How do liaison nurses feel when feedback from the consultee regarding their input is negative?
- How do they deal with isolation?
- What do they need in their professional lives to promote stimulation and to feel gratified?
- What do they do with their own anger, frustration, identification, or countertransference issues? And what stimulates them?
- To what degree are liaison nurses self-observant?

The degree of importance they place on their professional lives as sources of self-esteem and personal characteristics influences the responses to these questions.

Clinical mistakes are made even by the most experienced psychiatric liaison nurses. Assessing each situation, formulating a plan, and being prepared to accept responsibilities and consequences may be difficult. Yet they are essential. Liaison nurses try not only to recognize when contacting their supervisors and/or psychiatrists is necessary, but also to feel comfortable in asking for help. The most skilled supervisor and/or colleague can err. The ability to accept the reality that mistakes are inevitable is fundamental to recognizing the human elements in all areas of clinical practice.

The following list of behaviors may prove counterproductive to role implementation and development:

1. assuming the "expert-know-it-all" stance,
2. assuming a rigid stance,

3. saving time by not reviewing the patient's *old* and *present* medical records,
4. minimizing patients' physiologic status and its influence on his or her psychiatric status,
5. responding to the "urgent" request for help,
6. making unrealistic promises to patients and/or to the consultee(s),
7. pressing the consultee for detailed information that is unavailable or threatening,
8. interpreting the consultee's behavior,
9. interpreting the consultee's feelings,
10. setting expectations for the consultee(s),
11. failing to call for psychiatric back-up, and
12. utilizing the consultation process to work through personal issues.

As liaison nurses become more proficient in their practice and secure in their role, they become better able to avoid pitfalls. Even so, identifying the etiology of an unsuccessful consultation is not always a definitive process. Perhaps the liaison nurse, although careful not to use psychiatric jargon, is still explaining issues in a complex, theoretical manner that proves unhelpful. Liaison nurses may be unaware of administrative problems or intra-staff tensions on a ward, which negatively influence the consultation. In addition, they may be unaware of social relationships existing on a ward, which influence psychiatric interventions. Also inhibiting consultation are such factors as identification, as well as transference-countertransference issues among health care team members, the patient, and the liaison nurse.

To provide competent psychiatric nursing consultation, liaison nurses remain aware of the potential problematic issues that have been discussed. As their role develops, problems are acknowledged. Absolute resolution is an unrealistic goal. Problems may be addressed with humor, silence, confrontation, apology, or negotiation. Clinical supervision is an appropriate forum for further examination of the inherent complexities and difficulties in consultation-liaison work. By thoughtfully analyzing and observing the implementation and development of their role, psychiatric liaison nurses can experience personal and professional growth.

references

1. John Locke, "An Essay Concerning Human Understanding," in *The English Philosophers from Bacon to Mill*, edited by Edward Burtt (New York: The Modern Library, Random House, Inc., 1939), p. 242. Reprinted with permission.
2. Jack Zusman and David Davidson, *Practical Aspects of Mental Health Consul-*

tation (Springfield, Ill.: Charles C. Thomas, Publisher, 1972), p. 30.

3. Z. J. Lipowski, "Consultation-Liaison Psychiatry: Past, Present and Future," in *Consultation-Liaison Psychiatry*, edited by R. O. Pasnau (New York: Grune & Stratton, Inc., 1975), p. 4.

4. Mary O'Neil Mundinger and Grace Dotterer Jauron, "Developing a Nursing Diagnosis," *Nursing Outlook* 23:2 (February 1975): 94–98.

5. Murray Levine, "The Practice of Mental Health Consultation: Some Definitions from Social Theory," in *Practical Aspects of Mental Health Consultation*, edited by J. Zusman and D. Davidson (Springfield, Ill.: Charles C. Thomas, Publisher, 1972), p. 13.

6. Jack Zusman, "Mental Health Consultation: Some Theory and Practice," in *Practical Aspects of Mental Health Consultation*, edited by J. Zusman and D. Davidson (Springfield, Ill.: Charles C. Thomas, Publisher, 1972), p. 31.

7. Thomas Hackett and Ned Cassem, *Massachusetts General Hospital Handbook of General Hospital Psychiatry* (St. Louis: The C. V. Mosby Company, 1978).

8. ———, pp. 1–14.

9. Ida Jean Orlando, *The Dynamic Nurse–Patient Relationship* (New York: G. P. Putnam's Sons, 1961), p. 36.

10. E. Brenner, *An Elementary Textbook of Psychoanalysis* (New York: International Universities Press, Inc., 1973).

11. G. Blanck and R. Blanck, *Ego Psychology Theory and Practice* (New York: Columbia University Press, 1974).

12. J. C. Nemiah, *Foundations of Psychopathology* (New York: Oxford University Press, 1961).

13. Sigmund Freud, "Beyond the Pleasure Principle," in Vol. XVIII of *The Standard Edition of the Complete Psychological Works of Sigmund Freud* (London: The Hogarth Press and The Institute of Psycho-Analysis, 1955), p. 12.

14. E. Kris, *Psychoanalytic Explanations in Art* (New York: International Universities Press, Inc., 1965), p. 105.

15. E. H. Erikson, *Childhood and Society*, 2nd ed. (New York: W. W. Norton & Co., Inc., 1950), pp. 247–274.

16. S. Freud, *The Ego and The Id* (London: The Hogarth Press, 1927).

17. G. S. Engel, *Psychological Development in Health and Disease* (New York: W. B. Sanders Co., 1962), p. 289.

18. H. Selye, *Stress of Life* (New York: McGraw-Hill Book Company, 1956).

19. E. Meyer and M. Mendelson, "Psychiatric Consultations with Patients on Medical and Surgical Wards: Patterns and Processes," *Psychiatry* 24:197 (1961): 197–220.

20. A. Weisman and T. Hackett, "The Organization and Function of a Psychiatric Consultation Service," *The International Record of Medicine and General Practice Clinics* 173 (1960): 306.

21. J. J. Sandt and R. Leifer, "Psychiatric Consultation," *Comprehensive Psychiatry* 5 (1964): 409.

22. W. Gray, F. J. Duhl, and N. D. Rizzo, eds., *General Systems Theory and Psychiatry* (Boston: Little, Brown & Company, 1969).

23. L. von Bertalanffy, "General Systems Theory," *Main Currents in Modern Thought* 11 (March 1955): 75–83.

24. A. D. Hall and R. E. Fagan, "Definition of a System," in *Modern Systems Research for the Behavioral Scientist*, edited by W. Brekley (Chicago: Aldine Publishing Co., 1968), p. 81.

25. Thomas Hackett and Ned Cassem, *Massachusetts General Hospital Handbook of General Hospital Psychiatry* (St. Louis: The C. V. Mosby Company, 1978).

26. M. Knowles, *The Modern Practice of Adult Education* (New York: Association Press, 1970), p. 39.

27. M. E. Hazzard, "An Overview of Systems Theory," *The Nursing Clinics of North America* 6:3 (September 1971): 393.

28. J. J. Schwab and W. A. Bradnan, "Life Phases in Health and Illness," in *The Psychiatric Clinics of North America* (August 1979): 277–288.

29. G. Caplan, *An Approach to Community Mental Health* (New York: Grune & Stratton, Inc., 1961), p. 18.

30. H. M. Lefcourt, *Locus of Control Current Trends in Theory and Research* (Hillsdale, N.J.: Lawrence Erlbaum, Assoc. Publishers, 1976), p. 3.

31. C. B. Bilodeau and Suzanne O'Hara O'Connor, "Role of Nurse Clinicians in Liaison Psychiatry," in *Massachusetts General Hospital Handbook of General Hospital Psychiatry*, edited by Thomas P. Hackett and Ned H. Cassem (St. Louis: The C. V. Mosby Company, 1978), pp. 508–523.

32. S. Goldstein, "The Psychiatric Clinical Specialist in the General Hospital," *Journal of Nursing Administration* (March 1979): 34–37.

33. H. A. Jackson, "The Psychiatric Nurse as a Mental Health Consultant in a General Hospital," *The Nursing Clinics of North America* 4 (1969): 327–340.

34. B. S. Johnson, "Psychiatric Nurse Consultant in a General Hospital," *Nursing Outlook* 2 (1963): 728–729.

35. L. J. Weinstein, M. M. Chapman, and M. A. Stallings, "Organizing Approaches to Psychiatric Nurse Consultation," *Perspectives in Psychiatric Care* 17 (1979): 66–71.

36. M. Kramer, *Reality Shock* (St. Louis: The C. V. Mosby Company, 1974), in S. A. LaRocio, "An Introduction to Role Theory for Nurses," *Supervisor Nurse* (December 1978): 41.

37. J. Levy and A. Lewis, *A Model Job Description* (Unpublished, 1980).

38. M. Hennig and Anne Jardim, *The Managerial Woman* (New York: Doubleday and Company, Inc., 1976), p. 12. Reprinted with permission.

39. M. Hennig and Anne Jardim, *The Managerial Woman* (New York: Doubleday and Company, Inc., 1976), p. 12. Reprinted with permission.

40. J. S. Howard, "Liaison Nursing," *Journal of Psychiatric Nursing Services* (April 1978): 35–37.

41. F. Lehmann, "Liaison Nursing: A Model for Nursing Practice," in Gail Stuart

and Sandra Sundeen, *Principles and Practice of Psychiatric Nursing* (St. Louis: The C. V. Mosby Company, 1979).

42. H. A. Jackson, "The Psychiatric Nurse as a Mental Health Consultant in a General Hospital," *The Nursing Clinics of North America* 4:3 (September 1969): 527–540.

43. J. Nelson and D. Davis, "Referrals to Psychiatric Liaison Nurses: Changes in Characteristics Over a Limited Time Period," *General Hospital Psychiatry* 2:1 (March 1980): 41–45.

44. G. E. Flynn, "The Romance of Consultation," in *Practical Aspects of Mental Health Consultation*, edited by J. Zusman and D. L. Davidson (Springfield, Ill.: Charles C. Thomas, Publisher, 1972), pp. 126–127.

bibliography

books

BELAND, I. L. *Clinical Nursing: Pathophysiological and Psychosocial Approaches*. New York: The MacMillan Company, 1965.

BENNIS, W. et al. *Interpersonal Dynamics*, 3rd ed., Homewood, Ill.: Dorsey Press, 1973.

BION, W. R. *Experience in Groups*. New York: Ballantine Books, Inc., 1974.

BOLES, R. C. *Theory of Motivation*. New York: Harper & Row, Publishers, Inc., 1967.

BOWDEN, C. L. and BURSTEIN, A. G. *Psychosocial Basis of Medical Practice*. Baltimore: The Williams and Wilkins Company, 1974.

BURGESS, ANN WOLBERT and BALDWIN, BRUCE. *Crisis Intervention Theory and Practice*. Englewood Cliffs, N.J.: Prentice-Hall, Inc., 1981.

BURGESS, A. and LAZARE, A. *Psychiatric Nursing in the Hospital and the Community*. Englewood Cliffs, N.J.: Prentice-Hall, Inc., 1981.

CAPLAN, G. *The Theory and Practice of Mental Health Consultation*. New York: Basic Books, Inc., Publishers, 1970.

DUBOS, R. *Man, Medicine and Environment*. New York: Frederick A. Prager, 1968.

ENGEL, G. L. *Psychological Development in Health and Disease*. New York: W. B. Sanders Co., 1962.

FAULKES, S. H. and ANTHONY, E. J. *Group Psychotherapy: The Psychoanalytic Approach*, 2nd ed. England: Penguin Books Ltd., 1965.

GRAY, W.; DUHL, F. J.; and RIZZO, N. D., eds. *General Systems Theory and Psychiatry*. Boston: Little, Brown & Company, 1969.

HOFLING, C. K.; LENINGER, M. M.; and GREGG, E. *Basic Psychiatric Concepts in Nursing*, 2nd ed. Philadelphia: J. B. Lippincott Company, 1967.

JACO, E. G. *Patients, Physicians and Illness*. Glencoe, Ill.: The Free Press, 1968.

KOHNKE, M. F. *The Role for Consultation in Nursing Designs for Professional Practice*. New York: John Wiley & Sons, Inc., 1978.

LAPLANCHE, J. and PONTALIS, J. B. *The Language of Psychoanalysis*. New York: W. W. Norton & Co., Inc., 1973.

LAUGHLIN, H. P. *The Ego and Its Defenses*, 2nd ed. New York: Jason Aronson, Inc., 1979.

LIFF, Z. A., ed. *The Leader in the Group*. New York: Jason Aronson, Inc., 1975.

LINDZEY, G. and ARONSON, E., eds., *The Handbook of Social Psychology*, Vol. 1. Reading, Mass.: Addison-Wesley Publishing Co., Inc., 1954.

LOOMIS, M. E. *Group Process for Nurses*. St. Louis: The C. V. Mosby Company, 1979.

MERENESS, D. A. and TAYLOR, C. M. *Essentials of Psychiatric Nursing*. St. Louis: The C. V. Mosby Company, 1978.

PARAD, H. J. *Crisis Intervention: Selected Readings*. New York: Family Service Association of America, 1965.

PASNAU, R. O. *Consultation-Liaison Psychiatry*. New York: Grune & Stratton, Inc., 1975.

PHARES, E. J. *Locus of Control in Personality*. Morristown, N.J.: General Learning Press, 1976.

SACKETT, D. H. and HAYNES, R. B. *Compliance with Therapeutic Regimens*. Baltimore: Johns Hopkins University Press, 1976.

SCHWAB, J. J. *Handbook of Psychiatric Consultation*. New York: Appleton-Century-Crofts, 1968.

SKIPPER, J. K. and LEONARD, R. C. *Social Interaction and Patient Care*. Philadelphia: J. B. Lippincott Company, 1965.

STRAIN, J. and GROSSMAN, S. *Psychological Care of the Medically Ill: A Primer in Liaison Psychiatry*. New York: Appleton-Century-Crofts, 1975.

STUART, G. and SUNDEEN, S. *Principles and Practice of Psychiatric Nursing*. St. Louis: The C. V. Mosby Company, 1979.

TRAVELBEE, J. *Interpersonal Aspects of Nursing*, 2nd ed. Philadelphia: F. A. Davis Company, 1971.

USDIN, G. and LEWIS, J. *Psychiatry in General Medical Practice*. New York: McGraw-Hill Book Company, 1979.

WAELDER, R. *Basic Theory of Psychoanalysis*. New York: International Universities Press, Inc., 1960.

YALOM, I. D. *The Theory and Practice of Group Psychotherapy*. New York: Basic Books, Inc., Publishers, 1975.

ZINBERG, N. E., ed. *Psychiatry and Medical Practice in a General Hospital*. New York: International Universities Press, Inc., 1964.

articles

BAKER, BETTY and LYNN, MARY. "Psychiatric Nursing Consultation: The Use of an Inservice Model to Assist Nurses in the Grief Process," *Journal of Psychiatric Nursing and Mental Health Services* (May 1979): 15–19.

BARTON, D. and KELSO, M. T. "The Nurse as a Psychiatric Consultation Team Member," *International Journal of Psychiatry in Medicine* 2 (1971): 108–115.

BLAKE, P. "The Clinical Specialist as a Nurse Consultant," *Journal of Nursing Administration* 7 (1977): 33–36.

BROWN, W. A. and JACOBSON, E. M. "Consultation-Liaison Psychiatry: Current Responsibilities," *American Journal of Psychiatry* 133:3 (March 1976): 326–328.

BURGESS, A. C. and LAZARE, A. "Nursing Management of Feelings, Thoughts and Behavior," *Journal of Psychiatric Nursing and Mental Health Services* (November–December 1972): 7–11.

CALHOUN, G. and PERRIN, M. "Management Motivation and Conflicts," *Topics in Clinical Nursing* 1:3 (October 1979): 71–88.

CANTER, A. et al. "The Frequency of Physical Illness as a Function of Prior Psychological Vulnerability and Contemporary Stress," *Psychosomatic Medicine* 28 (1966): 344–350.

DARBONNE, A. "Crisis: A Review of Theory, Practice, and Research," *International Journal of Psychiatry* 6 (1968): 371–379.

EISDORFER, C. and BATTON, L. "The Mental Health Consultant as Seen by His Consultees," *Community Mental Health Journal* 8:3 (1972): 171–177.

FREEMAN, C. K. "Transactional Analysis: A Model for Psychiatric Consultation in the General Hospital," *Nursing Forum* 18:1 (1979): 43–51.

GEIST, R. A. "Consultation on a Pediatric Surgical Ward: Creating an Empathic Climate," *American Journal of Orthopsychiatry* (1977): 432–444.

GOLDSTEIN, S. "The Psychiatric Clinical Specialist in the General Hospital," *Journal of Nursing Administration* (March 1979): 34–37.

GREENBERG, I. M. "Approaches to Psychiatric Consultation in a Research Hospital Setting," *Archives of General Psychiatry* 3 (December 1960): 139–145.

GRINKER, R. "Anxiety as a Significant Variable for a Unified Theory of Human Behavior," *Archives of General Psychiatry* 1 (November 1969): 537–547.

HOLLISTER, W. G. and MILLER, F. T. "Problem-Solving Strategies in Consultation," *American Journal of Orthopsychiatry* 47:3 (July 1977): 445–450.

HOLMES, T. H. and RAHE, R. H. "The Social Readjustment Rating Scale," *Journal of Psychosomatic Research* 11 (1967): 213–218.

HOWARD, JOAN STOLTZ. "Liaison Nursing," *Journal of Psychiatric Nursing and Mental Health Services* (April 1978): 35–37.

JACKSON, H. A. "The Psychiatric Nurse as a Mental Health Consultant in a General Hospital," *The Nursing Clinics of North America* 4:3 (September 1969): 527–540.

JANSSON, D. "Student Consultation: A Liaison Psychiatric Experience for Nursing," *Perspectives in Psychiatric Care* 17 (1979): 77–82.

KARASU, T. B. "Psychotherapy of the Medically Ill," *American Journal of Psychiatry* 136 (January 1979): 1–11.

KARASU, T. B. and HERTZMAN, M. "Notes on a Contextual Approach to Medical Ward Consultation: The Importance of Social System Mythology," *International Journal of Psychiatry in Medicine* 5:1 (1974): 41–49.

KARASU, T. B.; PLUTCHIK, R.; STEINMULLER, R.; CONTE, H.; and SIEGEL, B. "Patterns of Psychiatric Consultation in a General Hospital," *Hospital and Community Psychiatry* 28:4 (April 1977): 291–294.

KARASU, T. B.; WALTZMAN, S.; LINDENMAYER, J. P.; and BUCKLEY, P. "The Medical Care of Patients with Psychiatric Illness," *Hospital and Community Psychiatry* 31:7 (July 1980): 463–471.

KASL, S. V. and COBB, S. "Health Behavior, Illness Behavior, and Sick Role Behavior," *Archives of Environmental Health* 12 (April 1966): 531–541.

KIMBALL, C. P. "Conceptual Developments in Psychosomatic Medicine: 1939–1969," *Journal of Internal Medicine* 73 (August 1970): 307–316.

———. "Liaison Psychiatry of Approaches and Ways of Thinking about Behavior," *Psychiatric Clinics of North America* 2:2 (August 1979): 201–210.

KNABLE, J. and PETRE, G. "Resistance to Role Implementation," *Supervisor Nurse* (February 1979): 31–34.

KREUTER, FRANCES. "What Is Good Nursing Care?" *Nursing Outlook* 5 (May 1957).

LIPOWSKI, Z. J. "Review of Consultation Psychiatry and Psychosomatic Medicine III, Theoretical Issues," *Psychosomatic Medicine* 30 (July–August 1968): 395–422.

———. "Physical Illness, the Individual and the Coping Process," *International Journal of Psychiatry in Medicine* 1 (1970): 91–102.

————. "Consultation Liaison Psychiatry: An Overview," *American Journal of Psychiatry* 131 (1974): 623–630.

McBRIDE, A. G. "How Attribution Theory Can Shape Therapeutic Goal-Setting," a paper presented at the biannual meeting of the American Nurses' Association, Houston, Texas (June 1980).

McGEE, T. "Some Basic Considerations in Crisis Intervention," *Community Mental Health Journal* 4 (1968): 319–324.

MEYER, E. and MENDELSON, M. "Psychiatric Consultations on Medical and Surgical Wards," *Psychiatry* 24 (1961): 197–220.

MOHL, PAUL. "A Review of Systems Approaches to Consultation–Liaison Psychiatry," *General Hospital Psychiatry* 3 (June 1981): 101–110.

————. "A Systems Approach to Liaison Psychiatry," *Psychosomatics* 21:6 (June 1980): 457–461.

NELSON, J. and SCHILKE, D. "The Evolution of Psychiatric Liaison Nursing," *Perspectives in Psychiatric Care* 14 (1976): 61–65.

NUCKOLLS, KATHERINE. "The Consultation Process: A Reciprocal Relationship," *Maternal Child Nursing* (January–February 1977): 11–16.

PATI, BARBARA. "Nursing Consultation: A Collaborative Process," *Journal of Nursing Administration* (November 1980): 33–37.

PEPLAU, H. E. "Professional Closeness," *Nursing Forum* 8:4 (1969): 342–360.

RAHE, R. et al. "Social Stress and Illness Onset," *Journal of Psychosomatic Research* 8 (1964): 35–44.

ROBINSON, L. "Liaison Psychiatric Nursing," *Perspectives in Psychiatric Care* 6 (1968): 87–93.

SCHWAB, J. J. "The Psychiatric Consultation: Part I," *Journal of Continuing Education in Psychiatry* 40:2 (February 1979): 17–27.

————. "Psychiatric Consultation Part II, Potential for Therapy," *Journal of Continuing Education in Psychiatry* 40:3 (March 1979): 23–31.

SNYDER, J. C. and WILSON, M. F. "Elements of a Psychological Assessment," *American Journal of Nursing* (February 1977): 235–239.

STEVENS, BARBARA J. "The Use of Consultants in Nursing Service," *Journal of Nursing Administration* (August 1978): 7–15.

VAILLANT, G. E.; SHAPIRO, L. N.; and SCHMITT, P. P. "Psychological Motives for Medical Hospitalization," *Journal of the American Medical Association* 214:9 (November 1970): 1661–1665.

VAUGHN, BETH ANN. "Role Fusion, Diffusion, and Confusion," *The Nursing Clinics of North America* 8:1 (December 1973): 703–713.

VISOTSKY, H. M. et al. "Coping Behavior under Extreme Stress," *Archives of General Psychiatry* 5 (November 1961): 423–448.

VOLICER, B. J. "Patients' Perceptions of Stressful Events Associated with Hospitalization," *Nursing Research* 23:3 (May–June 1974): 235–238.

WOLFF, P. "Psychiatric Nursing Consultation: A Study of Referral Process," *Journal of Psychiatric Nursing* 16 (1978): 42–47.

WOODROW, MARY and BELL, JUDITH. "Clinical Specialization: Conflict between Reality and Theory," *Journal of Nursing Administration* (November–December 1971): 23–28.

3

the psychiatric liaison nurse in the health care delivery system

The dog barking at you from behind his master's fence acts for a motive indistinguishable from that of his master when the fence was built.

ROBERT ARDREY [1]

section 1 department of nursing

The *entire* institution of the hospital becomes the workplace for the psychiatric liaison nurse. Every system and subsystem is examined and considered as the liaison nurse becomes involved in the life of the hospital and in the delivery of care. Nurses are intimately involved in the world of the hospital. "As the only permanent members of the unit social system, nurses are its culture bearers and the primary socialization agent [2]." Sociologists in the 1940s and 1950s began to study the hospital as a social system. Yet these contributions, which examined both the influence of structure, role, and other factors on group behaviors and the influence of social factors on individual behaviors, have rarely been incorporated into practice [3]. In the undefined and complex environment, liaison nurses, with their knowledge of systems theory, attempt to carve out a place within a multidisciplinary model to meet the psychological needs of the hospitalized patient.

A focus for liaison nurses is the department of nursing of which they are members. As previously mentioned, consideration of the philosophy, goals, policies, and procedures of the department of nursing is primary. The liaison nurse's place on the organizational chart, along with the nursing department's relationship to other hospital departments, is recognized. Global trends and developments in the nursing profession and the resulting effects on the department of nursing are noted. Finally, the effects of societal, political, and economic pressures on the status of the nursing profession are of importance. Nursing is the largest health care profession in this country [4]. As liaison nurses implement, develop, and function in their positions, the department of nursing remains their base of operation. The strength, influence, and potential power of this base is frequently underestimated. As inevitable conflicts and problems arise, the support of the department of nursing becomes crucial.

Traditionally, nursing has defined its role in terms of the best interests of the patient. Obviously this orientation continues to be of utmost importance, but it must now be combined with increased political astuteness and protection of nursing's professional position within the health care system. Nurses, historically subservient, have viewed themselves as being in a powerless position. In turn, this view has decreased group cohesiveness and further weakened them. The struggle for unity has been hampered by confusion within nursing itself. This confusion, in part, emanates from basic nursing education. The educational preparations available vary and include an associate degree, bachelor's degree, and three-year hospital-affiliated program, any of which allows the student to take the same licensing examination for registration as a professional nurse. Other disciplines, as well as the general public, are confused by this. While the overall level of education in nursing has increased—that is, with masters and doctoral programs—nurses have become more cognizant of the need for, and better able to negotiate, a more powerful position in the health care system.

As liaison nurses attempt to establish themselves within the health care delivery system, they can seek identity with nurses in other specialties who are also struggling with chronic role confusion. Complicating the picture are some of the titles or descriptions applied to nurses: Extended (or expanded) role practice... nurse clinician... clinical specialist... nurse practitioner... nurse consultant are but a few. The status of nurses' roles in the institution has a direct bearing on the liaison nurse's functioning within that system. The sophistication and quality of the nursing staff, as well as the perceived power of the department of nursing, influences the liaison nurse's permission to practice and to succeed.

Nursing, as a predominantly female profession, has been directly affected by the changing status of women. "The role and place of the nurse in the total system correspond to the minor role assigned to women in American society as a whole [5]." The traditional (female) nurse as handmaiden to the (male) physician has been further complicated by the increasing number of female physicians. The roles are changing, and behaviors are frequently challenged. Confrontation, assertiveness, and aggression have become inappropriately identified with emancipation. As women struggle to become recognized as truly equal citizens, the tensions, anxieties, and frustrations are acted out in the social system of the hospital and within the nursing profession. Within this framework, competent, well educated, and qualified liaison nurses work toward integrating these societal struggles into their efforts toward collaborative, effective care for patients. This integration includes being politically aware, accountable, and assertive when appropriate.

> *Example:* As part of her clinical responsibilities, a liaison nurse, along with other members of the consultation-liaison team, provided emergency coverage. The negotiated arrangement with the team was that a psychiatrist would remain available to the liaison nurse for problems that might be beyond the scope of her practice. When the liaison nurse responded to an emergency with a surgical patient, the attending physician was adamant that he wanted a doctor, a psychiatrist. The liaison nurse, instead of trying to impress the surgeon with her qualifications or to confront his bias, explained the way the consultation-liaison service functioned. Confident of the support of the liaison psychiatrist, the liaison nurse again offered to proceed with the evaluation. The surgeon decided not "to make an issue" out of it and agreed. In subsequent requests for consultation, this issue did not arise.

The increasing awareness of the need for higher education for nurses is reflected in a general move toward requiring and acquiring more advanced degrees. Many states are now requiring validation of continuing education units for renewal of licensure. This trend meshes well with the liaison nurse's goal of educating staff to become increasingly knowledgeable and therapeutic in their interactions. This kind of climate within the nursing profession supports the liaison nurse. Nurses who do not assume responsibility for their continued professional education, but who rather expect it to be provided, are as outdated as black stockings and pinafores. Tuition reimbursement plans and opportunities for continuing education have aided the return of nurses to the classroom.

The changing status of women has stimulated more occupational opportunities. Computer technology, engineering, law, business, and other fields previously not as welcoming to women have become open and desirable. No longer are nursing, educational, secretarial, and social work the only routes to job security for women. In fact, nurses have become disillusioned with nursing and have discovered that it is not what they thought [6]. The problems of inadequate staffing, low salaries, long and/or inconvenient hours, the necessity of doing non-nursing tasks, and the lack of power and prestige have all contributed to this disenchantment. Changes in the entire health care delivery system, including consumer participation and increased skepticism regarding nurses, have transformed nurses from "angels of mercy" to "angels of death." Legal action against nurses, which was almost unheard of in the past, is no longer as uncommon [7]. Nurses must now more than ever consider the legal aspects of nursing care [8]. There is increased accountability for clinical practice both publicly and within the profession.

The problems facing nursing administrators have grown in complexity, as has the practice of nursing. Young graduate nurses now feel less bound to their jobs. Students, mothers, and those not wanting to be "tied down" are attracted to the upsurge of nursing agencies in metropolitan areas. These agencies allow nurses flexibility by permitting them to choose a day, a shift, and a clinical area in which to work. Liaison nurses must keep abreast of these changes, as well as their impact on patient care. When there is lack of consistency in the membership of the nursing staff, the teaching and implementing of principles of psychological care is more difficult.

The health care field is the third largest industry and the largest that is unorganized [9]. Emerging unions, by their very nature, have precipitated a new value system. Whether nurses are in agreement with these values or not, the changes are occurring and ultimately affecting patient care. Some departments of nursing must be involved in contract negotiations, grievances, and legal matters. The provision of psychological care is also affected by these issues and must be kept in its proper perspective for the welfare of the patient.

From this environment in the department of nursing, liaison nurses set out to fulfill their clinical objectives. Should they serve on nursing committees? Become involved in unions? Testify in legal cases? These are, needless to say, difficult questions. The guidelines are in an accurate assessment of the individual institution, coupled with each nurse's personal goals, qualities, and professional interests. A liaison nurse's decisions for involvement must be tempered by the commitment to multidisciplinary collaboration and to the viability of the psychiatric liaison nursing role.

section 2   multidisciplinary and interdisciplinary collaboration

Our capacities for sacrifice, for altruism, for sympathy, for trust, for responsibilities to other than self-interest, for honesty, for charity, for friendship and love, for social amity and mutual interdependence have evolved just as surely as the flatness of our feet, the muscularity of our buttocks, and the enlargement of our brains, out of the encounter of ancient African savannahs between the primate potential and the hominid circumstance. Whether morality without territory is possible in man must remain our final, unanswerable question [10].

A multidisciplinary approach to meeting the psychological needs of patients occurs across several hospital systems and departments. Many tasks in the health care delivery system cannot be carried out by one discipline. To provide optimal psychological care to the hospitalized patient, collaboration by the liaison nurse may extend to the following:

1. physical therapists,
2. social workers,
3. occupational therapists,
4. respiratory therapists,
5. pastoral counseling,
6. psychiatric-psychology staff,
7. medical-surgical staff,
8. vocational counseling,
9. continuing care coordinators,
10. dietitians,
11. recreational therapists,
12. volunteers,
13. language interpreters, and
14. neurology staff.

Multidisciplinary can be defined as members of diverse disciplines in the same setting, informally interacting [11]. This definition, for general purposes, would apply to this list. Each discipline becomes, by education and experience, a reliable evaluator of certain aspects of psychological adjustment. Occupational therapists, in their assessment, add a crucial dimension in predicting, for example, the chances of adaptive coping mechanisms for the fracture patient who must have prolonged bed rest. The physical therapist, experienced in working with amputees, becomes a vital evaluator of a patient's psychological course. When a team approach is used, not only is the assessment more accurate and thorough, but the team members become more involved and knowledgeable.

More likely, the disciplines that are closely related clinically have the potential for more role conflict and overlapping. When health care providers are threatened or rejected by their colleagues, they tend to become more territorial and rigid. Social work and liaison nursing, both predominately female professions, have the potential for conflict. Like other mental health professions, social work and psychiatric nursing flourished with the increased federal money of the 1960s, only to be threatened with its withdrawal in the 1980s. Social workers and psychiatric nurses within their own professional groups have faced a similar predicament. After completing masters level educational programs, both are facing the stress and uncertainty of certification and licensure. The commonality of their issues has, in some large academic centers, fostered a territorial struggle rather than stimulating professional cohesion. Psychiatric liaison nursing as a specialty within psychiatric nursing is identifying the management and psychological nursing care of the patient as its turf. In the past, social workers may have fulfilled this role in the very same institutions. Perlman described two aspects of socio-psychodynamic transactions that are considered the "turf" of social workers: (1) problems of social functioning of large numbers of people and (2) social environment [12].

The overlap between psychiatric liaison nursing and social work occurs as both struggle with their own identities. The evolution of liaison nursing has been addressed. As social work has moved from a scientific base of sociological theory to psychiatric theory, there have been changes in the educational process and in the focus of its practice. The educational division of psychiatric and medical social work no longer exists. Social work education is now focused on the treatment of people based on psychodynamic knowledge. These similarities may produce a breeding ground for territorial struggles. As each discipline provides its part of the care of the patient, an understanding and knowledge of intraprofessional issues provide a vital dimension in the quest for an honest collegial relationship.

In the multidisciplinary approach no one is required to relinquish power, authority, or territory. The approach is less formal, more familiar, and requires no binding commitment. Although both the multidisciplinary and interdisciplinary approaches are influenced by individual participants and the clinical situation, the former is easier to negotiate and accomplish.

An *interdisciplinary approach* to health care is described as members of different disciplines involved in formal team arrangements that maximize opportunities for educational interchange and the delivery of service [13]. Although the concept of teams is a familiar one now, it was not so prior to 1930. During World War II there was an increase in the use of the team approach. Although originally out of necessity, interdisciplinary collaboration encouraged professional growth and provided a new method of health care delivery. By the 1950s the literature indicated a continued need for teamwork as well as a need to study its effectiveness [14]. Brill has offered this definition of teamwork:

> A team is a group of people each of whom possesses particular expertise; each of whom is responsible for making individual decisions; who together hold a common purpose; who meet together to communicate, collaborate, and consolidate knowledge from which plans are made, actions determined, and future decisions influenced [15].

In the attempt to explore and encourage the collaboration of health care professionals, it is crucial not to become overenthusiastic about teams. The merits of an individual approach must not be overlooked. There certainly may be times when more effort is put into the team collaboration than into providing health care. Perhaps there should be caution in choosing this approach to care delivery, as well as in not discounting the value of a one-to-one relationship. Styles of nursing care delivery have phased in and out, running the gamut of total patient care, functional team nursing, specialization, and primary nursing. Teamwork may provide optimal care at certain times, but it is not a panacea.

A variety of health care providers working as a team to deliver service has been illustrated in the literature. The collaborative approach, for example, was fostered when physicians and nurses led a seminar, in a primary care setting, devoted to the psychological aspects of medical care [16]. The participation of nurses contributed to the success of the group due to their increased sensitivity to the psychological aspects of patient care.

A team consisting of a liaison psychiatrist, a chaplain, a social worker, and a psychiatric nurse consultant was used as a creative crisis intervention technique. Following a tank car explosion, the families of burned patients met in a group. The psychiatric nurse met with the nursing staff, and each team member contributed to the overall goal of dealing with the crisis through multiple family groups [17]. Leaders in liaison psychiatry have emphasized and supported the team approach [18]. An interdisciplinary consultation program— including representatives from psychiatry, psychology, social work, and nursing—illustrated the provision of psychosocial care in a general hospital [19].

Several factors should be addressed to increase the chance of success when applying the interdisciplinary team concept. This list is not inclusive but rather a guideline for liaison nurses in their professional practice with other disciplines:

1. *Professional responsibility:* As professionals work together in consultation-liaison teams they may tend to minimize their differences. Although they have common knowledge and skills, by clearly identifying their differences, each professional becomes more distinctive. The special territory that each member maintains enhances his or her identity and self-esteem. Furthermore, individual territories promote the growth of the group by making the members not interchangeable, but rather visible and responsible for their specialty. The members are divided by their interest and competence.

2. *Goals:* The team must share common values and goals. Basic agreements about the psychological needs in the institution, the method of delivery, and the philosophy of health care are the building blocks of an interdisciplinary team.

3. *Structure:* For an interprofessional team to work, group norms and standards, provided within an agreed-upon structure, are essential. These may include meetings, rounds, seminars, and the like. Members of the team must have an opportunity to interact so the team concept can develop. If there is no structure, there is no planned communication and probably, in reality, no team.

4. *Decision making and leadership:* Recognition of the authority and responsibilities of the leader of the group is essential. Clearly the team should be involved when there are decisions affecting the entire group. The nitty-gritty functioning of the team, however, is best allocated to a leader. When groups get stuck around the issues of power and control, their energy gets diverted into the struggle rather than channeled toward the delivery of service. Disagreement is encouraged and conflict is inevitable, but power or control struggles become destructive. To be a team, the group must function together both as role models and professionals.

5. *Autonomy:* In addition to functioning independently, accepting responsibility for decisions is fundamental. Furthermore, team members recognize their personal and role limitations. The "leader" of the team is not the protector but rather a colleague. The liaison nurse, along with other team members, must accept the consequences of autonomy to function in this type of team.

6. *Respect:* Each professional in an interdisciplinary team has made a commitment to invest energy in a collaborative and collegial model. Unless this commitment is coupled with personal and professional respect, the structure can slowly crumble without an obvious cause. Respect develops with a display of competence and humanism that is the core of the interdisciplinary approach.

Working together as a team may provide not only comprehensive care but also professional stimulation for the liaison nurse. As each professional clearly marks off his or her own territory, each may benefit through the promotion of a collegial relationship.

section 3   isolation—search for a peer group

Psychiatric liaison nurses are in a unique position within the general hospital setting. Usually in staff positions within the department of nursing, they may encounter many colleagues and very few peers. Peers have equivalent academic preparation and are engaged in similar work [20]. Although there may be other nurses functioning in expanded roles within the institution, such as clinical specialists, liaison nurses carefully consider the potential implications on consultation work and alliances if they choose to identify themselves with a specific group of nurses. In most other nursing roles, a legitimate, safe peer group is already established. Staff meetings, change-of-shift reports, and certain ward social activities provide group structure and peer support for staff nurses. Supervisory meetings and seminars afford similar benefits to nursing leadership personnel. Liaison nurses may be invited or requested to attend any of these gatherings; but their participation retains the flavor of the consultant–consultee relationship.

Clinical autonomy can breed isolation. Consultation-liaison work can prove to be exciting, stimulating, overwhelming, and anxiety-provoking. Liaison nurses move in and out of a variety of situations. James Strain describes the atmosphere of the medical environment, defining the fundamental task of consultants as the simultaneous assessment of the psychological processes of the patient, the consultee(s), and of themselves [21]. The degree of stress that liaison nurses continually encounter is so impressive that it is unrealistic to assume that they can remain truly neutral on all issues. The sources of stress are diverse. Usually they are founded in the three processes mentioned. Stress, exaggerated by isolation, stimulates both an awareness of and a search for peers. The awareness of the need for an appropriate peer group is as essential to successful role functioning as is clinical education, experience, and supervision.

The liaison nurse may be fortunate enough to be employed in a general hospital that has more than one psychiatric liaison nurse. This situation is probably the ideal circumstance for the creation of a peer group. In the majority of hospitals, however, such is not the case. The liaison nurse may be the only autonomous psychiatric practitioner in the institution. Perhaps psychiatric liaison nurses in nearby hospitals could be contacted. Consensual validation and support are crucial, especially during the first few years of clinical practice when anxiety is at its highest level.

The purposes of a peer group are:

1. To provide a safe and supportive environment in which to express confusion, anxiety, frustration, anger, and other feelings regarding consultations and the experience of being a psychiatric liaison nurse.
2. To provide a confidential opportunity to discuss clinical issues, to achieve greater understanding, to receive feedback, and to identify strategies for problem resolution.
3. To identify, in a collaborative manner, researchable areas of clinical practice and role expansion.
4. To promote professional identity, development, and collegiality.

A careful assessment of the department of nursing is important for the achievement of membership in an appropriate peer group. As previously mentioned, identification with specific nurses may be either hazardous or beneficial to liaison nurses. By the very nature of their position and work within the hospital, they are tremendously visible. Their words and behavior are subject to observation and misinterpretation. When looking for a peer group within the hospital, consideration is given to individuals, to their clinical specialties, and to their positions within the system. Some members of the department of nursing are safer to align with than other members. Consistently having lunch with nursing supervisors may be viewed by the staff nurse consultee as a validation that the liaison nurse has supervisory responsibilities. Such social relationships may also be regarded by the supervisors as an indication that the liaison nurse is interested in being included in supervisory issues and will share information accordingly. Sometimes the offering of "professional friendship" is merely a guise for "friendly therapy." Such may be the case when aligning with a nurse who is experiencing system-related professional and/or personal difficulties. Joining a group of nurses regarded by the consultees as "elite" may afford liaison nurses an appropriate peer group in terms of educational preparation and clinical functioning, but doing so may also result in their being viewed as distant and unapproachable. In addition, liaison nurses are aware that the system may look to their identified peer group to cover vacations, even though they are not theoretically and clinically educated to do so. If the peer group includes nurses from the hospital's psychiatric unit, this situation is more apt to occur.

Finding an appropriate nursing peer group within the hospital setting may prove to be more complex than initially apparent. It is not unusual to discover that certain individuals who may have been regarded as peers are very much consultees. Sharing anxiety with a member of the nursing staff who is also a consultee is detrimental to clinical effectiveness. The liaison nurse may experience a sense of peership with a psychologically minded head nurse and, in so doing, share some of her frustration in working with another resistant head nurse. Many months later, the liaison nurse may find not only that those two head nurses are friends, but also that the resistant head nurse has been promoted to clinical supervisor over the "peer" head nurse. Understanding the relationships among members of the department of nursing is a complicated and at times a consuming task. Caution and prudence in forming these relationships promote a clearer understanding of the consultation liaison role.

Keeping thoughts and feelings private can be burdensome, and at times it may be impossible. The ideal situation is characterized by a balance between self-containment and self-disclosure. Perfection in clinical work and professional behavior are unreachable goals. Just as liaison nurses may fall prey to misdiagnosing a consultation, the quality and intensity of their reaction to a given situation may cause them to respond in a way that they later regret. Nevertheless, self-control, along with unrelenting calmness and patience, is not only unrealistic, but, if achieved, it may cause the liaison nurse to be viewed in a magical, fantasy-filled light.

> *Example:* The consultees on a stressful medical ward had utilized a liaison nurse frequently during her first year at the hospital. Consultations were almost always quite difficult, focusing on complex patient situations. These situations were characterized by severe regression and demandingness in the identified patient, anger and frustration in the nursing staff, and poor communication among the members of the health care team. Problem resolution could not be adequately achieved. One of the goals of the liaison nurse's work with this ward was to aid and support the nursing staff in tolerating these circum-stances which, at this time, could not be altered. The response to the liaison nurse was quite positive, but she was aware of a hint of envy and magic that seemed to color her alliance with the consultees. They continually expressed admiration and bafflement at the liaison nurse's ability to remain "cool and professional." The liaison nurse employed humor when acknowledging the frustration that she shared in com-

mon with the nursing staff. At the end of a nursing conference, dealing with a patient management problem, the consultees presented the liaison nurse with a poster for her office. On the poster was a bright sun shining down on colorful spring flowers. Across the flowers was written the phrase, "Someday I will burst my bud of calm and blossom into hysteria." Obviously the consultees were saying a great deal about their own fears and possible expectations of themselves, as well as about their view of the liaison nurse and what might happen if she "really reacted."

Isolation is most painful when first beginning to do consultation-liaison work. Perhaps collegial support, intellectual stimulation, and professional relationships can be found within the departments of psychiatry, psychology, or social service. Yet the possible ramifications of establishing close relationships with the members of these disciplines should also be carefully weighed. Obviously, the purposes of a peer group cannot be fulfilled through such affiliations, but they can be helpful, to a degree, in combating isolation. The opportunity to share humor and the importance of a relationship with a member of the "in-group" cannot be overemphasized. In practical terms, it may help prevent distortions, misperceptions, exhaustion, or a defensive retreat.

The responsibility of liaison nurses is to decrease the isolation that they experience by introducing themselves to individuals within the institution, through psychiatric and nursing supervision, and by working directly with patients. When occupying a role in which clinical competency is challenged frequently by the system, by the consultees, and by themselves, liaison nurses may derive immediate gratification from direct patient contact. Working with patients and attending educational programs are some of the ways in which they can combat apathy and burn-out. If group membership and approval are needed within the general hospital milieu to feel personally and professionally valuable, liaison nurses are doomed to experience devaluation. A peer group can provide support, empathic criticism, intellectual stimulation, professional intimacy, identity, and reality.*

"Living with ambiguity and working with approximate answers is really the most important process in consultation [22]." When combined with the wish to be helpful and the vulnerability to misinterpretation, the need for a peer group becomes obvious. It behooves

---

*The authors are members of A Peer Group of Liaison Nurses/Greater Boston Area, which has proven to be an invaluable experience. See Chapter 2, Section 2, "Creating and Negotiating the Role" as one illustration of the peer group's contribution to this text.

liaison nurses to creatively utilize their diagnostic and consultative skills to develop such groups for themselves.

section 4   models of supervision

Regular clinical supervision is essential to the ongoing practice of the psychiatric liaison nurse. Models of supervision are identified and discussed in the context of principles of general psychiatric supervision, with emphasis on the application to liaison nursing.

Supervision is defined as a supportive, stimulating, and mutually educative process. During this process, various issues and problems encountered in clinical practice are presented to a more experienced clinician who possesses expertise in the appropriate area(s). The goals of supervision are:

1. the expansion of the knowledge base,
2. the development of clinical proficiency, and
3. the development of professional autonomy and self-esteem.

The supervisory process is characterized by certain beliefs and expectations. First, and perhaps foremost, is an awareness and agreement by both participants that supervision is not psychotherapy for the supervisee. Self-disclosure on the part of the supervisee is respectfully heard and not solicited. Personal issues and conflicts of the supervisee that may come to the attention of the supervisor are dealt with only in terms of their impact on clinical practice. The development of a supervisor–supervisee alliance, which is characterized by mutual respect, trust, and acknowledgement of the goals of supervision, is paramount. The supervisor serves as a role model and teacher. The supervisee's clinical strengths are emphasized, while weaknesses are identified and strategies developed. Both supervisor and supervisee remain willing to examine their relationship and its possible reflection of issues in clinical practice [23,24] and/or professional style. It is helpful for both supervisor and supervisee to evaluate actively their work together.

An "ideal" supervision situation has been described. The process is not always so smooth and the goals are not always agreed upon. Depending on the personalities, character styles, needs, and values of each participant, combined with the possible inclusion of an evaluation element, obstacles to effective supervision may develop. The establishment of a supervisor–supervisee alliance may be seriously jeopardized. If so, the effectiveness of the supervision itself will be significantly compromised.

Both parties may be involved in certain interactional games as a result of anxiety [25]. Identification, the projection of feelings of clinical inadequacy, the excessive use of jargon and cliches [26], idealization, and competition can color the embryonic supervisory alliance. The supervisee may become excessively dependent on the supervisor or rigidly argue away his or her recommendations. The supervisee may respond much like a helpless child to a controlling parent, and the supervisor may assume the role of the parent. Hopefully, individualization in therapeutic style is recognized and respected, while control/power struggles are acknowledged, resolved, or avoided. The combined clinical expertise, self-awareness, and investment in learning of the supervisor and the supervisee potentially results in the recognition of counterproductive games and their transformation into productive ones.

Selecting a qualified supervisor requires time, professional and personal investment, honesty, and understanding of the supervisory process. Each of these elements, as well as the expectations of supervision, may vary among supervisors. The urgency for help in knowing what to do in a clinical situation can stimulate any practitioner to approach the wrong person for clinical advice—including agreeing to have an unqualified supervisor. This is especially true of psychiatric liaison nurses. The responsibility of liaison nurses is to acknowledge their learning needs, to bring them to the attention of their employers, and to negotiate for appropriate psychiatric and nursing supervision. In some general hospitals these aims are easily accomplished, since clinical supervision is valued and qualified professionals are readily available. In other settings, supervision may or may not be regarded as an institutional priority, and/or qualified individuals may not be available. Nevertheless, liaison nurses must persevere in efforts to select a qualified supervisor. If, in reality, the system cannot provide them with adequate supervision, they may need to explore possible supervisory resources outside the hospital setting.

In considering formal psychiatric supervision, a familiar model is that of less experienced therapists regularly presenting their clinical work to more experienced practitioners within the same system. The supervisee is commonly a member of the same professional discipline as the supervisor, but this is not a requirement. The supervisor may assume clinical accountability for the supervisee and participate in an evaluation. Such may not be the case if the supervisor is outside the institution and under private contract with the supervisee. In this type of situation, the supervision process usually has no connection with evaluation of less experienced therapists, who are clinically accountable to themselves and to someone within the institution. This is not to say that the supervisors are free of clinical accountability. They merely have no formalized responsibility to the system in which the supervisee is employed.

During a supervision session, the supervisee may present material from a therapy session with clients or from a diagnostic evaluation. Written process recordings and tape recordings may also be employed in an effort to review, analyze, and increase understanding of the material. Supervisors may choose to "sit in" with the supervisee and the patient, or they may role model through more active participation. The supervisee may be encouraged, or expected, to formulate specific questions on which to focus during the supervision. Finally, reading material may be provided or suggested by the supervisor.

Another model is informal psychiatric supervision, which closely resembles the collaborative elements in consultation. In this situation, a contract for ongoing supervision has not been negotiated. The more experienced clinician is not accountable for the practice or evaluation of the less experienced clinician. In both formal and informal supervision, the more experienced practitioner is considered a resource as clinical or theoretical issues are discussed. Formal supervision is more commonly characterized by pressure being felt to carry out the supervisor's recommendations. As the role of the liaison nurse develops within an institution, the appropriate use of informal supervision increases.

Liaison nurses may identify opportunities for informal psychiatric supervision. A nursing peer group can serve as one source for such supervision. As a forum, the unique value of the group is founded in its nursing identity and clinical expertise. Other arenas for informal supervision include workshops and seminars, case conferences, and consultation-liaison rounds. Depending on the services offered in a hospital by the departments of psychiatry, psychology, and/or social service, teaching conferences and rounds may occur on a regular basis. These can serve as valuable educational opportunities for rich clinical discussion.

Professional opportunities to examine clinical practice should be used and enjoyed. Nevertheless, models and sources of supervision remain far easier to identify than the conceptualization of the supervision process itself. If liaison nurses are to obtain theoretically and clinically sound consultation-liaison supervision, they must be aware of its goals. This knowledge is applicable to both formal and informal supervision.

Psychiatric consultation-liaison work necessitates that supervision be provided by a colleague who has both theoretical and clinical knowledge of this specialty. The goals of consultation-liaison supervision are:

1. To develop the diagnostic, treatment, and teaching skills of the supervisee in the medical setting.
2. To increase the supervisee's understanding of the consultation-liaison process and its application.
3. To encourage a problem-identification/problem-solving approach to consultation, emphasizing crisis intervention and prevention.
4. To foster the clinical application of a clinical philosophy based on a holistic theoretical model and a multidisciplinary/interdisciplinary approach to clinical work.

By virtue of their clinical and educational experience, liaison nurses come to the work situation and to the supervision session with some knowledge, expertise, and familiarity with the process of supervision. Initially, it may be very stressful for clinicians to openly share their work and their clinical shortcomings. Rarely do liaison nurses not experience an urgency to be informative and helpful to their consultees and patients in the face of anxiety. Doing so, however, may result in presenting their concerns in a confusing fashion. The uniqueness of the stress that psychiatric liaison nurses may experience in supervision is based on several factors. The nature of the work itself necessitates that an enormous amount of theoretical and clinical material be processed and integrated. Other factors include the critical time limitations, the effects of their work being openly exposed in the hospital, and the element of unpredictability of the quantity of work.

Although the selection of a supervisor is a critical element in the success of the role of liaison nurses, they may not be able to exercise a great deal of choice. They may learn that a supervisor has been chosen for them or that only certain clinicians are available. For supervision to be meaningful and helpful, it is imperative that the supervisor selected has had clinical experience and expertise in consultation-liaison work. Presumably, the supervisor has provided these services in a general medical-surgical hospital setting. Ideally, the supervisor is presently or has previously worked in the same hospital as does the liaison nurse. Familiarity with the system in which consultation-liaison is being practiced is invaluable. Next, it is advantageous to liaison nurses if their supervisors are also clinically knowledgeable in physiological responses to illness and to general medical issues. For these reasons, liaison psychiatrists are frequently called upon to supervise liaison nurses. In some situations, the liaison psychiatrist may be fairly well versed in psychiatric nursing roles and principles and aware of nursing issues on the general hospital wards. Gaps in general nursing knowledge and practice may be filled in when the liaison nurse also has supervision with a member of the nursing department. This individual may be someone in an administrative position and/or an experienced psychiatric nurse. In addition to nursing supervision and support, liaison nurses are also kept abreast of policy changes, role-appropriate administrative concerns, and departmental objectives.

Travelbee believes that only nurses should supervise nurses. Members of other health care professions are not educationally qualified or sufficiently experienced [27]. Although supervision from related disciplines is beneficial, experienced psychiatric liaison nurses who are familiar with the supervisory process are the ideal supervisors. Familiar with the psychiatric liaison nursing role, they are successful practitioners. They bring to the supervision setting psychiatric expertise, nursing knowledge, and clinical sophistication. Supervision is enhanced by the commonality of the experiences. Liaison nurses as supervisors combine the pragmatic with the theoretical in fostering a meaningful supervisory alliance. It is further evidenced in their empathic understanding of the many trials and tribulations of psychiatric liaison nursing in a general hospital—the difficulties, the frustrations, and the joys.

references

1. Robert Ardrey, *The Territorial Imperative* (New York: Atheneum, 1966), p. 15. Reprinted with permission of Atheneum Publishers.
2. Paul Mohl, "A Systems Approach to Liaison Psychiatry," *Psychosomatics* 21:6 (June 1980): 458.
3. William Glazer and Boris Astrachan, "A Social Systems Approach to Consultation-Liaison Psychiatry," *International Journal of Psychiatry in Medicine* 9:1 (1978–79): 3–47.
4. Jerome P. Lysaught, "An Abstract for Action," *National Commission for the Study of Nursing and Nursing Education* (New York: McGraw-Hill Book Company, 1970), p. 26.
5. Marlene Grissum and Carol Spengler, *Woman Power and Health Care* (Boston:

Little, Brown & Co., 1976), p. 18. Reprinted with permission.

6. Marlene Kramer, *Reality Shock: Why Nurses Are Leaving Nursing* (St. Louis: The C. V. Mosby Company, 1974).

7. Massachusetts Appeals Court Advance Sheets (1980) Delicata v. Bourlesses, pp. 963–970.

8. Helen Creighton, *Law Every Nurse Should Know*, 3rd ed. (Philadelphia: W. B. Saunders Co., 1975).

9. N. Brill, *Teamwork: Working Together in Human Services* (Philadelphia: J. B. Lippincott Company, 1976).

10. Robert Ardrey, *The Territorial Imperative* (New York: Atheneum, 1966), p. 351. Reprinted with permission of Atheneum Publishers.

11. Bernard Bloom and Howard Parad, "Interdisciplinary Training and Interdisciplinary Functioning," *American Journal of Orthopsychiatry* 46:4 (October 1976).

12. Helen Perlman, "Confessions, Concerns and Commitment of an Ex-Clinical Social Worker," *Clinical Social Work Journal* 2:3 (Fall 1974): 221–229.

13. Bloom and Parad, p. 676.

14. Ralph Crawshaw and William Key, "Psychiatric Teams," *Archives of General Psychiatry* 5:3 (1961): 397–405.

15. Brill, p. 22.

16. J. Ludden, R. Winickoff, and S. Steinberg, "Psychological Aspects of Medical Care: A Training Seminar for Primary Care Providers," *Journal of Medical Education* 54 (1979): 720–724.

17. Thomas Campbell et al., "Use of Multiple Family Group for Crisis Intervention," *General Hospital Psychiatry* 2 (1980): 95–99.

18. Z. J. Lipowski, "Consultation-Liaison Psychiatry Past Failures and New Opportunities," *General Hospital Psychiatry* 1 (1979): 3–10.

19. Nancy Kaltreider et al., "The Integration of Psychosocial Care in a General Hospital: Development of an Interdisciplinary Consultation Program," *International Journal of Psychiatry in Medicine* 5:2 (1974): 125–134.

20. Mary F. Kohnke, *The Case for Consultation in Nursing Designs for Professional Practice* (New York: John Wiley & Sons, Inc., 1978), p. 81.

21. J. J. Strain, "The Medical Setting: Is It beyond the Psychiatrist?" *American Journal of Psychiatry* 134 (1977): 253–256.

22. Jack Zusman and David L. Davidson, eds., *Practical Aspects of Mental Health Consultation* (Springfield, Ill.: Charles C. Thomas, Publisher, 1972), p. 77.

23. Helen K. Gediman and Fred Wolkenfeld, "The Parallelism Phenomenon in Psychoanalysis and Supervision: Its Reconsideration as a Triadic System," *Psychoanalytic Quarterly* 49 (1980): 234–255.

24. David M. Sacks and Stanley H. Shapiro, "On Parallel Processes in Therapy and Teaching," *Psychoanalytic Quarterly* 45 (1976): 394–415.

25. A. Kadushin, "Games People Play in Supervision," *Social Work* 13 (1968): 23–32.

26. J. de la Torre and Ann Appelbaum, "Use and Misuse of Jargon in Clinical Supervision," *Archives of General Psychiatry* 31 (September 1974): 302–306.

27. Joyce Travelbee, *Intervention in Psychiatric Nursing: Process in the One-To-One Relationship* (Philadelphia: F. A. Davis Company, 1969), p. 215.

bibliography

books

ASHLEY, JO ANN. *Hospitals, Paternalism, and the Role of the Nurse.* New York: Teachers College Press, 1977.

CAPLAN, GERALD and KILLILEA, MARIE, eds. *Support Systems and Mutual Help: Multi-disciplinary Explorations.* New York: Grune & Stratton, Inc., 1976.

FREEMAN, HOWARD; LEVINE, SOL; and REEDER, LEO. *Handbook of Medical Sociology.* Englewood Cliffs, N.J.: Prentice-Hall, Inc., 1963.

HESS, A. K., ed. *Psychotherapy Supervision Theory, Research and Practice.* New York: John Wiley & Sons, Inc., 1980.

KELLY, LUCIE. *Dimensions of Professional Nursing.* New York: Macmillan, Inc., 1975.

REYNOLDS, B. C. *Learning and Teaching in the Practice of Social Work.* New York: Rinehart and Co., Inc., 1942.

RIEHL, JOAN and McVAY, JOAN, eds. *The Clinical Nurse Specialist: Interpretations.* New York: Appleton-Century-Crofts, 1973.

articles

AUSTIN, L. N. "Basic Principles of Supervision." Paper presented at the National Conference of Social Work, Chicago, Ill., May 1952.

BANDLER, BERNARD. "Interprofessional Collaboration in Training in Mental Health," *American Journal of Orthopsychiatry* 43:1 (January 1973): 97-107.

BENFER, BEVERLY. "Defining the Role and Function of the Psychiatric Nurse as a Member of the Team," *Perspectives in Psychiatric Care* 18 (July–August 1980): 166-177.

BERGER, I. L. "Resistances to the Learning Process in Group Dynamics Programs," *American Journal of Psychiatry* 126:6 (December 1969): 850-857.

BIBRING, GRETA. "Psychiatry and Social Work," in *Psychiatry and Medical Practice in a General Hospital,* edited by Norman Zinberg. New York: International Universities Press, Inc., 1964, pp. 28-40.

CHALLELA, MARY. "The Interdisciplinary Team: A Role Definition in Nursing," *Image* 11:1 (February 1979): 9-15.

DAMMANN, G. "Interprofessional Aspects of Nursing and Social Work Curricula," *Nursing Research* 21 (1972): 160-163.

DAVEY, J. C. "The Employee's Meaning of Supervision," *Supervisor Nurse* (May 1978): 93-94.

GIVEN, BARBARA and SIMMONS, SANDRA. "The Interdisciplinary Health-Care Team: Fact or Fiction?" *Nursing Forum* 16:2 (1977): 165-180.

GIZYNSKI, M. "Self Awareness of the Supervisor in Supervision," *Clinical Social Work Journal* 6:3 (1978): 202-210.

GROTJAHN, M. "Supervision of Analytic Group Psychotherapy," *Group Psychotherapy* 13 (1960): 161-169.

HALL, R.; GARDNER, E.; PERL, M.; STICKNEY, S.; and PFEFFERBAUM, G. "The Professional Burnout Syndrome," *Psychiatric Opinion* (April 1979): 12-17.

HAWTHORNE, L. "Games Supervisors Play," *Social Work* 20:3 (1975): 179-183.

HOLT, JACQUELINE. "The Struggles inside Nursing's Body Politic," *Nursing Forum* 15:4 (1976): 325-400.

HOWES, E.; LEVY, J.; LUONGO, S.; and MONTELEONE, M. "A Team Approach to Emergency Psychiatry," *Journal of Psychiatric Nursing and Mental Health Services* 17:8 (August 1979): 31–37.

IVANCEVICH, J. M. and MATTESON, M. T. "Nurses and Stress: Time to Examine the Potential Problems," *Supervisor Nurse* (June 1980): 17–22.

JONES, PAT. "Psychiatric Liaison Nurse for Neurosurgery: An Innovative Approach to Management of Chronic Pain," *Journal of Neurosurgical Nursing* 10:1 (March 1978): 160–165.

KADUSHIN, A. "Supervisor–Supervisee: A Survey," *Social Work* 19:3 (1974): 23–32.

KANE, ROSALIE. "The Interprofessional Team as a Small Group," *Social Work in Health Care* 1:1 (Fall 1975): 19–32.

LAKIN, M.; LIEBERMAN, M.; and WHITALAR, D. "Issues in the Training of Group Psychotherapists," *International Journal of Group Psychotherapy* 19 (1969): 307–325.

LEVIN, S. and KANTER, S. "Some General Considerations in the Supervision of Beginning Group Psychotherapists," *International Journal of Group Psychotherapy* 14 (1964): 318–331.

McGEE, T. F. "Supervision in Group Psychotherapy: A Comparison of Four Approaches," *International Journal of Group Psychotherapy* 18 (1968): 165–176.

MULLANEY, S. W.; FOX, R. A.; LISTON, M. F. "Clinical Nurse Specialist and Social Worker—Clarifying the Roles," *Nursing Outlook* 22:11 (1974): 712–718.

MULLINS, A. C. and BARSTOW, R. E. "Care for the Caretaker," *American Journal of Nursing* (August 1979): 1425–1427.

NADELSON, T. and NADELSON, C. "Reflex and Reflection: Defining Psychotherapy in Supervision," *Psychotherapy and Psychosomatics* 25 (1975): 207–216.

NORRIS, C. M. "A Few Notes on Consultation in Nursing," *Nursing Outlook* (December 1977): 756–761.

PETRILLO, MADELINE. "The Role of the Mental Health Team in Communicating with Patients and Staff," *ACCH Newsletter* (1973): 10–13.

RAE-GRANT, A. F. and MARCUSE, DANIEL. "The Hazards of Teamwork," *American Journal of Orthopsychiatry* 38 (1968): 4–8.

RICHARDS, J. F. "Integrating a Clinical Specialist into a Hospital Nursing Service," *Nursing Outlook* 17:3 (March 1969): 23–25.

SAMTER, JEANNE; SCHERER, MARY; and SHULMAN, DIANE. "Interface of Psychiatric Clinical Specialists in a Community Hospital Setting," *Journal of Psychiatric Nursing and Mental Health Services* (January 1981): 20–29.

SCHULDT, S. "Supervision and the Informal Organization," *Journal of Nursing Administration* (July 1978): 21–25.

SHUBIN, S. "Rx for Stress—Your Stress," *Nursing '79* (January 1979): 53–55.

SPAN, PAULA. "Where Have All the Nurses Gone?" *New York Times Magazine* (February 22, 1981): 70.

STICKNEY, SONDRA and HALL, RICHARD C. W. "The Role of the Nurse on a Consultation-Liaison Team," *Psychosomatics* 22:3 (March 1981): 224–225.

WEINSTEIN, LESLIE; CHAPMAN, MARY; and STALLINGS, MARY ANN. "Organizing Approaches to Psychiatric Nurse Consultation," *Perspectives in Psychiatric Care* 17:2 (March–April 1979): 66–71.

WHITE, ELIZABETH. "The Clinical Specialist on the Mental Health Team," *Journal of Psychiatric Nursing and Mental Health Services* (November 1976): 7–12.

WIECZOREK, RITA; PENNINGTON, ELIZABETH; and FIELDS, SYLVIA. "Interdisciplinary Education," *Nursing Forum* 15:3 (1976): 225–237.

WILLIAMS, M. "Limitations, Fantasies, and Security Operations of Beginning Group Psychotherapists," *International Journal of Group Psychotherapy* 16 (1966): 150–162.

WOODROW, M. and BELL, J. A. "Clinical Specialization: Conflict between Reality and Theory," *Journal of Nursing Administration* (November–December 1971): 23–28.

YALOM, I. D. "Problems of Neophyte Group Therapists," *International Journal of Social Psychiatry* 12 (1966): 52–59.

ZETZEL, E. "The Capacity To Be Alone," *The International Journal of Psycho-Analysis* 38 (July 1957): 416–420.

part two
the clinical
practice of the
psychiatric liaison
nurse

4

the consultation process

The process of consultation is complex but identifiable. The psychiatric liaison nurse, on request, helps to define the problem, "diagnoses the total consultation," makes recommendations, and helps to plan interventions. Included in this process is follow-up and/or reassessment of the patient whenever feasible. The consultation process described is in part based on consultation theory proposed by Gerald Caplan. Four types of consultation are described by Caplan:

1. client-centered,
2. consultee-centered,
3. program-centered administrative, and
4. consultee-centered administrative [1].

The emphasis in this text is on client-centered, referred to as "direct consultation," and on consultee-centered, referred to as "indirect consultation." Which type of consultation is to be provided remains flexible as the "total consultation" is diagnosed. Refer to Table 4-1 for a detailed description of direct and indirect consultations. A firm commitment to one type of consultation rarely occurs.

The proposed theoretical model is the framework for operationalizing the consultation process. Within this process, liaison nurses consider, as will be illustrated, the identified patient, the nurse, the milieu, and all other aspects of the consultation, and thus they "diagnose the total consultation."

The goals of psychiatric nursing consultation are, and remain, the framework for all clinical practice:

1. To demonstrate and teach mental health concepts and their application to clinical nursing practice.
2. To effect appropriate psychiatric and nursing intervention.

TABLE 4–1 MODELS OF CONSULTATION

Direct	*Indirect*
The patient and/or family are interviewed. Psychological treatment is provided by the liaison nurse as indicated.	A consultee-centered/case-centered meeting is held. The patient and/or family are not interviewed.
Specific nursing intervention is planned and may be initiated.	Specific nursing intervention is planned and initiated.
A consultee-centered/case-centered meeting is held with further intervention planned.	Further consultee-centered/case-centered meetings are held as needed.
The consultation is documented in the patient's record by the liaison nurse.	The consultation is documented in the patient's record by the patient's nurse.
Follow-up, reassessment, and evaluation are ongoing.	Follow-up, reassessment, and evaluation are ongoing.

3. To support nurses in continuing to provide high-quality nursing care.
4. To promote and develop the professional and personal self-esteem of the nurse.
5. To encourage tolerance among the members of the nursing staff of those situations in which immediate and/or effective intervention or resolution is unattainable.

section 1   the consultant

The psychiatric liaison nurse is prepared clinically and educationally to act in the best interests of the identified patient, of the consultee, and of the medical milieu. Usually the process itself is egalitarian. The liaison nurse, who is first a consultant with special skills in psychiatry, is invited by the consultee to participate in problem solving.

Liaison nurses may receive a request for consultation from a member of the nursing staff, a physician, other health care providers, or a patient. The request may be generated through other clinical work such as in-service programs done by the liaison nurses. The basic goals, as stated, continue to be the major focus, irrespective of the content of the request for consultation. Regardless of the source of the consultation request, liaison nurses communicate with the consultee/nursing staff, if at all possible, prior to engaging in the consultation. Communication occurs with the head nurse and with other members of the nursing staff involved, both before and after the consultation has been provided. During their interventions, liaison nurses remain acutely aware of their words and behavior. They thoughtfully and carefully explain the nature of their participation in a consultation, as well as their clinical thinking concerning the situation.

Crucial factors warrant examination in understanding the utilization of liaison nurses as part of the consultation process. The following clinical cases demonstrate three different types of consultations. These cases, which illustrate the consultation process, will be referred to throughout this chapter. One describes a patient problem, another a staff problem, and the last a mixed problem.

case I. a patient problem

The request for consultation was expressed as follows: "We have this patient in here, renal failure, on dialysis, who's been screaming since she woke up. She's the only girl in a family of four children, so she's probably really spoiled, but we can't have a kid screaming in here like this. Maybe you could see her or something."

The request for consultation is made via telephone by the head nurse of the pedi ICU. Through further telephone discussion and upon arriving in the ICU, the liaison nurse gathered the following information:

Six-year-old Sara was admitted to the pedi ICU three days ago in acute renal failure. She was semicomatose. Her parents reported that the child had been fine up until two days prior to her emergency admission, when she had become increasingly irritable and lethargic. Sara had been incontinent twice of small amounts of urine and had a low-grade fever. She was taken to her local pediatrician, and a diagnosis of probable urinary tract infection secondary to viral flu was made. Antibiotic treatment was started, but the child's symptoms worsened with vomiting, dehydration, increased fever, and changes in mental status.

When Sara, the youngest of four children, was admitted to the ICU, her parents were frantic. The patient's three brothers were present and quite upset. Peritoneal dialysis was begun immediately. In less than forty-eight hours, Sara was awake, alert, and screaming. The visiting policy in the ICU allows only parents to visit patients ten minutes per hour. After many hours filled with unsuccessful attempts at comforting Sara made by the patient's nurse and by her mother, the

liaison nurse was contacted. The patient's physician was in full support of the request for psychiatric nursing consultation, sharing the
frustration of the nursing staff.

case II. a staff problem

The request for consultation was expressed as follows: "I was
just thinking about you. Maybe you could help the nurses with Mrs.
Roth. She's in her early thirties—nice lady—severe heart disease with
a poor prognosis. It's got to be hard for them to go into that room."

The request is made by the male resident in cardiology. He
makes the referral when casually passing the liaison nurse in the corri-
dor. Through further discussion with the resident, more data is collected. Mrs. Roth is a 31-year-old mother of two girls, ages 7 and $2\frac{1}{2}$.
She was admitted on an elective basis to the cardiology service about
two weeks ago. She is bright, verbal, and pleasant to talk with. She is
physically attractive. Mrs. Roth had been an elementary school
teacher before having her children and occasionally works as a substitute teacher. Her husband is a quiet guy who works hard as a carpen-
ter and who visits his wife every evening. The patient was admitted
with a complaint of heart palpitations, weakness, pedal edema, and
syncope. A diagnosis of inoperable cardiomyopathy and pulmonary
hypertension was made—etiology unclear. A prophylactic trial of
medications was started, but the patient's symptoms have not improved.

case III. a mixed problem

The request for consultation was expressed as follows: "We
really need help with Mr. Andrews. He's a 62-year-old patient with
gastric CA. Prognosis could be OK, but he won't let the docs finish
their workup so they can treat him. He's really depressed, won't do
anything for himself, and just wants to sleep and not feel any pain. It's
really awful for all of us."

The request was made in the weekly nurses' group. The patient's
doctors have also ordered a psychiatric nursing consultation. The situation is introduced and presented by the patient's primary nurse. With
some guidance by the liaison nurse, the following information is
obtained. Mr. Andrews has been in the hospital for over three weeks.
He was admitted on an emergency basis, after coming in to the clinic
with severe epigastric pain, vomiting, and general malaise. Diagnostic
studies demonstrated a large, solid mass within the abdominal cavity,
pressing on and invasive to the stomach. His physician made a working diagnosis of stomach cancer and informed the patient. The
primary site of the cancer had not been identified. The patient was

asked to give permission for additional studies, specifically surgical exploration, so that appropriate treatment could be planned and administered. The patient refused. Mr. Andrews is three years away from retirement. His wife died of cancer eight years ago. He has two sons, both married with children, living in the immediate area. Mr. Andrews appears to be attentive to the information given to him by his physician. He seems to understand his nurse's attempts to keep him involved in his care and as independent as possible. After the diagnosis of cancer was discussed with him, his complaint of pain increased. He begs for more pain medication and is found weeping much of the time. Talking with his immediate health care providers does not seem to help. The staff views the patient's behavior as infantile and regressed, and they are annoyed that he is refusing potentially helpful treatment.

Each of these cases raises pertinent issues for the liaison nurse. The psychiatric liaison nurse's actions are based on the application of the holistic theoretical model to clinical practice, that is, "diagnosing the total consultation."

The consultation process is a series of identifiable steps: how each step occurs, how each is developed, and why each is important become significant components of the consultant-consultee relationship. These components are frequently reflected in the success or failure of nursing interventions as recommended by the liaison nurse. Therefore, each step requires careful consideration. The consultation process includes the following identifiable steps:

1. A consultation is requested.
2. The appropriateness of the consultation is considered.
3. Problem identification begins.
4. The need for direct or indirect service is determined.

As the consultant considers the consultation, his or her response is determined by both the overt and covert requests. What may seem at first like an inappropriate consultation may in fact be a reasonable request for help in a complicated patient care problem. At the least, each consultation request is an opportunity to further illustrate the role and/or to explore aspects of psychological care. Liaison nurses endeavor to create a collaborative environment in which they and the consultee can discuss the nature of their participation in the problem solving. As the consultation is diagnosed, an initial decision is made as to whether to intervene directly by interviewing the patient or indirectly by working with the nursing staff. The choice of the direct and/or indirect model encompasses other ramifications, such as hidden agendas, identification, and transference/countertransference issues (Chapter 7, Section 1). In an effort to strengthen the consultation alliance, a flexible plan is used that is based on the ongoing clinical observations of the patient rather than on a strict commitment to one model. With any request for consultation, liaison nurses follow the beginning steps in "diagnosing the total consultation" (Section 3). Expansion of these steps involves a progression in "diagnosing the total consultation" that is fluid and flexible.

- Who is requesting the consultation?
- What is the liaison nurse's previous consultation experience with the patient's unit and with the specific consultee making the request?
- How is the request being expressed? What specifically is the consultee identifying as a problem?
- What knowledge does the liaison nurse have of this ward, and of the significant people involved in the problematic situation?
- Is the consultation appropriate for the liaison nurse?
- What is the formulation of the consultation question(s)?

In the first clinical case, Sara, the consultation is requested by the head nurse. The stated problem is in terms of the patient. The request is for the liaison nurse to see the patient. The overt need seems centered around getting the child to stop crying. Some of the pertinent issues for the liaison nurse to consider are:

- Why is the head nurse contacting the liaison nurse, as opposed to the nurse caring for Sara?
- What must it be like in general to care for a screaming child who cannot be comforted?
- What measures have already been tried?
- How old is this child and in what stage of psychosocial development? Cognitive development? Previous illness and/or hospitalization experience for child and family?
- Why can't this child be comforted?
- What is the illness experience in renal failure? With dialysis?
- How is dialysis being administered? Can this patient be sedated?
- Is the visiting policy detrimentally affecting this child?
- Could other consultation questions have gone unexpressed?
- What are the learning needs of this staff?

In the second case, Mrs. Roth, the request for consultation is not from a member of the nursing staff, but from a cardiology resident. He identifies a need in terms of the nursing staff implying that the very nature of this case creates an uncomfortable experience for the nurses. This presentation may certainly be accurate. Perhaps the tragedy of this patient's situation, as well as the possible identification with the patient, creates a painful situation for the nurses. However, the liaison nurse also considers other issues.

- Why is the resident, rather than a member of the nursing staff, requesting consultation?
- Why might the nursing staff not request consultation?
- Is the resident asking for help himself? Is there a doctor–nurse problem?
- What might it really be like to care for this patient? For the resident? For the nurses?
- What is the significance of the patient's age, sex, and social status?
- What are the emotional needs of this patient? Are they being met? By whom?
- Do the head nurse and the staff know that the liaison nurse has been contacted?
- How can the liaison nurse become appropriately involved?

In the third case, Mr. Andrews, the patient's primary nurse is requesting the consultation. Both the patient and his health care team appear to be having difficulty. The patient is depressed, which is increasing the team's frustration. Again, important areas to consider are:

- What is the expectation of the liaison nurse? Why have the doctors requested a psychiatric nursing consultation? Does psychiatric nursing consultation have to be ordered by the physician?
- Why has the psychiatric nurse been consulted rather than the psychiatrist? The social worker?
- What are the consultation questions? Which ones are priorities to answer?
- What is it like for the various members of the team to be responsible for this patient and to go into his room?
- What is meant by an "OK prognosis"?
- How much physical pain does the patient have? Is he receiving appropriate medication?
- Does the patient have brain metastases? Is this patient psychotic or psychotically depressed?
- What is the role of the family? Are they available to the patient? What significance does the loss of his wife and the cause of her death have for this patient?
- What has the patient been told about his illness and his prognosis? What is his level of understanding?
- What meaning does the illness have for him?

There are a wealth of issues to consider when responding to a request for consultation. Many areas in which data gathering would be beneficial can usually be identified. However, the constraints of time, the varying availability of detailed information and significant people, as well as the urgency with which the request is made, may create a situation in which comprehensive data collection is a luxury and not a reality. "The nurse consultant must work within the existing channels of authority and communication already present in the ward [2]." As consultants, liaison nurses do not have primary clinical responsibility for the patient. They are responsible for the quality and content of the consultation, that is, for the recommendations they make and the interventions they develop. If they provide direct service, their clinical responsibility is extended. The nonjudgmental, confidential approach to all clinical work becomes paramount.

Expectations of the liaison nurse are identified and understood by her or him. Sometimes, in the process of gathering data with the consultee, direct discussion concerning expectations is helpful. For example, in Case I (Sara), the expectation is that the liaison nurse will be able to make the child stop crying. The liaison nurse may choose to verbally state the expectation to the consultee for the purposes of validation and clarification. Obviously, other areas need to be addressed in the context of this consultation. It may be very reasonable to discuss expectations with the consultee, but only in terms of the identified patient, Sara. In this discussion, it is important to validate exactly how long the child has been crying. More importantly, it is crucial to introduce the possibility that the crying may be adaptive and in service of the ego—as well as unpleasant for the unit and the nursing staff. Some preliminary "brainstorming" with the consultee —that is, why is this child so upset?—may serve the purpose not only of clarifying expectations of the liaison nurse, but also of providing useful information to the consultee. This technique is effective in two ways: (1) It strengthens the consultee–liaison nurse alliance, and (2) it dispels the myth that the consultant has magical powers.

At times the direct exploration of expectations with the consultee is not advisable due to the patient's medical condition. In addition, such direct exploration may be counterproductive. The hope is to create a situation in which the liaison nurse and the consultee mutually redefine the problem and explore possible solutions. Yet this interaction may only heighten the consultee's anxiety. The consultee's major affectual response toward the patient may be not only augmented, but also displaced onto the liaison nurse. For example, in terms of Case I (Sara), further discussions may be heard by the consultee as validation of her shortcomings; that is, "good nurses can comfort ill children." The consultee may also feel that her clinical performance is being criticized by the liaison nurse: "What's the matter with you, why can't you be empathic to a crying child?"

No formula predicts whether or not it would be helpful to directly acknowledge and to discuss the reasonableness of the consultation questions or the expectations of the liaison nurse. The essential question for liaison nurses to ask themselves is how the alliance with the consultee can be maintained and strengthened, in the process of identifying the problem and understanding these important issues. There are inherent risks. As the consultation request is evaluated, as information is collected regarding the problem, as the consultee's position becomes clearer, the answer to this question is more easily understood.

Health care professionals may profit from psychiatric consultation by better understanding their patients' illness experience and by working more effectively with them. Liaison nurses remain respectful of what they are told and of the consultee's desire to keep them informed. The authors recall many times when consultees would contact them to tell them of the various happenings on a specific unit, but with no specific request for consultation. A need to maintain contact with the liaison nurse was apparent through communication regarding the patient care experience, the number of deaths during a week, Mr. X.'s biopsy results, or the admission of a schizophrenic with a medical problem. In these examples, the liaison nurse did not have any previous knowledge of the patients mentioned. There appeared to be an indirect request for support on the part of the consultee, along with the message, "Please stand by, because we might need you." Liaison nurses also remain respectful of the "unidentified," as well as the "identified," patients and anxieties within the hospital milieu. In Case III, the staff had, in their attempts to "help" Mr. Andrews, been less aware of their own feelings of helplessness. It is sometimes difficult for nurses, especially in acute care hospitals, to give up the "fight for life."

Although experienced in terms of applying mental health principles to general nursing practice, the presence of a liaison nurse may not be comforting to the consultee. The consultee may believe that he or she has failed with the patient and that his or her lack of clinical ability is clearly exposed. The consultee may test the liaison nurse in an attempt not only to validate the latter's ability, but also to measure the risk involved when asking for consultation. Regardless of the nature of the motivation behind the consultation request, the consultee's personal and professional self-esteem is respected, preserved, and maybe even developed. Liaison nurses strive to remain aware of their own feelings and reactions to the consultee, in an effort to separate these issues from the consultation process (Chapter 7, Section 1).

section 2   defining the problem

The request for consultation frequently reflects a concern for the patient's suffering, a diagnostic clarification, an aspect of patient care, or a sense of helplessness. Meyer and Mendelson have identified other precipitating circumstances under which psychiatric consultation may be requested by a physician. "Some part of the patient's total behavior strikes the physician as being inappropriate or abnormal or the physician feels a sense of responsibility for the abnormal behavior [3]." These authors go on to describe that "the perception of the behavior as sufficiently irrational to warrant calling the psychiatrist cannot be understood only in terms of behavioral acts, diagnostic psychiatric categories, or psychodynamic formulations of behavior. It is best understood as a state of active alienation in the doctor–patient relationship [4]." The reference in this quotation to the "physician" could easily be changed to "consultee."

To effectively intervene, the liaison nurse must identify the problem. The most thorough assessment and psychiatric examination of the patient may not be helpful if there is no agreement and discussion as to the nature of the problem. When attempting to achieve consultation goals, liaison nurses direct their clinical skill and energies, formulating interventions based on the identified problem.

Liaison nurses, aware of the limits and boundaries of their clinical expertise, remain open to a multidisciplinary/interdisciplinary approach to patient care. Collaboration with the social worker, the psychiatrist, and other health care providers is helpful. In addition, they are clear as to which colleague they should consult in terms of a specific situation. Social workers, psychiatrists, alcohol counselors, drug specialists, occupational therapists, or any other professionals within the hospital setting may be needed for their expertise. Effective intervention necessitates knowledge about resources.

Problem identification will be illustrated by continuing the discussion of Case I (Sara), Case II (Mrs. Roth), and Case III (Mr. Andrews) from Section 1.

The consultation question can be expressed in several ways:

• In terms of the patient: Is his behavior normal? What does his behav-

ior mean? (Sara—"We have this kid screaming in here.")
- In terms of the consultee: Are we doing what should be done for this patient? (Mrs. Roth—"Nice lady, poor prognosis—hard to go into that room.")
- In terms of both patient and consultee: This patient isn't coping well, and we don't know what to do. (Mr. Andrews—"We need help. He's really depressed—it's awful for all of us.")

The actual presentation of the need, however, is not always overt, and what the consultee is identifying as the problem may not be the problem at all. Liaison nurses apply their knowledge of the possible meaning of behavior in such a way as to support consultees and further their professional development. For example, instead of telling the consultee that she or he is behaving inappropriately toward the patient as a result of oedipal issues that the patient is stirring up in her or him, it is more appropriate and profitable to suggest that patients like Mr. X have a way of knowing just how to get us angry at them.

It is rarely appropriate to initiate discussion or comment on the psychodynamics of the consultee and how they interact with those of the patient. The liaison nurse attempts to maintain a patient care focus. On rare occasions, when identification has become so intense or behavior so dangerous that it dramatically interferes with safe nursing care, a more direct or active intervention may be warranted. These situations, characteristically manifested by abuse or neglect of patients, should be approached thoughtfully and carefully, with sensitivity and discretion (Chapter 7, Section 1).

The key element in this discussion is the patient care focus of the psychiatric liaison nurse's clinical work. Again, defining the problem provides the necessary foundation on which this focus is maintained.

section 3 diagnosing the total consultation

In a medical setting, the assessment of the patient becomes only one, albeit an important, aspect of the evaluation. "Diagnosing the total consultation" is the framework for practice. Johnson, in writing about the psychiatric nurse consultant in the general hospital, emphasized that the request for consultation was related to more than just the degree of the patient's disturbance [5]. Schiff and Pilot examined the manner in which psychiatric consultation was requested and the background of each situation. They made the assumption

that every psychiatric consultation stemmed from the referring physician's concerns, which were not always explicitly stated [6]. The
premise is that patients' psychological symptoms can be fully understood only as related to their medical illness, their environment, and
their care providers. This relationship is the basis of understanding
the meaning of a total consultation. Strain and Grossman describe a
model of the expanded psychiatric interview, which includes:

1. evaluating the requests for psychiatric consultation,
2. evaluating the doctor,
3. evaluating the chart,
4. evaluating the nurse,
5. evaluating the family,
6. evaluating the ward culture, and finally
7. interviewing the patient [7].

This is validation for extending the evaluation beyond the scope of
interaction between consultant and patient. We have termed this
process "diagnosing the total consultation."

Kucharski and Groves describe an "inappropriate" psychiatric
consultation that emanated from intrapsychic conflicts in the staff.
They further explore how the behavior or illness may arouse conflictual feelings [8]. The real skill is not in the recognition of the conflicts
and the defenses employed by staff, but rather in knowing how to
acknowledge—or, if possible, to resolve—them sufficiently for both
staff and patient to function effectively and with minimal stress. The
liaison nurse is often the mental health professional requested when
the problem is unclear. Skill is required in recognizing this phenomenon. Liaison nurses are expected to "think on their feet," because
they have little opportunity for reflection.

Accurate "diagnosis of the total consultation" is the precursor to
effective intervention. The holistic theoretical model, based on our
clinical experience as liaison nurses, is coupled with the expanded
psychiatric interview [9]. It is important to note that, to emphasize
the other crucial elements in "diagnosing a total consultation," the
direct evaluation of the patient is omitted at this time. Although the
patient interview as an assessment tool is more familiar to psychiatric
liaison nurses, it may or may not be utilized in "diagnosing the total
consultation." For clarity we have chosen to discuss direct patient
intervention in a separate chapter (Chapter 5, Section 3).

The following comprehensive illustration demonstrates the elements in "diagnosing the total consultation," omitting a discussion of

direct patient assessment. A clinical case will also be presented to demonstrate this further.

1. Evaluating the *request* for consultation: Is the liaison nurse being actively sought out by the consultee? Or is the request an after-thought? For example, the liaison nurse is paged, as opposed to walking on a ward and being greeted with, "I probably should have called you." Are there several consultees or only one? For example, "All the nurses are having difficulty with Mrs. D." Or, "I'm having a problem dealing with Mrs. D." Is the individual presenting the problem to the liaison nurse actually the consultee? As an example, "I have no problems with Mr. X, but the evening charge nurse ..." Is the request expressed with humor, anger, sarcasm? Is it expressed as a dare? For example, "Do we have a patient for you!" What is the scope of the problem presented? And what is the consultee asking for?

2. Evaluating the (nurse) *consultee*: What is your relationship and clinical experience with the consultee? What is the consultee's experience in nursing and/or on this particular ward? Length of employment? Education? Does this staff member usually have problems with this type of issue? Is the consultee under personal stress? How does this nurse usually function within the medical team? Is the nurse in conflict with the doctor, the patient, the nursing supervisors, or you?

3. Evaluating the *doctor*: Does the doctor view the problem differently from the nurse? Is the physician in conflict with the nurse or with some other part of the hospital system? Does the physician feel discouraged or hopeful about the medical condition? Is there evidence of personal conflict with the patient? How clinically experienced is the physician? What is your relationship and clinical experience with this person? How does the doctor view psychiatry and psychiatric nursing consultation?

4. Evaluating the *ward*: Is it a specialized setting, such as an ICU? Is the medical and/or nursing staff under stress? Are there acute medical problems with other patients? What is the tolerance of this ward for this kind of patient? Is there strong nursing leadership? What is your relationship to the ward? Do they usually have difficulty managing patients? What is the relationship between the doctors and nurses on this ward? Has the patient been placed under any stress because of the setting, occurrences with a roommate, a medical emergency on the unit, dissatisfaction with an inadequate physical environment?

5. Evaluating the *family*: Is the presence or absence of family contributing to distress? Are ongoing family conflicts adding to the stress for the patient? Is the illness exacerbating a pre-morbid problem? Is anger being directed at the family inappropriately? Does the family have support? What is the relationship between the family and the nursing staff? Between the family and the medical staff?

6. Evaluating the *medical illness*: Are there particular patterns of behavior, thoughts, or feelings that occur more frequently with this illness for the patient, the family, and/or the members of the health care team? Is there special meaning for the patient? Is the behavior possibly related to physiological processes? Are treatment, medications, or the lack thereof precipitating the behavior?

7. Evaluating the *chart*: Have there been a succession of invasive procedures? Have there been many changes in treatment? Are there notes about the patient's behavior or mood? Who is documenting this? Are there discrepancies? Has the patient been moved between rooms or wards? Does the patient have a primary nurse or consistent nurse and/or doctor? Is there anything to read "between the lines" to raise suspicion? Is there a nursing assessment? Is the chart lacking in information?

clinical illustration

The request for consultation was expressed as follows: "Mr. Hall is really depressed, and I don't blame him. He's had a rough time. Maybe you could help him."

The consultee, the nurse: Miss Ross, a young, new graduate referred her first patient to the liaison nurse. The consultation question, as stated, was not clear, illustrating her inexperience.

The doctor: The intern felt that the patient was appropriately depressed but not presenting any particular problem. He felt that the patient was discouraged from his long hospitalization, but that he was actually fortunate in terms of prognosis. His symptoms pointed to cancer of the pancreas, but he had only an ulcer. Although he had some complications (paralytic ileus), the medical staff felt positive about his recovery. The intern supported the liaison nurse's intervention for "support."

The ward: After many years of poor leadership with several head nurses, a new, well qualified, competent head nurse had been appointed two weeks prior to the request. The quality of psychological care to patients had suffered during the previous period. Mr. Hall had spent two weeks in a semiprivate room on a medical ward prior to admission to this four-bed room on a thirty-bed surgical acute care ward. The new head nurse supported the liaison nurse's intervention; she sensed the patient's stress.

The family: No visitors were noted at any time. There were no cards, flowers, or other signs of family or friend involvement. The patient, a childless widower, only told his landlord about his admission and preferred not to have anyone see him "like this."

The medical illness: Mr. Hall's diagnostic workup and surgery resulted in extended hospitalization and immobility. There were invasive, uncomfortable, and embarrassing procedures, including upper and lower GI series, hyperalimentation, chest PT, and the like. His movement was restricted.

The chart: The documentation indicates numerous tests and procedures. There is minimal social history. The patient is consistently described as "depressed." There is no indication that he had refused treatments, and no evidence of sleep disturbance. He requested to leave the hospital on several occasions but never did for reasons that were unclear.

How does the liaison nurse decide the most effective way to handle Miss Ross's request? After a "diagnosis of the total consultation," a decision is reached and the need for direct versus indirect service is determined. The decision about appropriate intervention is based on all the factors combined, and it is arrived at thoughtfully, rationally, and with clear clinical judgment. Hippocrates said, "First do no harm." To carry that thought further, do no harm not only to the patient but to the milieu, to the consultee, to the consultant, to the family, or to the relationship of patients and their health care providers. Sometimes the most sensible action might be to do nothing. In Mr. Hall's case, doing nothing would not have been helpful.

The consultation question regarding Mr. Hall was unclear. A decision to interview the patient, that is, a direct intervention, was made for the following reasons. The consultee was inexperienced, somewhat overwhelmed, and unable to formulate the question. Role modeling seemed more appropriate. The climate on the ward made this an opportune time for the liaison nurse to help the new head nurse in a concrete way, that is, to do the work. Furthermore, the patient was having a prolonged hospitalization and had no family or outside support. Mr. Hall's desires to leave the hospital precipitously were an indication of his frustration, fear, or anger, all of which were probably a result of his illness and personality style. In a direct intervention, the liaison nurse worked with the staff and the patient, while consulting the social worker.

The following brief note was written in the chart after discussing the case with the head nurse and the consultee, Miss Ross:

Mr. Hall, a widowed, childless, recently retired self-employed businessman is overwhelmed by his illness which has been characterized by repeated complications. An independent man, who has lived alone for twenty years, Mr. Hall is experiencing difficulty being dependent. He is struggling to gain control of his illness. Mr. Hall states that he likes everything "just so" and prefers to be alone. Suggestions:

1. If possible, transfer Mr. Hall to a private room where he states he would feel less stressed.
2. Whenever possible, encourage the patient's involvement in his care to decrease his sense of dependency. (For example, taking responsibility for tabulation of his intake and output.)
3. Try to obtain portable I-Vac, since the freedom to ambulate will probably help.
4. Follow-up by the liaison nurse.

The significant parameters that liaison nurses can utilize in "diagnosing the total consultation" have been illustrated and discussed. These parameters aid in identifying and understanding overt and covert consultation questions, defining the scope of the problem, clarifying expectations, determining the need for direct versus indirect services, and planning nursing interventions.

Liaison nurses may be contacted in different ways for a variety of problems. They are aware of the issues to listen for and the consultee behaviors to observe in providing consultation. They may share certain steps of the diagnostic process with consultees, to develop their psychological assessment skills, as they engage in joint problem solving.

section 4   interventions and recommendations

Interventions and recommendations are based on the total consultation. Unless consultants make practical suggestions, their efforts may be futile. Interventions should begin simply and progress as needed. Many times the involvement of the liaison nurse aids in clarifying the problem, and with very minor changes all parties involved are able to interact more productively. Interventions are not static; they are evaluated and changed when needed.

It is important to note here that behavior described as "irrational" may or may not be irrational. Patient behavior that is viewed as necessitating psychiatric consultation is usually behavior that consultees believe is either beyond the scope of their clinical expertise or, for some unknown reason, not responding favorably to their clinical intervention. The behavior is usually actually or potentially disruptive to the workings of the ward and/or to the care of the patient.

"Introducing into the situation a person who 'knows about' and 'can manage' disturbed (or disturbing) behavior is in itself, a tension-reducing event, quite independent of anything he may really know, say, or do [10]." Over time, as liaison nurses work with consultees, this tension-reducing influence can be not only demonstrated, but also utilized in building the consultee-liaison nurse alliance.

Caution is taken, however, to emphasize the theoretically based clinical approach to the problem to avoid the guise of magic and omnipotence. This distortion of the liaison nurse's abilities can be demonstrated by the consultee's asking, "How did you know that about Mr. X? I never thought of it that way. How do you think of these things?" The potential for the consultee to harbor a fantasy about the liaison nurse, or about psychiatry and psychiatric nursing, may be present. It is helpful for this impression to be openly acknowledged and dispelled, lest it be inappropriately regarded as flattery by the liaison nurse. It may also be experienced as an unrealistic facet of the liaison nurse by the consultee.

Liaison nurses, however, can realistically acknowledge with their nursing colleagues their areas of expertise and competence without having it seem magical. The psychiatric nurse may recognize ventricular tachycardia on the cardiac monitor with ease but feels less confident in understanding the cause. The medical nurse recognizes that the patient's depression is interfering with recovery but feels less confident about how to uncover the cause. Each nurse has specialized clinical skills. A mutual respect and acceptance form the basis of the consultant-consultee relationship.

There are several factors to consider in addition to those previously mentioned before planning the intervention. Is this situation presently a psychiatric emergency, or is it pending? Is the urgency a function of the psychiatric status of the patient or of the tolerance of the staff? Is the identification of the nurse or nurses with the patient so intense that it should be diffused? Or is the staff perhaps unsure of what to do or say? Sometimes the staff may want validation of their own skills. A comparison can be made to the staff nurse asking a more experienced nurse to check an IV that may have infiltrated. The nurse may be asking to have the hopelessness of the depressed patient checked.

Liaison nurses may find that a particular intervention allows them to demonstrate principles or to serve as a role model. One of the long-term goals is to further develop the staff nurses' ability to provide psychological care to patients. Therefore, good teaching opportunities should be utilized.

If the decision is for indirect or consultee-centered consultation, liaison nurses discuss the intervention with the consultee, provide support, and reassess as indicated. Sometimes the problem being presented for consultation is clearly one in which seeing the patient would not prove helpful. For example:

- The patient, for a variety of physiological reasons, may not be able to verbalize.
- The patient may already be involved with a psychiatrist or with a social worker.
- An interview may be disruptive for the patient and/or for the family.
- A direct patient interview may also be the undoing of the liaison nurse's collegial relationship with particular members of the health care team.
- A consultative approach may be more reasonable than a direct interview with the patient and/or family.
- The problem may be consultee-centered rather than patient-centered.
- The consultee may not want the liaison nurse to see the patient and/or family.

The list of possible circumstances that would contraindicate the feasibility of such an interview is potentially lengthy. Yet a decision not to interview contains inherent risks. The greatest risk is that the liaison nurse, in effect, may be misdiagnosing the consultation. In the process of providing the consultation, liaison nurses reassess the situation and, if necessary, can alter their decisions. If the decision is to provide indirect service, a patient care conference helps to clarify pertinent issues, as well as to develop and plan appropriate nursing intervention. Follow-up, reassessment, and evaluation would inevitably become the next steps, regardless of whether direct or indirect service was provided.

Sometimes the continued willingness of liaison nurses to be involved is all that consultees need. Time and time again this effect has been demonstrated in clinical practice. With a liaison nurse as a support and a role model, there may be a change in consultees' attitudes regarding the problem. This change of attitude may often result in a new approach to the problem and produce a therapeutic change in the patient–nurse relationship.

The decision to make a direct intervention may be based on one factor in the consultation or more often on a combination of several. Some factors to consider are:

1. Do the words and behavior of the patient match?

2. Is the behavior of the patient out of proportion to reality?
3. Are the nurses' interventions working?
4. Is the problem still unclear after indirect service has been provided?
5. Is there a strong desire by the consultee for the liaison nurse to interview the patient?

Through "diagnosis of the total consultation," a decision is reached, and the need for direct versus indirect service is determined. If the patient and/or family are seen by the liaison nurse, it may be helpful to conduct the interview in conjunction with the consultee. Yet even at times when the interview is best handled if the liaison nurse does not include the consultee, it is advantageous for the consultee to be at least a nonparticipant observer, for the dual purpose of teaching through role modeling and illustrating the team concept to the patient. After the patient interview, specific nursing interventions can be planned and initiated. When needed, a patient care conference with the specific health care providers can be held. The interview is documented in the patient's record by the liaison nurse. Recommended interventions are added to the nursing care plans in the Kardex by the patient's nurse.

The philosophy of the practice of psychiatry, along with the role and availability of the psychiatrist, influences the practice of the liaison nurse. The psychiatric responsibilities of liaison nurses vary among institutions. Pragmatic factors, such as the special interest of the consultant, the present case load, or the needs or interests of the psychiatric service when making intervention decisions, are also considered. As a general rule of thumb, the following circumstances would require a psychiatrist's intervention or consultation:

1. a legal issue (competency, suicide or homicide risk, commitment),
2. the use of psychotropic drugs,
3. a complicated medical-psychiatric interface and differentiation,
4. a severe psychiatric illness necessitating clinical supervision, or
5. a total consultation so complicated and intervention needs so great that the liaison nurse needs support and/or assistance.

An appropriate intervention may be to refer a specific problem to a social worker for direct intervention with the family. Again, the role and philosophy of the department of social service within the institution is considered. Often patients have concerns about their families, home situations, finances, or employment benefits, all of which can be effectively resolved by the social workers. Social

workers have a valuable perspective and can make an important contribution to the total problem.

A valuable and effective intervention technique is the involvement of a nurse clinical specialist. It is not uncommon for "unacceptable" patient behaviors to be labeled "psychiatric" or "emotional"
when they are more a reaction to the stress of illness or hospitalization. The confusion lies in defining the appropriate intervention. The
following example illustrates this point:

> Mrs. Davis is a 25-year-old primipara who had an incredibly
> complicated pregnancy requiring a long hospitalization at five months
> gestation. After four months of bed rest at home, she delivered a
> healthy baby boy. She was initially referred to the liaison nurse when
> hospitalized during her pregnancy. The staff immediately became
> overidentified with the patient and expressed concern regarding the
> patient's adjustment to the prolonged hospitalization and bed rest. In
> the process of "diagnosing the consultation," the liaison nurse identi-
> fied that Mrs. Davis was well supported by her family and seemed
> able to approach her problem realistically. She clearly had strengths.
> After her Caesarian section, her medical problems became even more
> complicated, and she became a very sick and discouraged young
> woman.
>
> But an interesting thing happened. The nurses on the gynecology
> service were so empathic that, as a result, they experienced great diffi-
> culty providing routine postoperative care. The liaison nurse clinically
> assessed that the patient and staff did not need more attention to, or
> discussion about, their thoughts and feelings. A postoperative surgical
> plan was indicated to demonstrate to the patient that she *was* making
> progress, and to demonstrate to the staff that they could indeed help
> Mrs. Davis. The liaison nurse and surgical clinical specialist met with
> the staff to help them redirect their efforts back to the physical care
> that had become emotionally a problem for them. The firmness and
> direction that Mrs. Davis received from the nurses helped her to feel
> that she was getting better. As she regained her health, her depression
> lifted. Because discussion of feelings about this patient proved to
> inhibit the delivery of nursing care, a follow-up conference to explore
> these feelings was held after Mrs. Davis was discharged.

Other services or departments within the hospital may be consulted or used as a source of referral. Interventions may include these
as needed. Examples are occupational therapy, dietary, volunteer
service, physical therapy, and the like.

Interventions are clinically sound nursing actions based on

"diagnosing the total consultation." The liaison nurse begins with the least intrusive interventions and observes, reassesses, and recommends further actions as are clinically indicated. There is neither a "cookbook" approach to the formulation of interventions, nor are interventions based on "gut" feeling. They must be scientifically and clinically based, and can be learned. Patients' responses to interventions are no mystery nor are they mystical. They are as predictable as any intervention based on diagnosis.

This chapter began with three clinical cases illustrating the type of problems presented in the consultation questions posed. Looking back at Case I (Sara), Case II (Mrs. Roth), and Case III (Mr. Andrews), and incorporating the discussion of the total consultation, the interventions that will be described can be more fully understood.

case I. a patient problem

The request for consultation was expressed as follows: "We have this patient in here, renal failure, on dialysis, who's been screaming since she woke up. She's the only girl in a family of four children, so she's probably really spoiled, but we can't have a kid screaming in here like this. Maybe you could see her or something."

The following factors determined for the liaison nurse that a direct intervention would be required:

1. the disruption of the screaming to the ICU,
2. the frustration of staff and the failure of their interventions,
3. the gravity and suddenness of medical illness, and
4. the opportunity for role modeling and teaching.

The patient's chart was reviewed to gather more information covering the child's past birth history, medical history, and present course of illness and prescribed treatment. Discussion with the head nurse, with the patient's nurse for the day, and with the pediatric resident also took place as part of the data-gathering process. Approximately fifteen minutes were spent in observing Sara, particularly in terms of her interaction with the nurse, the physician, and her mother. The liaison nurse was then introduced to the mother and child. A brief developmental history was taken from the mother. Sara's apparent physical discomfort and fear were verbally acknowledged by the liaison nurse. Sara was repeatedly assured by her mother and by the liaison nurse that the latter was there to visit and would not hurt her. Slowly, the liaison nurse was able to engage Sara in play around a doll that her mother had just purchased. Sara told the liaison nurse that she didn't feel good and that she "just got sick." She also mentioned that she had an old doll at home. In the process of talking about the "old doll," the liaison nurse learned that Sara missed her, but, according to the patient, had left the old doll home because "she was bad for wetting her pants." It was also learned that Sara's brothers, again according to the patient, "had to stay home." Sara could not explain the reason for this.

It was observed, both prior to and during the interview, that Sara was extremely anxious and baffled over her illness and hospitalization. Intervention by medical and nursing staff seemed only to heighten her fears, and she could not hear any of their attempts to comfort her. She was not able to identify when a treatment or procedure was over, but rather she kept her eyes closed while screaming and pulling away from the "assailants." Although she looked to her mother desperately, she appeared unable to understand why protection was not forthcoming.

These observations were discussed privately with the mother. The normalcy of the patient's anxiety and behavior was stressed. A diagnostic formulation of acute anxiety reaction and regression in the face of fears regarding body integrity and possible punishment was made. On the basis of this assessment, the following interventions were suggested and implicated.

1. The mother to visit more frequently, since separation anxiety was experienced by the patient.
2. The mother encouraged and permitted to physically hold the child. During this time the mother, in essence, would be "protecting" Sara and keeping her safe, since no aspects of care were to be carried out until the child was returned to her bed.
3. Consultation with the play therapist to help Sara understand her illness and the required medical care, as well as to encourage the "safe" expression of her anger and anxiety.
4. Familiar objects from home, including the "old doll," to be brought in, along with pictures of the family, the home, and so on. The purpose was to reintroduce important objects and to reassure Sara that her life outside the hospital continued to exist and was waiting for her to return.
5. Brothers allowed to visit. Preparation for the visit was to be done by Sara's nurse with the assistance of the liaison nurse.
6. Social service consultation, offered to the parents for additional support.

7. Consistency in nursing assignments to Sara, which would possibly aid in building a relationship between the patient and her nurse and in decreasing the patient's fear by increasing the continuity of care.
8. Suggestion of anti-anxiety medication, to be determined by the pediatrician and to be administered prior to any invasive procedure.

case II. a staff problem

The request for consultation was expressed as follows: "I was just thinking about you. Maybe you could help the nurses with Mrs. Roth. She's in her early thirties—nice lady—severe heart disease with a poor prognosis. It's got to be hard for them to go into that room."

The following factors determined the intervention:

1. The referral by the cardiology resident was most unusual and needed to be checked out with the nursing staff.
2. This ward appropriately utilized the liaison nurse, and it seemed unusual that they did not mention the patient.
3. It seemed that there was a lack of communication between the doctors and the nurses.
4. The nurses perhaps wanted to say that they didn't need help.

The liaison nurse discussed with both the head nurse and the patient's nurse the information she had gathered from the cardiology resident, and in so doing the source of the consultation request was acknowledged. The patient's chart was reviewed. The nurses were clearly angry at the cardiology resident. Through informal discussion, the liaison nurse learned that the nurses felt that everyone was having difficulty in caring for this patient. The general opinion was that they all just had "to live through it." They were not sure how the liaison nurse might be helpful. The patient did have a strong family support system and had refused both social service and psychiatric intervention, viewing these as unnecessary.

In learning this information, a formulation of acute hopelessness was made by the liaison nurse in terms of the patient's health care team. The major symptom seemed to be a generalized sense of helplessness, that is, having to "live through it." The degree of identification with Mrs. Roth was unclear. The quality of the communication among members of the health care team was unclear. Finally, whether or not an avenue for effective psychiatric nursing intervention was needed and/or existed was also unclear. On the basis of this assessment, the following interventions were indicated:

1. A milieu meeting was held for the nursing staff and other members of the health team involved with this patient. The purpose was to review the patient's case and hospitalization course, to express concerns and feelings about the patient, to identify needs of staff, if any, and to promote communication among members of the health team.
2. Discussions concerning this patient continued to occur in the weekly nurses' group. Acknowledgement of the nurses' difficult role helped them to "go back into the room."
3. The liaison nurse remained available to the entire health care team.

case III. a mixed problem

The request for consultation was expressed as follows: "We really need help with Mr. Andrews. He's a 62-year-old patient with gastric CA. Prognosis could be OK, but he won't let the docs finish their workup so they can treat him. He's really depressed, won't do anything for himself, and just wants to sleep and not feel any pain. It's really awful for all of us."

The following factors determined the intervention:

1. The anxiety was very high in the group.
2. There were drastic behavior changes.
3. The fact that this physician requested a nursing consultation was unusual.
4. The ward had a history of dealing effectively with problems of this type and were now bewildered.
5. The patient refused treatment.

The following interventions transpired:

1. The patient's medical record was reviewed, and the patient's physician was contacted to gather additional medical information—illness cause, treatments, prognosis, and a view of the patient's understanding.
2. The patient was interviewed with the primary nurse. The purpose was to make a psychological assessment of the patient and to strengthen the relationship with an important caretaker.
3. Psychiatric consultation was recommended by the liaison nurse to further evaluate the depression and to differentiate its organic versus functional origins, as well as to evaluate for antidepressant medication.
4. Discussion with the patient's physician resulted in a CAT scan, to rule out brain metastases and to consult the pharmacist for assistance in achieving pain control.
5. A supportive relationship with the liaison nurse, and the beginning of grief work.

6. A lawyer was contacted by the family to aid the patient in settling his affairs.
7. A minimal expectation was placed on the patient at this time to be independent.
8. Socialization was encouraged with the nurse and with the family.
9. Half-hour checks at night.
10. Weekly conferences with the health care team to evaluate and to plan care.

As illustrated, the interventions in each case were individualized. The suggestions themselves help to redirect the nurses toward more beneficial interactions.

section 5 follow-up and reassessment

When the clinical work is consultation, follow-up and reassessment cannot be overemphasized. The liaison component of the clinical work makes it more essential. As the three major cases discussed in this chapter illustrate, without follow-up, evaluation, and reassessment, further intervention cannot occur.

case I. a patient problem

Both the head nurse and Sara's mother were receptive to the interventions suggested by the liaison nurse. The child's distress was acutely apparent as well as terribly disruptive to the ICU. The interventions were carried out quickly, and Sara's response was positive. Sara was comforted by the increased availability of her mother. She was relieved to see her brothers and closely held her "old doll," especially when treatments and procedures were administered. The head nurse had designated an experienced member of the staff to be responsible for preparing the sibling visit. On reassessment, the liaison nurse learned that Sara's brothers were not sufficiently prepared. Upon leaving the unit, the brothers had many feelings and reactions that might have been prevented. Education in this area to the consultee was needed.

Five days after the psychiatric nursing consultation, Sara was transferred to the pediatric ward. Her acute renal failure had been reversed, and she was discharged home a few days later.

case II. a staff problem

The milieu meeting was held and all members of the health care team attended. The cardiology resident who had initiated the consultation arrived late, stating that he had forgotten the time of the meeting. Discussion ensued regarding the patient's prognosis, her emotional needs, and those of her family. It became clear that the health care team was providing Mrs. Roth with both excellent physical care as well as emotional support. It was very important for this fact to be shared. As mentioned previously, additional supports had been offered to the patient but were refused. From all reports, it did not appear that such interventions were needed. Mrs. Roth had told her nurse that, if and when she needed assistance from social service and/or psychiatry, she would be able to ask for it. Yet it became apparent, during the initial case presentation, that the degree of crisis in Mrs. Roth's family life was not fully acknowledged by her. Although Mrs. Roth was refusing additional supportive interventions, the consultees could benefit from discussions centering on speculation of family dynamics and the meaning of a crisis to a family.

A second meeting was held a week later with excellent attendance. Shortly thereafter, the patient was discharged home to be followed by the VNA and the cardiology resident.

case III. a mixed problem

Mr. Andrews's scan was negative. Consultation with the psychiatrist validated a diagnosis of reactive clinical depression secondary to the cancer diagnosis, as well as unresolved grief work regarding Mrs. Andrews. No psychosis was found, and Mr. Andrews was not felt to be suicidal. A supportive relationship and short-term therapy, rather than antidepressant medication, were indicated. Consultation with the pharmacist did result in effective pain management. Mr. Andrews became more responsive to his nurse's efforts to support his independence. In reassessing the consultation, Mr. Andrews requested to see a lawyer in order to settle family affairs. He continued to refuse treatment, but he was clearly competent. The health care team was able to accept his decision while utilizing the psychiatrist and the liaison nurse for support. Mr. Andrews remained in the hospital until his death, approximately three weeks later.

The feelings that the consultees experienced while allowing the patient to remain regressed were more available for discussion, because the consultees had been supported by the liaison nurse in caring for this difficult patient.

The goal of closure in terms of a specific consultation cannot be attempted unless there is follow-up. Liaison nurses cannot rely on the consultee to initiate the feedback process. Certainly there are many instances when consultees contact liaison nurses to inform them of the success or the failure of their recommendations. They may alert liaison nurses to changes in the patient's physical or emotional status. Most commonly, however, feedback does not occur, and liaison nurses may become aware of such important information long after any further intervention can be initiated. Liaison nurses are clinically responsible not only for consultation, but also for communicating with the consultee and with any other significant health care providers involved with the patient. There is a clinical responsibility for reassessment. Liaison nurses' interactions remain dynamic and dependent on the present situation.

During the process of reassessment, the liaison nurse has the opportunity to observe the effect of suggested interventions. Have they been carried out? Have they proved successful? Why? Have they achieved nothing? Why? Why not? If successful, is it possible to generalize interventions that were made so that the process of integrating mental health skills is enhanced? In Case II, the nursing staff discovered that communicating with each other and sharing the sad feelings about Mrs. Roth made it more bearable to care for her. The liaison nurse might generalize that to other patients. However, if the intervention failed, then generalizing may or may not be possible. Did the interventions fail because there was a misdiagnosis of a hidden agenda? Liaison nurses guide consultees in learning about generalizing mental health concepts.

Liaison nurses adjust the frequency of follow-up as indicated. They might check for documentation and care plans to assure that there is continuity among other nursing shifts. If the staff communication is weak, it may indicate a lack of acceptance of the suggestions made by the liaison nurse. Continued observation and involvement are the hallmarks of successful intervention. They also present opportunities to learn more about what is effective.

In addition to the development and initiation of effective psychiatric nursing intervention, the consultation is goal-directed toward teaching consultees mental health principles. It is not uncommon to discover that the teaching, rather than the actual nursing intervention, was unsuccessful. The consultee may have carried out the prescribed recommendations, and the patient may have even improved, but the learning needs of the consultee went unmet. This is not to say that the liaison nurse did not teach. He or she probably did, but, due to a variety of factors, the consultee failed to understand the clinical basis for the interventions. Perhaps anxiety was too high for learning to occur; perhaps the liaison nurse utilized too much psychiatric jargon; perhaps the consultee's wish and/or ability to learn was overestimated; or perhaps the liaison nurse "misdiagnosed the total consultation." Through the vehicles of follow-up and reassessment, the teaching/learning component of psychiatric nursing consultation can be reviewed and, if necessary, reinstituted. Liaison nurses benefit from this process as well. Patient- and consultee-centered follow-up and reassessment are opportunities for gaining further understanding of the milieu in which consultation is being provided, as well as of the consultee with which the liaison nurse must collaboratively work. This is a time when both negative as well as positive feedback regarding liaison nurses and their clinical work can be gathered. It is a time when liaison nurses can incorporate what they have learned about the milieu, the patient, the consultee, and themselves to stimulate their own professional growth.

Although there are inherent difficulties in describing and in evaluating the role of liaison nurses, the major focus remains on the quality of their clinical practice. Their ability, however, to build on rapport and to establish and strengthen professional alliances can influence their effectiveness. The ability to accept the frequent reality of insufficient data, to make a formulation and alter it if necessary, to develop and initiate interventions, to take clinically sound risks, and to be respectful of the needs of the consultee are the cornerstones of clinical practice. Nevertheless, the strength and validity of these elements are reflected in the process of follow-up and reassessment. Through these processes, liaison nurses can illustrate their concern about the problems identified and the consultee. It is important that they remain visible so that, after the consultation, the consultee does not feel alone with the problem. If physically returning to the ward is not immediately possible, a follow-up telephone call is a useful way of providing support, while demonstrating continued involvement. Only by maintaining professional contact with the consultee can liaison nurses preserve their invitation to continue to consult on the ward.

references

1. Gerald Caplan, *The Theory and Practice of Mental Health Consultation* (New York: Basic Books, Inc., 1970), pp. 32–35.
2. Betty Johnson, "Psychiatric Nurse Consultant in the General Hospital," *Nursing Outlook* (October 1963): 728.
3. Eugene Meyer and Myer Mendelson, "Psychiatric Consultations with Patients on Medical and Surgical Wards: Patterns and Processes," *Psychiatry* 24 (1961): 199.
4. Meyer and Mendelson, p. 216.
5. Johnson, p. 729.
6. Sheldon Schiff and Martin Pilot, "An Approach to Psychiatric Consultation in the General Hospital," *Archives of General Psychiatry* 1 (1959): 349–357.

7. James Strain and Stanley Grossman, *Psychological Care of the Medically Ill* (New York: Appleton-Century-Crofts, 1975), pp. 11–22. Reprinted with permission.

8. Anastasia Kucharski and James Groves, "The So-Called 'Inappropriate' Psychiatric Consultation Request in a Medical or Surgical Ward," *International Journal of Psychiatry in Medicine* (1976–77): 209–220.

9. Strain and Grossman, pp. 11–22.

10. Meyer and Mendelson, p. 214.

bibliography

books

BURGESS, ANN. *Psychiatric Nursing in the Hospital and the Community*. Englewood Cliffs, N.J.: Prentice-Hall, Inc., 1981.

CAPLAN, GERALD. *The Theory and Practice of Mental Health Consultation*. New York: Basic Books, Inc., Publishers, 1970.

KOHNKE, MARY F. *The Case for Consultation in Nursing Designs for Professional Practice*. New York: John Wiley & Sons, Inc., 1977.

MACKINNON, ROGER and MICHELS, ROBERT. *The Psychiatric Interview in Clinical Practice*. Philadelphia: W. B. Sanders Company, 1971.

NEILL, J. R. and SANDIFER, M. G. *Practical Manual of Psychiatric Consultation*. Baltimore: Williams and Wilkins, 1980.

ROBINSON, LISA. *Liaison Nursing Psychological Approach to Patient Care*. Philadelphia: F. A. Davis Company, 1974.

STRAIN, JAMES and GROSSMAN, STANLEY. *Psychological Care of the Medically Ill*. New York: Appleton-Century-Crofts, 1975.

WOOLDRIDGE, P. J.; SKIPPER, J. K.; and LEONARD, R. C. *Behavioral Science, Social Practice, and the Nursing Profession*. Cleveland: The Press of Case Western Reserve University, 1968.

articles

ANDERS, R. L. "Program Consultation by a Clinical Specialist," *Journal of Nursing Administration* (November 1978): 34–38.

BARTON, DAVID and KELSO, MARGARET. "The Nurse as a Psychiatric Consultation Team Member," *International Journal of Psychiatry in Medicine* 2 (1971): 108–115.

BATMAN, ROBERT H. "Consultation as an Educational Technique in Psychiatric Nursing," *Mental Hygiene* 52:4 (October 1968): 617–621.

BERLIN, I. N. "The Theme in Mental Health Consultation Sessions," *American Journal of Orthopsychiatry* 30 (1960): 827–828.

BLAKE, P. "The Clinical Specialist as Nurse Consultant," *Journal of Nursing Administration* (December 1977): 33–36.

BURSTON, BEN. "The Psychiatric Consultant and the Nurse," *Nursing Forum* 2:4 (1963): 7–23.

DORWART, NANCY. "A Model for Mental Health Consultation to the General Hospital," *Journal of Psychiatric Nursing and Mental Health Services* (March 1979): 26–33.

GANS, JEROME S. "The Consultee-Attended Interview—An Approach to Liaison Psychiatry," *General Hospital Psychiatry* 1:1 (April 1979): 24–30.

HEDLUND, N. L. "Mental Health Nursing Consultation in the General Hospital," *Patient Counseling and Health Education* (Fall 1978): 85–88.

HOLSTEIN, SHIRLEY and SCHWAB, JOHN. "A Coordinated Consultation Program for Nurses and Psychiatrists," *Journal of the American Medical Association* 194:5 (1965): 491–493.

JACKSON, HARRIET. "The Psychiatric Nurse as a Mental Health Consultant in a General Hospital," *The Nursing Clinics of North America* 4:3 (September 1969): 527–540.

KOLSON, GAIL. "Mental Health Nursing Consultations: A Study of Expectations," *Journal of Psychiatric Nursing and Mental Health Services* (August 1976): 24–32.

LEHMANN, F. G. "Liaison Nursing: A Model for Nursing Practice," in *Principles and Practice of Psychiatric Nursing*, edited by G. Stuart and S. Sundeen. St. Louis: The C. V. Mosby Co., 1979, pp. 518–532.

LIDZ, THEODORE and FLECK, STEPHEN. "Integration of Medical and Psychiatric Methods and Objectives on a Medical Service," *Psychosomatic Medicine* 12 (March–April 1950): 103–107.

MILLER, WARREN B. "Psychiatric Consultation: Part I. A General Systems Approach," *International Journal of Psychiatry in Medicine* 4:2 (Spring 1973): 135–145.

————. "Psychiatric Consultation: Part II: Conceptual and Pragmatic Issues of Formulation," *International Journal of Psychiatry in Medicine* 4:3 (Spring 1973): 251–271.

NORRIS, C. "A Few Notes on Consultation in Nursing," *Nursing Outlook* (December 1977): 756–771.

PETERSON, S. "The Psychiatric Nurse Specialist in a General Hospital," *Nursing Outlook* 17 (February 1969): 56–58.

POLLAK, O. and VINCENT, P. A. "Human Relations in Nursing Consultation," *Nursing Forum* 9:1 (1970): 85–89.

REYNOLDS, JANIS and LOGSDON, JANN. "Assessing Your Patients' Mental Status," *Nursing '79* 9:8 (August 1979): 26–33.

ROBBINS, P. R. and SPENCER, E. C. "A Study of the Consultation Process," *Psychiatry* 31 (1968): 362–368.

SCHWAB, JOHN J. "The Psychiatric Consultation," *Journal of Continuing Education in Psychiatry* (February 1979): 17–27.

SEDGWICK, RAE. "The Role of the Process Consultant," *Nursing Outlook* 21:12 (December 1973): 773–775.

SEVERIN, N. K. and BECKER, R. E. "Nurses as Psychiatric Consultants in a General Hospital Emergency Room," *Nursing Digest* (January–February 1976): 44–46.

SOCHET, B. R. "The Role of the Mental Health Counselor in the Psychiatric Liaison Service of the General Hospital," *International Journal of Psychiatry in Medicine* 5 (Winter 1974): 1–16.

SNYDER, S. and WILSON, M. "Elements of a Psychological Assessment," *American Journal of Nursing* (1977): 235–239.

STRINGER, L. A. "Consultation: Some Expectations, Principles and Skills," *Social Work* 6 (1961): 85–90.

TERMINI, M. and CIECHOSKI, M. "The Consultation Process," *Issues in Mental Health Nursing* 3:1–2 (January–June 1981): 77–88.

WOLFF, PEGGY. "Psychiatric Nursing Consultation: A Study of the Referral Process," *Journal of Psychiatric Nursing and Mental Health Services* (May 1978): 42–47.

5

the experience of illness and hospitalization

section 1   the hospital ward

A variety of authors have discussed and researched the multiple components that combine to create the uniquely stressful environment of
a hospital. Sociological, psychological, and systems theory orientations have been utilized in examining the experiential factors and
ramifications of being hospitalized. "In nursing, hospitalization (for
the patient) is usually referred to as 'distressing.' In psychological
terms, it might be described as 'ego threatening,' in sociological
terms, 'disorganizing' [2]." It is helpful for psychiatric liaison nurses
to incorporate into their clinical practice a knowledge of the hospital
ward and its impact on the patient/family. Comprehensive and effective consultation necessitates an appreciation of this environment.

The hospital may symbolize a variety of hopes, fears, and
beliefs. For some individuals, the hospital may be a frightening, controlling, death-tinged place, to which admission should be avoided at
all costs. For others, the hospital may be a safe, powerful, magical
place, where admission validates the hope for comfort and cure. The
patient/family's previous knowledge and/or experience with hospitals, along with the meaning of illness for them, influences the sym-
bolism of the hospital. In addition, the psychological stance that the
patient assumes in reference to being "ill" serves to further influence
the images of the hospital. Hospital life can be both unbelievable [3]
and dehumanizing [4]. The preponderance of humor and jokes associated with life in the hospital is an attempt by both providers and
consumers to integrate the effects of life in the hospital. The hopes,
fears, and beliefs regarding the hospital that the patient/family hold
to be true may be validated, shaken, or destroyed during the process
of hospitalization.

The nature of the hospital itself in terms of its type, size, and reputation may connote various meanings. When patients enter a hospital within their own community, they may feel reassured and comforted by professionals whom they know in another context. Patients may also believe that their illnesses are not severe. The admission to a chronic care hospital may be relief for patients, either validating their belief that their illnesses are incurable or serving as an acceptance that they will not improve. When patients enter large medical centers as the last stop on their search for a miracle, the hospital becomes associated with the final verdict. The hospital then represents the saviour or the failure.

The world of the hospital is unlike the world outside its doors. The highly intimate contact and often intrusive actions of health care providers would not be sanctioned elsewhere. This difference may be illustrated in terms of urinary catheterization, which is a necessary medical procedure sanctioned and practiced within the hospital. If nurses were required to provide this care in patients' places of work or business, consider how awkward and inappropriate things would seem. The policy and procedure that characterize the institutional functioning of the hospital influences health care staff and affects the patients. The results may be reflected in the patients' degree of cooperation with health care staff. Prescribed roles and behavioral expectations of the hospital staff, the patients, and the families frequently leave little room for flexibility and individualization.

This rigidity alone can precipitate problems for patients and affect the success of the hospitalization. In one hospital Mr. L, a young business executive who had suffered multiple fractures in an automobile accident, was conferring with his business staff in his private room. Without consideration of the impact of this conference on the patient, the visitors were asked to leave because the dinner trays had arrived on the ward. Mr. L had a wired jaw, and his dinner tray consisted of an eggnog and a frappe.

"The hospitalized patient is perhaps the prototype of the 'non-responsible' person [5]." Within the social and administrative organization of the hospital, the professional and nonprofessional employees have designated responsibilities and work assignments. Directly or indirectly, these "in-group" [6] members contribute to the overtly patient-centered focus of the institution. Covert institutional agendas are related to financial, social, administrative, and clinical policy and procedures. Patient care is also indirectly influenced by contract negotiations, personnel policies, and grievance procedures. The patient/family may be familiar with these issues, since they are characteristic of large bureaucratic organizations. Yet, unlike other highly technical institutions, the manifest product of the hospital is an exceedingly personal and subjective human experience, that is, the care of the patient. Knowledge of the workings of the hospital, however, does not provide patients with membership. They and their families are, by their very status, outsiders in the hospital. Others have found this to be unchallengeable [7], but clinical evidence has illustrated that pseudo-membership is allowed to patients with a knowledge of the system, prior experience, and social skills. Is the nature of ward membership different for the patient who orders Chinese food for the staff? Is it different for the patient who helps the staff feed other patients? The degree to which patient/family participation is expected, welcomed, and/or encouraged varies from hospital to hospital and from ward to ward.

"The nurse is the chief surgeon during major phases of the operation which changes people into patients [8]." The head nurse and his or her philosophy of clinical nursing practice set the tone on the ward and, more often than not, the expectation and definition of a therapeutic relationship between nurses and patients. Patients enter the hospital, and the transformation begins. With the completion of the paperwork and the application of a name band, individuals are designated as patients and outsiders. They may begin to feel that they are merely objects or numbers. When having a name band placed on her wrist, a young female patient was heard to say, "What could happen to me if this band was wrong?" Hospital staff may refer to a patient as "the admission in 306," even though the patient's name and personal data are readily available. The atmosphere of the hospital breeds crisis. Patients enter a world of sights, smells, and sounds that may be familiar, frightening, embarrassing, depressing, or stimulating. The geographical location, the type of hospital, and its philosophy all influence nursing care. Medical orders may be determined and written by interns and/or by residents, who are not known to the patient. In contrast, in some hospitals, the patient's private physician directs all care efforts. The regularity with which patients and/or their families have direct contact with the physician(s) may also vary.

> The liaison nurse was requested to aid the nursing and medical staff in working with the mother of a 4-year-old boy admitted to the intensive care unit with acute hemolytic anemia. The mother was described as "absent" since she had not been in to visit her son. When the physician called the mother on her son's third hospital day, she was further described as "hostile." Upon "diagnosing the consultation," the liaison nurse learned from the mother that some of her affec-

tations and behaviors related to her unmet expectations of hospital staff. Because she was unfamiliar with the workings of a large teaching hospital, she assumed that she would not be allowed to visit her son while he was in the intensive care unit. The mother had not been allowed to visit her own mother many years earlier when she had been in an intensive care unit. She also assumed that the doctors would call her regarding her son's condition, just as her mother's doctor had done.

The pace of the ward, the demands on health care providers, the seriousness of the patients' illnesses and their care needs can all influence the frequency and quality of contact with health care providers. The number of physicians and physician assistants per ward, the method of nursing care delivery, the philosophy and leadership skills of the head nurse, and the number and staffing pattern of the professional nurses, LPNs, nursing technicians, and nurses' aides on a unit may determine with which health care providers patients most consistently interact. This arrangement may or may not be acceptable to the patient and family. If the patient/family's expectations of hospital personnel, of care delivery, and of their relationships with care providers are unmet, then serious conflict can occur. Such factors as the age, sex, religion, color, and intellectual capacities of both staff and patient may also influence the giving and receiving of care. Identification and transference/countertransference issues between patients and their health care providers, which may or may not be clearly apparent, are also significant factors in the care of the patient (Chapter 7, Section 1).

The prehospital environment and lifestyle of patients warrant acknowledgement since they can influence adjustment to the hospital. Patients' perceptions of and reactions to the hospital are also altered by anxiety. In addition, the physical structure of the hospital and the ward deserve consideration when attempting to understand the environment and its impact on the individual patients and their families. The psychiatric liaison nurse considers these issues as well as the observable facets of the environment. The location of the nurses' desk in relation to a patient's room is a factor to be noted. Although many factors influence the decision to place a patient in a certain room, the possible meaning to and the effects on the patient are considered. For example, how isolated is this room? What kind of call system is used? How quickly can response be provided? Is there a window in the room? Where are the windows in reference to the patients? Are there separate bathrooms? If not, how many patients must share such facilities? Finally, what do the bath facilities include?

Is the patient in a private room or with a roommate(s)? Who is the roommate(s) in terms of age, religion, color, vocation, language, number of visitors, and so on? How similar or dissimilar is the roommate(s) to the patient? How visibly ill is the roommate(s)? How might the roommate(s)'s symptomatology affect the patient? What are the comparative care needs of all of the patients in this room?

The impact of a roommate in the course of the hospitalization is often underrated and ignored as a significant factor in the possible traumatic effect of hospitalization. The acceptance and progress of medical treatment, as well as the emotional adjustment of patients, may be influenced by roommates or by other patients.

> Lisa, a 23-year-old woman with cerebral palsy was sharing a room with another cerebral palsy patient. Although the roommate was fourteen years older, Lisa's disease was markedly more severe. At the request of the nursing staff, the psychiatric liaison nurse interviewed Lisa because her demanding behavior had become problematic. During the interview, Lisa stated that her fear and anxiety were not due to the upcoming orthopedic surgery. She was hopeful that the surgery would improve her ability to ambulate. But she was very upset about sharing a room with a woman whose disease would probably progress similarly. Lisa was very uncomfortable in the room and was positive that her roommate was equally upset, although they never spoke. Lisa not only felt that she was the negative picture of what was to come for the roommate, but at the same time, she felt angry with the roommate for not being "as debilitated." The roommate was described by the nursing staff as extremely quiet and cooperative.

Other important issues relate to hospital policy and to geographical location. Are there telephones at each bedside? Are they shared? Or are public telephones located on the ward? Does the hospital provide televisions and/or radios? Is it permissible for patients to bring in their own? Does the hospital provide recreational and/or diversional activities for patients? When are meals served? What is the quality of the food and the degree of flexibility in ordering food? Where is smoking permitted? Where is the coffee shop? What is the hospital's policy regarding visitors, and is there a margin of flexibility? Does the hospital provide a brochure describing hospital services? Where are parking and hotel facilities? How costly are they? In what kind of area is the hospital located? How available and safe is public transportation? For some individuals the issues just described have little significance. The structure of the ward matters little to the person who regards admission to the hospital as the ultimate priority.

> Mr. R was a 36-year-old paraplegic who lived in a nursing home and who was periodically admitted to the hospital for decubitus care and skin grafting. He was observed destroying his graft, probably to prolong his hospitalization. Unable to adjust to his physical limitations following an auto accident at age 26, Mr. R gradually became embittered and isolated from his family. He sought hospitalization as a pleasant and stimulating environment, as compared to the nursing home. He feared improvement and discharge, as opposed to illness and admission to the hospital.

Multiple pertinent issues reflective of the hospital ward exist. Any of the issues mentioned may hold special or no significance for individual patients. Some of the realities may be acceptable, while others may prove intolerable and thus serve to heighten the anxiety that they may be already experiencing. Regardless of the content and intensity of the patient/family's reactions to the hospital environment, the importance of recognizing and understanding these reactions and their etiology is emphasized. Patients and their families have entered a significant and powerful environment. By considering the impact of the environment on the patient—in conjunction with data regarding the patient's beliefs, feelings, and responses to the experience of being ill—psychiatric liaison nurses have a broader frame of reference. They utilize this in understanding consultees, the consultation questions, patients, and their families. The ramifications are evidenced in the quality and effectiveness of the consultation. "It matters little that the rules are made by hospital administration or the orders written by the physician. It is the nurse who makes patients of people [9]."

section 2   the patient's illness

Individuals experience a great deal more than the realities of the hospital environment when assuming a patient identity. They also experience a series of perceptions, expectations, and assumptions from their health care providers and families. These viewpoints are slowly revealed as patients share and demonstrate the special meanings that illness and hospitalization have for them. Influenced by many factors, emotional and behavioral responses unfold that belong to the patients. This individuality of patients remains a point of reference.

Their responses are not merely a reflection of the physiological experience and social/personal implications of illness and hospitalization. They are also a reflection of developmental issues, responses to illness, the meaning of illness, personality, defensive style, and the patients' cognitive abilities. Responses to certain types of illnesses can, in part, be predicted [10]. Generalized and common categories of response to illness, as well as possible meanings of illness, can also be formulated [11]. Psychiatric diagnostic categories may prove helpful in understanding and appropriately utilizing these generalizations [12]. When interacting with each health care provider, a unique situation and pattern of response can be observed.

Perceptions, expectations, and assumptions regarding patients comprise generalized concepts that health care providers may adopt, both consciously as well as unconsciously. The delineation of each of these concepts can prove helpful in understanding certain aspects of "diagnosing the total consultation." For purposes of clarity and consistency, each will be discussed separately and described in terms of patient motivations and behaviors. Health care providers are usually quite skilled in differentiating realistic from unrealistic beliefs about patients. However, the highly emotional atmosphere of a hospital, combined with the quality and quantity of clinical demands placed on care providers, may create a situation in which unrealistic perceptions, expectations, and assumptions remain unconscious. The reader is reminded of the importance of thoughtfully appreciating the individual personalities and character styles of each provider. Possible identification and transference/countertransference issues between patients and their care providers also deserve consideration in the diagnostic and intervention processes of consultation-liaison work.

Perceptions refer to the health care provider's intellectual and emotional understanding of patients. Perceptions are often based on subjective reactions that individuals symbolize by virtue of being patients. The professional and personal response to this understanding influences health care providers' interactions with patients, whom they recognize as persons seeking care, although in reality, they may or may not want or need care. The hospitalization may have been precipitated to avoid known personal responsibilities or as the result of some unconscious conflict. Patients are initially regarded as persons who are able and willing to assume the appropriate patient role. Comfort and care are most commonly felt to be patients' major priority. An example to the contrary is the patient who refuses to maintain bed rest, even though it is clinically indicated and imperative. Patients are further understood as persons who cannot effect their own comfort and cure. Health care providers may regard admission to the hospital as concrete validation that patients and/or their families are cognizant that professional assistance is needed to achieve the restoration of health or an adaptation to chronic ill health. Patients are also regarded as presently suffering some type of disruption in their usual life patterns and social/family roles.

Expectations comprise the kinds of anticipated emotional and behavioral reactions that health care providers believe their patients should and will demonstrate. These reactions are often viewed as being "normal" reactions to illness and hospitalization. For example, it is frequently expected that patients suffering alopecia post chemotherapy will become depressed or angry at times. However, it is also anticipated that such behavior is motivated by a wish for comfort and cure. It is expected that their depression and/or anger, because it is "normal," will subside as their physical condition improves. It is expected that they value their lives more than their hair. Therefore, it is anticipated that they will continue to try and cooperate with prescribed care and to participate in their care in accord with their physical and intellectual capacities. At times, their emotional status may influence the degree of their cooperation and participation. Nevertheless, regression, although anticipated, is expected to occur in such a way as to jeopardize neither the patients' health nor the care efforts of their doctors and nurses. It is expected that most of the time, these patients will try to maintain age-appropriate behavior and to demonstrate some degree of concern and interest in their own well-being.

Assumptions refer to certain beliefs concerning patients, that is, premises that are closely associated with the definition of the role of patient. It is assumed that patients will try their very best to provide accurate medical histories. It is not assumed that they and/or their families will deliberately withhold pertinent information. This is not to say that health care providers are unfamiliar with the possibility that socially or personally embarrassing information—such as alcohol abuse, cigarette and drug usage, or a sexual history—may be minimized or only partially revealed. Certainly, it is clearly recognized that, when under stress, patients may forget to report important information. However, it is assumed that, in most instances, upon remembering information, patients will report it to the health care team. In the majority of cases, it is further assumed that patients and family members regard health care providers as professionals whose work is goal-directed toward the restoration and preservation of the highest level of health possible. With the exception of some pediatric patients, most patients realize that doctors and nurses are not omnipotent and that tests and procedures usually are in the best interest of the patient. It is assumed that most patients will formulate appropriate relationships with their health care providers and that they will understand the one-sided intimacy that connotes a professional relationship. Yet patients do inquire about the nurses' personal life. It is further assumed that most family members will not inhibit care delivery and are usually quite concerned about the patient, as well as his or her health and comfort. But what does it mean when the family gives the patient fluids when they know he or she is NPO?

Obviously, there are multiple exceptions to these perceptions, expectations, and assumptions. Not every adult behaves as an adult when hospitalized, and not every pediatric patient regresses similarly. Certainly there are hospitalized patients who are not seeking comfort and cure, as well as others who want much more than a professional relationship with their health care providers. Not every family is supportive, let alone interested in the health of the patient. In terms of the "in-group" of the hospital, exceptions to these generalities also exist. Not every doctor and/or nurse can be consistently empathic to patients and families. Some doctors and/or nurses may feel omnipotent in that they may feel responsible for certain patient care outcome, when in reality these events are beyond their control [13]. Appropriate behavior on the part of health care providers is also needed in order to establish and preserve a professional patient-centered relationship.

The inherent danger in generalizing is without question. Psychiatric liaison nurses would forfeit an opportunity to gather more data and thus provide more effective consultation if they failed to identify and understand each individual's beliefs and the exceptions to them. These are all too frequently taken for granted or personalized. Health care providers may proceed in ministering care to their patients as if the patient and family are not only cognizant of these beliefs, but reacting in agreement with them. Clearly, when conflict occurs, a variety of reactions may be evoked in health care providers and in their patients. Anger, frustration, disappointment, surprise, and confusion are but a few of the possible responses. One of the more subtle clinical responsibilities of psychiatric liaison nurses is to assist the consultee in identifying the possible etiology of the conflict, that is, which belief has been disproven. Promoting understanding of this kind is critical. It is more successfully achieved if the liaison nurse refrains from supporting or stimulating discussion that is focused on the "right or wrong" of the patient/family's reaction and behaviors. It is more profitable to channel discussion in such a way as to stimulate collaborative brainstorming as to why such reactions and behaviors in patients seem to make care delivery difficult and/or appear contrary to the norms and mores of the "patient/family role" within the hospital.

Although generalizations are avoided, certain behaviors typify persons who are experiencing alterations in their physical health. Broad definitions support a nonjudgmental approach to care. *Illness behavior* is any activity, undertaken by persons who feel ill, to define the state of their health and to discover a suitable remedy. *Sick-role behavior* is the activity undertaken, for the purpose of getting well, by those who consider themselves ill [14].

The patient/family also have beliefs regarding the members of the health care team. These beliefs are founded on a variety of issues that hold a personal significance for the patient and family. Joyce Travelbee describes ten factors that influence patients' perceptions of illness and their responses to a diagnosis of illness. In attempting to understand the special meaning of illness and the illness experience, it is necessary to consider these factors.

1. Cultural beliefs about illness.
2. Symptoms and their meaning.
   a. previous knowledge (whether true or not).
   b. amount of pain, discomfort, inconvenience.
   c. extent to which symptoms interfere with customary way of life.
3. The area of the body involved and the symbolic meaning.
4. The extent to which signs or effects of illness are visible to others.
5. The individual's habitual manner of coping with stress and the degree to which the self is threatened.
6. Preconceptions and assumptions about physicians (and other health workers) and the nature of the assistance they can offer.
7. Physician's interpretation of:
   a. the nature of the illness.
   b. its duration and probable course.
   c. symptoms.
   d. measures which must be taken to control symptoms or cure illness.
   e. probable prognosis.
8. Amount of personal concern or interest shown by the physician.
9. The way in which family, friends, and others react toward the ill individual.
10. The way in which health workers perceive the ill individual, i.e., whether as an illness, room number, category, stereotype or as a human being [15].

A few additional factors are important. The quality of concern and interest demonstrated by nurses is another important element contributing to the perception of and response to illness. "The behavior of the nurse stimulates the patient to see and thereby to develop further his own competencies to understand situations and problems [16]." Although overstated, the nurse spends the majority of time with the patient. The nurse not only skillfully carries out the care prescribed by the physician, as well as the necessary nursing care, but also assesses daily the illness behavior demonstrated by the patient. The liaison nurse recognizes the potential clinical expertise of staff nurses in assessing illness behavior and encourages them to further develop their skills. By virtue of their clinical and theoretical education, nurses can serve as an effective deterrent to the potential trauma that patients face in the hospital. "Quality nursing care is primarily determined and directed by the patient's immediate needs, both physiologic and psychosocial, an integral part of that care is crisis intervention [17]." Sometimes, for the health care provider, the patient's illness holds a special meaning, which may directly or indirectly influence the quality and quantity of care delivered, as well as influence the patient's perception of the illness. What is the nurses' professional experience in treating this illness and in caring for this type of patient? How "serious" an illness do they believe it to be and what kind of illness behavior on the part of the patient/family is anticipated and acceptable? Also noted are identification issues as they relate to patients and families.

What is the personal experience with a particular illness? A second-year medical resident was described by the nurses as "extremely interested and invested" in a patient with hepatitis. The resident was very cautious in writing medical orders regarding the patient's care and wrote copious progress notes on the patient's chart. Upon discussing the patient with the resident, the liaison nurse learned that the resident also was concerned about the "possibility of depression" in the patient. The liaison nurse also learned of the resident's "frightening experience with hepatitis" when in medical school.

The significance or meaning of the illness and of the hospitalization to patients and families, their responses to illness, and their subsequent degree of compliance are all taken into consideration. Some patients and/or families tend to deny or to minimize illness. Others regress severely under the strain of illness. Some patients and/or families become fearful, depressed, angry, euphoric, or even psychotic in the face of illness. Others become very concrete, rigid, and utilize intellectualization to master the experience. Some patients seek strength, comfort, and rationale for illness in religion or philosophy. "In general, physical disease constitutes psychological stress that tends to evoke the patient's characteristic ways of dealing with stresses of life in general [18]." To understand how and why the patient and family demonstrate a specific style of illness behavior, the special meaning of the illness and the significance of the stress it creates must be acknowledged. What is the focus of the patient/family's fear and anxiety? What is the real and fantasied nature of the threat posed by the illness?

Illness is a personal and social crisis. It is a private as well as public experience. For example, patients in physical pain may be able to describe their pain with the appropriate medical jargon, that is, as a jabbing pain, a stabbing pain, throbbing pain. Nevertheless, although the physician and the nurse may observe patients' pain, examine patients, and take note of the significant physiological signs that indicate discomfort (vomiting, increased blood pressure, tachycardia, increased respirations, pallor, clenched teeth), the pain experience for patients is a private affair. How the pain feels, what it means, the thoughts, emotions, and fears brought to mind are an intrapsychic, physiological, and a cultural phenomenon [19]. Variation in terms of feeling invulnerable is associated with self-esteem [20]. How powerful and self-sufficient patients view themselves as being in reality is helpful for the liaison nurse to identify and to compare with patients' views of themselves in fantasy. What does it mean for patients to depend on and trust the health care team? Can they appropriately reality-test the extent to which they require professional assistance? And are their object relations such that they can allow themselves to be cared for by persons designated as health care providers? What are the patients' perceptions, expectations, and assumptions of themselves, their families, and their health care providers?

Lipowski has described eight categories of subjective meanings of illness—"illness as a challenge, as an enemy, as punishment, as weakness, as relief, as strategy, as irreparable loss or damage, and as value [21]." The subjective meaning of illness, the coping strategy evoked as a reflection of the patient's individual character style, creates a situation that is unique to every patient. "Human experience is unconsciously, preconsciously, and consciously constructed as a story or a series of stories in which we are the hero. It is this story and its cogency that provides our sense of being a unique individual [22]." The patient may be triumphant with cure, relieved with comfort measures, hopeful in the face of treatment, compliant or cooperative with care efforts, or distraught and victimized by unrelenting illness.

A multiplicity of factors influence patient compliance. Providing information to patients regarding their illness and health care needs is no longer viewed as a major factor that affects cooperation and compliance. The manner in which illness and wellness are viewed by patients, as well as how they are viewed within their families and culture, often sets the tone for the degree of compliance. Whether patients defend against feeling dependent by denying illness, view themselves as being in control of their fate, or assume a fatalistic view has much to do with illness behavior. Both the unconscious meaning of illness and its cognitive appraisal influence compliance. Economic realities are also taken into consideration, as the cost of health care may be either prohibitive or regarded as less a priority than paying other debts, acquiring material items, going on vacations, and so on. There has been increased attention in health care circles to this problem of compliance. Unless the patients' view of illness is thoughtfully considered and included in any treatment plan, there is a high risk of noncompliance [23]. Effective medical care mandates patient involvement.

A useful theoretical framework that liaison nurses can employ in diagnosing this aspect of the total consultation is knowledge of personality development [24]. The stages of the life cycle in their diagnostic application help liaison nurses to clarify and understand the nature of some of the psychological stresses associated with health and illness. "Conceptualizing the patient's emotional distress as an aspect of personality development is of educational value for the staff and enriches consultation-liaison work [25]." During the provision of psychiatric nursing consultation to consultees who are clinically responsible for pediatric patients and to those who are clinically responsible for adult patients, the authors have been consistently impressed with the following observation. A developmental approach to understanding illness behavior appears to be utilized by the physician and nursing staff with some degree of regularity with pediatric patients, but it appears to be minimally employed in clinical efforts to understand illness behavior in adult patients. The potential emotional trauma of separation for mother and child is common knowledge. The significance of separation for the adult patient receives less attention.

The chronological age of the patient can greatly influence the behavioral expectations placed on the patient. For example,

Donna, an 11-year-old girl with leukemia, was to begin chemotherapy treatment. She was told that she would lose all her beautiful, long, dark hair. Donna usually wore her hair in braids. The mother and primary nurse convinced Donna to allow them to cut her hair. Although tearfully consenting, the child insisted on keeping her braids tacked to the bulletin board in her hospital room. The consultees agreed that the presence of the braids made it very difficult to enter the room, let alone administer chemotherapy. Most children did not save their hair. Those who did usually sent it home with their mothers. The consultees were empathic to Donna's angry statements and bulletin board display. They regarded both as indications of the degree of the child's distress, as well as of her view that they were responsible for her hair loss. Because Donna was 11 years old, the nurses were able to tolerate her behavioral response to the ramifications of her leukemia.

When a 37-year-old woman with leukemia initially refused chemotherapy due to her fear of alopecia, the liaison nurse was requested to evaluate the patient. Although this patient also tearfully agreed to accept the chemotherapy and the suggested trimming of her hair, the narcissistic injury that she experienced failed to evoke empathy in her health care providers. The expectation was that a grown woman should have behaved more reasonably in considering her alternatives.

The broader the theoretical frame of reference from which liaison nurses can draw in understanding a specific response to illness and hospitalization, the greater the possibility of their accurately formulating the consultation. Teaching a developmental appreciation of patients' responses to illness, regardless of their age, not only improves the quality and effectiveness of the consultation, but also enhances the consultees' knowledge of normal and abnormal responses to usual life stresses. This information can then be applied to knowledge previously learned regarding the well documented stresses of illnesses and hospitalization.

Developmentally assessing patients can enhance understanding of their responses to illness and hospitalization. The intensity of emotional conflict experienced by patients can be altered by their health care team's ability to appreciate that most patients do strive to maintain social roles and age-appropriate behavior. A thorough developmental view of patients necessitates an assessment of their families. The patient/family's intellectual and emotional appraisal of the stress of illness and hospitalization is significant. Their fantasies and fears regarding the healing and hurting powers of physicians and nurses warrants consideration not only in the context of their individuality, but also in terms of the family system. Patients and family members have beliefs and expectations regarding each other's affective and behavioral responses to illness and hospitalization. The individual's cognitive appraisal of stress is also noted.

Zilbach has carefully described the stages and characteristic components of family development [26]. The individual personalities and character styles of all the family members, the manner in which roles are assumed and carried out, as well as the patterns of communication, interpersonal relationships, and coping strategies utilized by the family, are all significant. These factors indicate not only the developmental stage of the family, but also the degree of emotional and social health and maturity of each of its members. It is important to note the position of the identified patient within the family system. What is the patient's usual role within the family? How is he or she regarded? What is the quality of the interaction with other family members? What does it mean to the family, both as a system and as individuals, to have this particular member ill? What kind of burden, stress, or sense of relief is the family experiencing? The meaning of illness and subsequent illness behavior must be understood in the context of the patient's family system.

The delicate balance between independence (autonomy) and dependence (regression) is related to the individualized and family responses to illness and hospitalization. Again, the importance of a developmental assessment is apparent. Both patient and family participate in some way in defining this balance. At times, the family's definition is not in keeping with the patient's. The patient's appraisal of and reaction to the illness may differ from those of the family. At other times, patients and their families may agree. The balance between independence and dependence is also prescribed for patients by their health care providers. Presumably, the members of the health care team agree upon an individualized definition of independence and dependence for the patient, and this definition is clearly communicated to patients and their families in terms they can understand. The patient/family may or may not agree with this. When is it therapeutic to encourage patients to feed themselves? When is it therapeutic to have their nurses or family feed them? Can the age of patients, their medical condition, or their prognosis always serve as criteria for determining this balance? Food and feeding hold a variety of meanings for patients and their families. When combined with the meaning of and response to illness, defining the balance becomes very complex.

It is crucial, yet often difficult, for health care providers to understand and support patients' efforts to maintain psychological equilibrium. Three psychological stages of illness have been identified.

1. transition from health to illness,
2. period of illness, and
3. convalescence [27].

With illnesses requiring hospitalization, the stages of transition and convalescence may occur in or outside of the hospital. The period of illness becomes the focal point of the liaison nurse's work. Clearly, the most prominent psychological feature of the medically ill is regression.

The unspoken expectation by health care providers is patients' ability and willingness to regress to a "safe level," that is, to a dependent enough level to tolerate having things done to them yet independent enough to assume some responsibility for their illness. With the appropriate balance of dependence and independence, patients can curl up in the fetal position for a lumbar puncture and remain perfectly still. When the LP is completed, they can assume responsibility for lying perfectly flat for the requisite number of hours. In this example, adult patients are placed in a social environment reminiscent of childhood. The belief is that adults have completed the psychological tasks of that period. If not, they may be unable to tolerate the challenge to their autonomy. By contrast, pediatric patients are placed in a social environment in which their continued attempts to understand and to master the world, in order to become autonomous, are interrupted.

Patients respond to the childlike world of illness and react with behavior reminiscent of their own childhoods. The main features of such behavior are:

1. egocentricity,
2. constriction of interests,
3. emotional dependency, and
4. hypochrondriasis.

These behavioral features are psychologically necessary to "work through" the illness. They exemplify the combined effort of the psychological and the physiological. The environment of the hospital, which fosters helplessness, also forces patients to respond in some way to their illness. They then respond by directing all their psychological energy on the illness. By shutting out the outside world, their focus of attention is on themselves. To survive, patients commonly become egocentric. Ambulatory patients who request a cold drink from the nurse, who is obviously involved in the complex medical care of another patient, appear egocentric. Patients who relate a highly detailed account of their sleeping patterns or bowel movements are demonstrating a constriction of interests.

Illness work is like grief work. Physiologically the bodily processes are retarded during the grieving process [28], just as the psychological process is in a state of regression during the period of illness.

Superimposed on the three psychological stages of illness, of transition to illness, and of illness and convalescence are the psychological tasks of each stage. As previously stated, the perceptions, expectations, and assumptions of patients, together with their responses to illness, developmenal levels, personalities, and defensive style, all comprise the essence of the transition from health to illness. Upon admission to the hospital, patients most commonly accept that they are ill. In accordance with their aforementioned beliefs and styles, they enter the world of the sick, which mandates psychological reorganization and regression. They may be fed, changed, and told when to ambulate, as well as when to sleep and where to void. Patients to varying degrees behave like children. The "good" patient is similar to the "good" child. Spirited children may be seen as feisty patients.

The third stage of illness, convalescence, has similar characteristics to the developmental stage of adolescence. Most adults can gradually relinquish their dependency on the health care providers and regain the level of independence they held prior to their illness. The health care providers become the "parents" of the adolescent (patient), slowly relinquishing control, as appropriate, yet offering guidance and support. This phenomenon is evident by the process of ambulation following abdominal surgery. The patient is first assisted as necessary, then encouraged to walk alone with the nurse very close by, and finally set free to ambulate as desired. Patients may re-enact their struggle for independence by accelerating or retarding their return to full ambulation.

When the illness becomes chronic, this process is interrupted. The self-centeredness characteristic of serious illness interferes with the re-entry of the chronically ill person into the world of health. Illness groups serve, often temporarily, to reconnect the chronically ill to the world through contact with others in the same situation. At this juncture, the long-term effects of the narcissistic injury may be explored. Regression in the hospitalized chronically ill is a phenomenon influenced by a variety of factors, and it should be recognized as separate from regression in the acutely ill. Influenced by many variables is the continuum from acknowledging illness and seeking professional assistance, to accepting diagnosis and treatment, to engaging in grief work, convalescence, and/or adaptation to chronic ill health and terminality. Both the continuum and the variables that are particularly applicable to the individual patient/family deserve careful examination. To provide thoughtful, intelligent, humane care, nurses must understand the intangible concept of illness as an experience [29].

Nurses are sensitive to the illness experience of their patients/ families. Awareness of the components and of the possible impact of illness and hospitalization is somewhat automatic and reflected in nursing care. Many patients are able to maintain the emotional balance necessary to restore or stabilize their health. "A significant proportion of all normal medically ill patients manifest adverse psychological reactions, of varying severity, to their illness and hospitalization that may impede their treatment and recovery [30]." The clinical responsibility of the psychiatric liaison nurse is to assist the consultee in understanding the patient's experience when the balance is not maintained, and to intervene directly with the patient when clinically indicated.

section 3 assessment of the patient

The range of psychological adaptations to illness and to the experience of hospitalization, coupled with the physiological responses to illness, may at times exaggerate what might otherwise be a minor problem. This exaggeration may result in a disruption of the overall emotional balance previously described as needed to restore or stabilize health. Utilizing the assessment process, liaison nurses clarify the issues and create a foundation on which interventions can be planned. After "diagnosing the total consultation," they may decide that interviewing the patient is indicated. The psychiatric skill of liaison nurses in this direct intervention is based on the assumption of proficiency in interviewing techniques and clinical competence. The authors therefore wish to emphasize areas of particular importance that liaison nurses attend to in psychologically assessing the patient in a medical-surgical milieu. The assessment of the patient by liaison nurses will be described in this section and illustrated by a clinical case.

Liaison nurses utilize nursing diagnosis in the psychiatric assessment of the patient. Substantial efforts have gone into the development of standard nomenclature for nursing diagnosis. When the problem-solving process is used in a patient-centered approach to nursing practice, the explicit statement of the patient's presenting problem to be addressed by nursing constitutes the *nursing diagnosis* [31]. The First National Conference on the Classifications of Nursing Diagnosis was held in October 1973. The publication of *Nursing Diagnosis and Intervention in Nursing Practice* in 1978 is an example of the organized efforts in developing identifiable nursing problems, with subsequent plans to initiate independent nursing treatment. There is a need to psychologically assess the patient in a systematic manner. Based on this data collection, a nursing diagnosis can be made. Reynolds and Logsdon, recognizing the problem of assessing patients psychologically, developed a "no-nonsense, jargon-free form for an accurate mental assessment of the general patient [32]." The following factors are crucial and directly applicable to the practice of liaison nursing:

1. Patient problems are identified in nursing rather than in medical terms.
2. Patient problems are analyzed.
3. A nursing diagnosis is made.
4. Intervention is planned.
5. Evaluation occurs.

The process of nursing diagnosis can be illustrated by comparing a wound infection to a reactive depression to illness. In both instances, for treatment to be effective, intervention should be based on assessment and diagnosis. Some of the nursing tools for accurately diagnosing wound infection include the observation of increased pain, redness, swelling, exudate, and fever. Some of the nursing tools for accurately diagnosing a depressed affect include identifying the meaning of illness, possible precipitants, results of the mental status examination, general behavior, and involvement of the patients in their care. In each situation, there are often possible "sources of infection." But just as guessing at the pathogen for the wound infection would be clinically unsound, so is guessing at the "pathogen" for depression.

The Standards of Psychiatric-Mental Health Nursing Practice, published by the American Nurses Association, are reprinted in the

Appendix. These standards of practice, which include both rationale and assessment, are the building blocks for the psychiatric nurse. The clinical setting may change, but the basic assessment is simply adapted appropriately. It is not essentially changed. Factors that are especially germane to the general hospital setting are stressed and emphasized. The assumption is that there is familiarity and competence in the assessment of patients.

Numerous books and articles have been written about interviewing patients and about the psychiatric interview [33,34]. In the hospital, with its unique environment, the techniques are adapted, but the essential principles remain the same. The interview is influenced in the medical setting primarily by the constraints of the environment and by the medical status of the patient. The unique feature of this interview is interweaving the medical data with the psychological data. As previously discussed, the request for nursing consultation may be presented in a variety of ways. Listening and assessing are ongoing processes that begin when psychiatric nursing consultation is requested. When the problem is initially identified by the liaison nurse, the assessment continues even though the decision for direct intervention may be delayed. There is often contradictory data presented by the consultee, which becomes grist for the mill and which aids in the assessment when a direct intervention is required. A flexible approach is maintained regardless of whether there is direct or indirect intervention. Modes of intervention may change as the psychological status of the patient changes. After the interview by the liaison nurse, the treatment of choice may be an intervention by the primary nurse and indirect involvement by the liaison nurse. Yet liaison nurses continue to follow patients individually after their initial assessment only if it is clinically indicated.

In emergency situations or in instances of impulsive acting-out (wishing to leave the hospital, pulling out tubes), there is often limited time to obtain information. These situations warrant immediate intervention. They are no different from any medical emergency. The most important things are done first, while the patient's safety is maintained. When the patient is stabilized, the situation is further assessed. These situations are often confusing diagnostically due to the influence of medical illness. Even with this confusion, the liaison nurse's willingness to remain involved is helpful.

The format of a thorough assessment is presented to enhance the understanding of the consultation process. It is flexible, adaptive, and dynamic. The process of direct assessment of the patient begins with a careful perusal of the patient's chart, including medication, laboratory values, history, or indications of drug or alcohol abuse. Also included is a review of the old record to substantiate history. The interview of the patient can then begin with a data base, although prior information should be kept in some perspective to insure the objectivity of the interview. The medical background of the liaison nurse is an advantage in helping to integrate the relationship between the mind and body. A general understanding of the patient's medical status is a portion of the assessment. Is the patient having an anxiety attack or experiencing a hypertensive episode? Is the patient closing his or her eyes due to fear or pain?

Upon entering the patient's room, the liaison nurse may be initially distracted by the medical apparatus. However, an initial priority for patients is the identity of the liaison nurse. Although patients do not usually request mental health intervention, our experience has shown that patients suffering from emotional stress in the general hospital are more relieved than threatened by the liaison nurse. Usually sufficient is a forthright, simple introduction such as, "I am a nurse working with the staff who is especially interested in patients' adjustment or reaction to the hospital." The interaction may then be viewed as an extension of nursing care, which is more acceptable to patients. In this context the assessment develops. The responsibility to be vigilant in uncovering significant psychopathology is implicit. The following illustrates this:

> Mr. S, who was admitted for surgery, was mentioned casually to the liaison nurse as being cooperative and pleasant, but "weird." As the consultee further described the patient's actions, the behavior seemed less understandable. Within the context of defining the problem it was agreed that the liaison nurse would at least initially meet the patient and observe the "weird" behavior. It readily became apparent that the patient was probably schizophrenic, having recently broken treatment and discontinuing his medications.

The format of the psychiatric interview in the general hospital follows. Usually the interview would rarely exceed an hour and is most often about thirty minutes. Occasionally it can require only ten minutes and prove profitable. Although it is assumed that all aspects of the interview should be considered, those of particular importance in the general hospital are stressed.

Even though the environment may not be conducive to an interview, efforts are made to be seated within view of the patient and with as much privacy as possible. As liaison nurses assure the comfort of patients and themselves, they can utilize this time to visually absorb the environment. Are there many get-well cards? Is there reading material or a TV? Is there a telephone or any other evidence of socialization? As the liaison nurse becomes acquainted with the patient, he or she can explore the course of hospitalization. Attention is given to the patient's general physical appearance, evidence of pain or discomfort, and sense of illness and/or well-being. As issues are explored, the offers of help and the concern of the staff are communicated.

The following format is provided as a review of the content of a thorough interview. The interview is adapted by liaison nurses to the various clinical situations.

1. *Past hospital experience:* Stress may result from a lack of familiarity or an association with past hospital experiences. Examination and review of past hospital experience can provide data that is useful in understanding presently experienced stress. Liaison nurses carefully inquire about coping strategies that may have been successful in the past.

2. *Support system:* A brief family history, as well as a knowledge of social supports, aids in further understanding patients and their present experience in the hospital. The ongoing stresses in patients' lives warrant attention since they may be the basis for problem behavior in the hospital. Family support systems may need further exploration for which social workers' assessments are most valuable.

3. *Past psychiatric history:* Liaison nurses listen for and/or ask about psychiatric history. This past history is extremely important and may direct the course of the interview. Information is obtained regarding past psychiatric hospitalization and utilization of psychotropic medications. If the patient is in psychiatric treatment, this may be an appropriate time to explore the progress or status of that therapy.

4. *Alcohol and drug abuse:* The awareness of the prevalence of these abuses, coupled with their interaction medically and psychologically, makes their inclusion, when indicated, a vital part of the assessment.

5. *Observation of behavior, personality style, defense structure:* Throughout the interview, liaison nurses continually observe behavior, characteristics of personality style, defense mechanisms, and coping strategies. There is a delicate balance between intrusion and gathering information. In this setting there is rarely permission for interpretation, and it is usually nonproductive. Much of the for-

mulation is based on observation. However, behaviors are easier to observe in patients under stress because they are often exaggerated. Any changes in a characteristic personality style can be important clinical symptoms. While noting the degree of stress and its effect on behavior, it is wise to consider the possibility of pharmacological intervention.

6. *Mental status examination:* The mental status exam is a relatively formal organization of observations about patients' behavior, thoughts, and feelings. In this setting it is usually most helpful when it is interwoven with the data collecting of social, psychological, and medical history. The extent of the mental status examination is determined by the purpose of the evaluation and observations by the liaison nurse during the interview. Much of the information can be skillfully obtained during the interview without rigidly following the mental status examination format. Questions concerning patients' knowledge and views about their illness are an effective way, in the general hospital, to assess memory and function. There are certainly instances when a thorough and extensive mental status exam would be indicated, for example, in differential diagnosis or confusional states.

The professional responsibility of liaison nurses, like psychiatric nurses, is to provide the most appropriate psychiatric intervention for patients. If psychiatric illness becomes evident, appropriate treatment should be instituted. For example, if the patient shares with the liaison nurse suicidal thoughts that require intervention beyond the liaison nurse's scope of practice, some form of consultation with and/or referral to a psychiatrist would be indicated.

7. *The present hospitalization:* Liaison nurses explore with patients their views and perceptions of their illness and hospitalization. They gather information to assist in understanding the reason for and the timing of admission. Patients' degrees of understanding are influenced not only by their intellectual ability, combined with what they have been told, but also by their capacity to accept their illness. It is important to note what patients identify as physically and emotionally stressful and how they describe and experience it.

Throughout the entire interview, but especially in the context of this segment, the original consultation question and the problem(s) identified at that time are kept in mind. Comparing the patient's experience with the problem(s) precipitating the consultation is useful in "diagnosing the total consultation." At some point, usually at the end of the interview, an opportunity may be provided for the patient to ask questions.

8. Formulation: This is a descriptive summary of the clinical observations and data about the patient. Clinical thinking is shared with the consultee(s), and possible nursing diagnoses are proposed.

9. Impression: Although diagnostic labels are avoided, a brief statement is helpful. For example, "Probable regressive behavior associated with decreased stimulation and acute separation anxiety."

10. Recommendations or suggestions: These are clear, concrete clinical suggestions that are both sensible and realistic. Whenever possible, define the liaison nurse's ongoing involvement in the suggestions, including follow-up. Be specific and brief. Just as in the management of colitis, in which a conservative medical approach is utilized first, it is also more sensible to try the more conservative psychological treatment first. A liaison nurse's willingness to continue to observe, to evaluate, and to modify the treatment recommendations must be conveyed. Again, it is both alliance-building and professional to communicate to other health care providers that the essence of psychological assessment is clinical and not mystical.

11. Reassessment and follow-up: Re-evaluation is an essential and integral part of the assessment process. The complexities of the general hospital can, on occasion, present a "slice of life" that is atypical, bizarre, or, more importantly, an issue to be "left alone." Due to the type of crisis precipitated for patients who have been hospitalized, they may momentarily be "out of control." If such a case is assessed during the initial interview, it may prove more beneficial to have a very brief initial interview and to re-evaluate the patient in a few hours or the next day. Remembering that one goal of consultation is to achieve a reasonable hospitalization for the patient, liaison nurses tailor the interview and the intervention to the patient's needs, not to their own formats. The following example illustrates this point:

> Mrs. Sanford, admitted for abdominal surgery in the morning, was pacing the corridors, becoming increasingly agitated because her TV set had not arrived. Upon assessing the situation, the nursing staff felt that her behavior was inappropriate. The patient had numerous social problems for which she was being treated by a social worker on an out-patient basis. The nursing staff therefore viewed her as a risk for psychological decompensation. Although the patient was willing to discuss her feelings about surgery and her problems at home with the liaison nurse, Mrs. Sanford clearly knew that the distraction of TV was what she needed and wanted. After a brief interview by the liaison nurse and the arrival of a TV, Mrs. Sanford adapted, became very cooperative and pleasant, and had a successful hospitalization. This

outcome was evaluated several times by the liaison nurse during her hospitalization. Being respectful of Mrs. Sanford's point of view, while listening to and encouraging her participation in the solution to her problem, was a useful tool in planning effective intervention.

This is obviously an extreme, but true, example of a "slice of life" that did not require a "million-dollar workup" psychologically. Ten minutes and a TV set were needed and proved effective.

The goals of consultation and the medical status of the patient are the key factors to consider when planning interventions. Although the crisis of the patient's illness and hospitalization imposes limits, it also provides a unique opportunity for psychological intervention. As liaison nurses assess the illness experience of patients, they also assess the potential for psychological growth. The opportunities for psychological insight for patients during a crisis are an important source of professional satisfaction for liaison nurses. The consultee can also benefit in terms of professional development by learning about the psychological care of patients. This knowledge promotes an ability to understand, generalize, and apply psychological insight to the care of other patients.

The following case serves as an example of a liaison nurse's interventions.

> *Problem:* The primary nurse discussed with the liaison nurse her concerns and sadness about Mrs. Martin, a 32-year-old high school teacher who was scheduled for a mastectomy in the morning. Although the primary nurse felt that she had established a good relationship with Mrs. Martin, she also realized that Mrs. Martin's psychological needs at this time might be extensive. Furthermore, she thought that Mrs. Martin was "too good" about accepting her diagnosis. She had told Mrs. Martin about the liaison nurse, and Mrs. Martin seemed very interested in consultation, but wanted it after surgery.
>
> *Assessment:* The primary nurse, a competent, experienced, and sensitive clinician, had in the past expressed a special interest in mastectomy patients. Although the request for "help" from the primary nurse was vague, what was communicated was a need for support for both the nurse and the patient. The liaison nurse agreed to talk with the patient after surgery. The plan also included a discussion with the surgeon, to promote collaboration.
>
> Perusal of the chart revealed nothing further except that Mrs. Martin was the private patient of a surgeon who in the past had been either unpredictable or negative about agreement for psychological intervention. What was not discussed initially was the emotional involvement that the primary nurse was experiencing with this young,

charismatic woman. The first task seemed to be to demonstrate, as a role model, for the primary nurse, the appropriate clinical intervention even when one might feel overidentified.

The primary nurse discussed with the surgeon the plans for the liaison nurse's intervention. In addition, the liaison nurse discussed the case with the surgeon before interviewing the patient and prior to her discharge. The surgeon viewed the patient as stable, supported by a "solid" husband, and adjusting well to her cancer. He felt that the nursing staff was having the problem. The liaison nurse agreed that patients such as Mrs. Martin did create certain emotional entanglements for nurses, but Mrs. Martin also had communicated her need for more psychological assistance to the staff to help her to integrate this overwhelming experience. The liaison nurse believed that the surgery might precipitate an opportunity for crisis intervention.

Two days post-op, upon request of the primary nurse, the liaison nurse interviewed the patient. Mrs. Martin eagerly welcomed the liaison nurse. She was progressing well surgically, resuming normal physical activities, and tolerating her hospitalization well. Mrs. Martin had no previous significant hospitalizations and no past psychiatric, drug, or alcohol history. She was the oldest of three children, married for seven years to a writer, and childless by choice. As a high school music teacher, she was the wage earner. Ten years ago, her mother, with whom she had a close and warm relationship, died of cancer. Her father was living but chronically ill from multiple CVAs. After graduation from college, Mrs. Martin cared for her mother during her mother's last year of life. Mrs. Martin's mother, who had not sought medical help until her cancer was far advanced, urged Mrs. Martin to get on with her own life immediately after her demise and not to remain in their home town. Mrs. Martin complied with her mother's wishes, but she did not take time to grieve. For many years after, she had nightmares and then a delayed grief reaction five years after her mother's death, which resulted in a severe depression. Her husband was her support, and she did not seek professional assistance at that time.

Mrs. Martin, a bright, trim, and pleasant-looking woman, had a magnetic charm that probably contributed to her strong support system of family and friends. She was articulate, socially active, and very perceptive. Her charisma was clearly evident on the ward. As an active woman she used her activity to ward off anxiety. She described this by revealing, "When I get upset I might paint a room in one night." In the hospital her speech was pressured, and she seemed somewhat hypomanic. However, with all her verbosity she clearly avoided discussion of her thoughts or feelings except superficially. She consistently used projection, "I'm worried about my students and their reaction, my sister, my husband, and so on."

Mrs. Martin bombarded the liaison nurse with questions that many post-mastectomy patients may consider over time. These questions included issues such as body image, sexuality, informing people, exercise, returning to work, contacting Reach to Recovery, Inc., and similar inquiries.

Formulation: An intelligent, active, well-supported, young, married woman, Mrs. Martin is overwhelmed by a malignant illness —is struggling for adequate coping strategies. Viewing herself as strong and usually in control, she is experiencing difficulty obtaining the "help" she really needs. Her past history of delay in grieving her mother's death is of concern.

Impression: Difficulty grieving loss of breast. Potential for delayed grief reaction.

Intervention:

1. Follow-up mental health counseling arranged through primary physician as discussed with patient.
2. Nursing staff's continued involvement and provision of concrete information was encouraged to help physical adjustment.
3. Close follow-up by the surgeon, as planned, crucial to patient's adjustment. She views him as very supportive.
4. Daily follow-up by liaison nurse during hospitalization.

Reassessment—follow-up: Mrs. Martin, as she became more physically active, was able gradually to reassume her sense of control. After discussion with the liaison nurse, Mrs. Martin arranged a meeting with her high school principal and decided how to tell the students about her surgery and agreed upon a realistic length of time for her absence from work. She had very much wanted to return to work immediately and not tell anyone.

Not wanting to relive the tortures following her mother's death, she was very accepting of professional help both for herself and her husband. Just prior to discharge, she told the liaison nurse that she had not been revealing her true feelings to anyone.

The follow-up in this case involved both the nurses and the surgeon. An important consultation goal in working with the primary nurse and the entire nursing staff was to promote their professional development. They knew Mrs. Martin needed something more but experienced difficulty in adequately assessing the patient. Understanding that her appealing character style served as a defense against fear and anxiety was made apparent. Through discussions in the nurses' group, the sadness and "involvement" of the staff with Mrs. Martin were shared and subsequently channeled into helpful interventions. Mrs. Martin clearly needed psychiatric intervention.

Discussion with the surgeon was focused on the impact of physical rehabilitation on Mrs. Martin's emotional adjustment. The liaison nurse discussed the patient's quest for factual information as an added support to her acceptance. For example, her concerns about her sexual functioning were not only premature, but they also constituted an attempt to keep the staff from her feelings of grief. The liaison nurse told the surgeon about Mrs. Martin's questions so that in his continued contact he could follow them up and provide the information she needed.

This case, where the issues are rather clear, can be used time and again to demonstrate the interplay between illness and emotion. It illustrates how a brief intervention by a psychiatric liaison nurse can make a significant difference in the course of adaptation for the patient. Regardless of the course of action by the patient after discharge, there are significant ramifications of this case:

1. The patient was afforded an opportunity to learn about ways of looking at and dealing with grief.
2. The consultees were afforded an opportunity to learn about such behavior precipitated by illness.
3. The climate for future consultations was further enhanced since some of the goals of consultation were met.

section 4 medical psychology as a basis for intervention

Interventions with patients are based on the synthesis of multiple factors. The perceptions, assumptions, and expectations of staff and patient/family are often very different. Although this interplay is seemingly obvious and simplistic, it is understandable that health care providers may underestimate or forget about it. In reality, it is fairly easy to recognize the existence of problems, yet more complicated to develop an appropriate intervention. The patients' experience and views of hospitalization have been discussed previously. Certainly one aspect of intervention is related to these factors. For many patients, interventions are adequately based on assessments and a "diagnosis of the total consultation." Special attention to patients' experience with hospitalization is emphasized. Nevertheless, sometimes this is not sufficient. Because patients may demonstrate behavior anywhere along the psychological continuum, from adaptation to maladaptation, an appreciation of personality and defensive styles is necessary for therapeutic intervention.

The psychological continuum from adaptation to maladaptation can be illustrated by the extremely angry hostile woman signing out against medical advice, by the cooperative, interested, involved patient, or by the quiet withdrawn man who is dutiful and submissive. Along the continuum, the following types are also recognized:

- the dutiful but questioning patient,
- the pleasant, helpful patient who is sensitive to the nurses' plight,
- the popular, socially adept patient,
- the seductive, provocative patient,
- the argumentative but cooperative patient,
- the inconsistently compliant patient, and
- the nontrusting, abusive patient.

Uncooperative patients are easily identified by the staff and often brought to the attention of the liaison nurse.

> A 48-year-old gentleman was described by the nursing staff as "demanding and manipulative." His behavior seemed to escalate as the day progressed, with late evening and nighttime being the most difficult. The patient would constantly ring for the nurse, requesting that she rearrange his bedside table, pour water for him, change the TV station, and perform other chores. The patient had been admitted for an emergency appendectomy and was three days post-op. Although progressing medically, he refused to ambulate, complained of a variety of aches and pains, and was requesting to be fed. The patient's behavior was very much like that of a small child, frightened to be alone, frightened of the dark, and wanting mothering. This kind of behavior, demonstrated by an adult, was difficult for the staff to accept. Did this illness and resulting separation hold unrecognized significance for this patient? What about his perceptions, assumptions, and expectations?

The patient who is compliant appears cooperative while experiencing feelings that may be similar and/or as intense as those of the uncooperative patient.

Liaison nurses are rarely consulted regarding cooperative patients unless the patients carry their behavior to an extreme. Although the nursing staff is aware of such patients, they do not pose a nursing care management problem. In the context of teaching concepts of psychological care, this patient may be identified. Liaison nurses may suggest or offer to interview "nonproblem" patients on the ward to illustrate their less obvious response to illness. It is helpful for some of the consultees to attend the interview.

Mrs. Nesson, a 35-year-old woman, recovering from her second kidney transplant, was described by the nurses as "very cooperative and quiet." During the interview, the patient's private distress and anxiety were illustrated. Although compliant, Mrs. Nesson was terrified about the status of her new kidney. She was fearful of moving, lest she jeopardize it. Mrs. Nesson was convinced that the first kidney transplant had failed because she was too mobile. Mrs. Nesson felt trapped between her beliefs and the mandate from her doctor and nurse that she ambulate.

As defined by Webster, *psychology* is the science of mind and behavior [35]. The authors define *medical psychology* as the interaction of illness, mind, and behavior. It is a valuable tool when formulating the therapeutic intervention. If a patient has a psychiatric diagnosis, it may be viewed separately from a formulation. Patients may have problems with dependency/independency, as hospitalized patients, in addition to manic-depressive illness. Using medical psychology, the issue of dependency/independency for individual patients is more fully understood, and, based on this understanding, a therapeutic intervention is planned.

Nurses, in their clinical practice, are constantly assessing patients. Being familiar with the possible ways patients may feel about illness, they listen to the process, observe the patients, and intervene accordingly. Nurses recognize anxiety demonstrated in frequent questions, joking, increased or decreased physical activity, intellectualization, hostility, and in other ways. When the usual interventions prove unsuccessful, this lack of response may be a result of the patient's unresolved conflict, of the interaction with an individual staff member, or of an inadequate or inaccurate assessment of the process. This is frequently the point at which the liaison nurse is consulted.

With this in mind, it may now be necessary for interventions to progress from the more simple to the more complex. A multifaceted intervention is required based on both the "diagnosis of the total consultation" and a knowledge of medical psychology. A therapeutic intervention is a clinical approach resulting from a recognition of patients' personality styles, defensive structures, and psychological statuses as integral parts of their adaptation to stress. It is not enough to assess patients' problems and make formulations. The intervention or plan of approach also incorporates their views. "The data [interviews] suggests that the behavior of patients is, at least in part, a function of their preconceptions of and reactions to hospital reality and not solely a function of 'emotional disturbances' [36]."

Kahana and Bibring describe variations of "personality types," which aid in conceptualizing character styles. "The dependent, over-demanding patient; the orderly, controlled patient; the dramatizing patient" are but a few of the personality categories and types described in the literature [37]. Recognizing personality styles is a useful adjunct to developing appropriate interconnections. Not every patient fits a category exactly. Nevertheless, consideration of the meaning of physical illness in terms of the individual's basic needs, the nature of the perceived threat, the ego defenses mobilized, and the quality of the behavior that is intensified as a result of stress is paramount.

The identification of defense mechanisms as used by the patient and the consultee is helpful in understanding the quality of their individualized responses to each other and to the illness experience. Defense mechanisms are unconscious psychic processes adopted by the ego in response to a preconceived threat or danger. Regardless of whether the threat or danger is real or imagined, it is regarded by the ego as potentially intolerable. Defense mechanisms are employed by the ego as a method by which to cope with the impending threat. These mental operations, either adaptive or maladaptive, are mobilized spontaneously in response to the perceived threat or danger. The work of George Vaillant regarding the ego mechanisms of defense is particularly helpful in gaining a broader understanding of specific patient/family and consultee behaviors [38].

The cognitive and emotional significance of the body part or area in which the illness is focused greatly influences illness behavior and coping styles. Conflicting issues, sources of gratification, and narcissism are frequently associated with certain parts of the body [39].

Recognizing patterns and understanding them aids in developing interventions based on the medical psychology of the patient. Knowledge of medical psychology, as stated, is a precursor to therapeutic intervention. As liaison nurses attempt to understand patients' presenting behavior, they also attempt to formulate interventions that improve patients' psychological adaption to help meet the ultimate goal of adequate medical care.

Mr. Davis, a middle-aged man who had suffered a myocardial infarction three days prior, was found at the foot of his bed repeatedly lifting the bed off the floor. This patient, who was trying to convince himself of his masculinity and potency, was denying his illness. After assessing the dynamics involved, the liaison nurse as a therapeutic intervention suggested to Mr. Davis that *any* man could defy medical orders but a really "tough guy" would be able to follow the proposed regimen. In fact, it was further suggested that Mr. Davis might not be "tough enough" to do the most difficult job of all, which was staying in bed. Mr. Davis rose to the challenge and, now viewing himself as strong, was able to accept the temporary limitations of bed rest.

Another illustration of therapeutic intervention, based on an understanding of the medical psychology of the patient, is with the unmotivated patient.

> Miss O'Brion, a 52-year-old single, compliant, and very quiet woman, was admitted to the hospital with an abscess of the perineum that she had neglected medically. Miss O'Brion said she let it "go too far." Her guilt, passivity, and lack of self-esteem made her unresponsive to attempts by the staff at encouraging her cooperation. The liaison nurse, after her assessment, recommended that the staff ask Miss O'Brion to cooperate for their sake—that is, not to make it hard for the nurses to do their job—or they would be criticized if treatments were not completed. Miss O'Brion responded and improved because it was easier for her to do for others (help the nurses) rather than for herself.

Liaison nurses recognize, in the hospital setting, patients' ambivalence just as ambivalence is recognized in psychotherapy. It is both appropriate and effective to play to the positive side of the ambivalence to effect a therapeutic intervention. Sometimes a paradoxical approach is used.

> Mrs. Stone, admitted for congestive heart failure, was presented to the liaison nurse because she seemed so discouraged about her life situation. She felt she was ill and abandoned by her family and friends. Mrs. Stone's complaints were endless, and any attempts to "encourage" her were met with an increase of complaints. Joining the patient, that is, agreeing with her that her situation is indeed the most horrible, allowed her to see the other side. The response from Mrs. Stone was that it really wasn't *that* bad. This approach was a therapeutic intervention.

These types of interventions are certainly not curative, but they are helpful and extremely effective in the medical setting.

In Section 3, the assessment process was illustrated with the case example of Mrs. Martin, a 32-year-old teacher who had a mastectomy. The hospital experience was less significant for her. Mrs. Martin would closely fit Kahana and Bibring's classification of the dramatizing, emotionally involved, captivating (hysterical) personality.

Clearly, Mrs. Martin was able to involve staff by her "charisma." She repeatedly expressed concerns about her body image and her felt need to remain attractive and active. Similar to Kahana and Bibring's description of the meaning of illness for the dramatizing, emotionally involved kind of person, Mrs. Martin felt defective, unattractive, and unsuccessful. She felt threatened by her changed body image, and she compensated by special attention to her appearance and dress. Mrs. Martin's struggle against her anxiety was demonstrated by increased efforts to gain admiration, and by being "too good" about accepting her diagnosis. Her efforts to gain control were illustrated by her bombarding the liaison nurse with questions.

The work of the liaison nurse in this case is twofold: first, to assist Mrs. Martin in thinking about and identifying that which would be helpful to her in adjusting to her stress, both physically and emotionally; second, to assist the nursing staff in recognizing that understanding, ventilation, support, and empathy are vital aspects of basic nursing care. However, therapeutic intervention has the potential of carrying that process even further. When Mrs. Martin sought reassurance about the attractiveness of her new bathrobe, instead of only commenting positively on the color or style, recognition of her need to be attractive was also important. Verbalizing such recognition would have been appropriate and therapeutic for Mrs. Martin.

What about Mrs. Martin's courage? Was it a cover-up for her anxiety? Or was she so frightened that she channeled her energies into being "attractive" to the staff? Why did she worry about her students' reaction rather than her own? The comment about painting a room when she was upset would correlate with her desire to return to work two weeks post-operative. For Mrs. Martin, activity served to contain her anxiety.

The identification and/or staff's countertransference reaction to the patient is intimately involved with the therapeutic intervention. It is useful for nurses to be increasingly cognizant of the quality and intensity of their identification with the patient. As illustrated in the case of Mrs. Martin, it is not only negative, angry, hostile reactions that can interfere with a therapeutic intervention.

What about patients who feel superior, entitled, and powerful? They may demand attention from the head nurse, humiliate the student nurses, and request special privileges. What is certain is that they will most likely antagonize the staff. Probably their characteristic narcissistic behavior has become intensified under the threat or reality of illness. "But this very 'entitlement,' repulsive as it may be, is resorted to by the patient in an effort to preserve the integrity of the self in a world that seems hostile or during an illness that seems terrifying [40]." The recognition by staff that patients may be very frightened is the beginning of wisdom. The staff's getting angry, annoyed, withholding, or threatening is the beginning of disaster. Therapeutic intervention may progress along a continuum from simply an awareness on the part of staff to direct psychiatric intervention. The most clinically sound approach is to begin with the least intrusive intervention, to observe, to reassess, and to modify interventions as necessary. The importance of reassessment cannot be overemphasized.

Therapeutic intervention is also influenced by the medical reality of the patient. Decompensation of the psychological status of hospitalized patients in some instances must be tolerated by professionals, just as decompensation of the physical status is endured. The resulting stress for both is impressive. Regardless of the etiology of the decompensation, interventions remain reasonable, appropriate, and directly related to the clinical assessment of the patient.

The psychological status of patients may be determined and/or greatly influenced by their physiological status. In these instances, nurses are encouraged to be tolerant and supportive, while recognizing that a purely therapeutic intervention may be limited. With an electrolyte imbalance and an elevated BUN, a patient's mental status and behavior is better managed with tolerance and with appropriate medical management, as opposed to therapeutic intervention as previously defined. The visibility and ongoing support of the liaison nurse in these frustrating nursing management problems becomes obvious.

As nurses, each expectation that we have for our patients and ourselves must be recognized, understood, and evaluated. The concept of reassurance as intervention serves as an illustration. Gregg, through examples of nurses' conversations with patients, suggested that "patients feel reassured when they are helped to use their own skills to work with problems that seem overwhelming at the outset [41]." If patients are valued as individuals and listened to, they are more likely to feel reassured. In the hospital situation, the physical presence of family members may be reassuring. Accurate, clear information may reassure them. For others the competence of the health care team members may be sufficiently reassuring.

Nurses believe that patients are probably frightened, anxious, and unhappy about their illness. But is that always true? Is it the same for everyone? What about the woman who has structured her family around herself in the sick role? Or the man who is lonely living alone and who enjoys the excitement and attention in the hospital? Before nurses reassure patients, they must accurately assess them and plan a therapeutic intervention appropriate for the patient. It is easy to fall prey to offering patients reassurance while failing to recognize its hollowness.

> Mr. Angelo, a 65-year-old retired Italian man, was successfully recovering from abdominal surgery, yet he refused to get out of bed. The physicians and nurses repeatedly reassured him and encouraged him to increase his activities. His family was supportive, very attentive, and reassuring. However, he always had an excuse for not complying with the prescribed activity schedule. The more he was reassured, the more adamant he became that he was not well enough to move out of bed. The nursing staff became frustrated and annoyed. The family became frightened. The intern persisted in his attempts at reassuring the patient by guaranteeing his return to good health. The liaison nurse was consulted. As she gathered data it was unclear what was interfering with Mr. Angelo's convalescence. Even after talking with many health care providers and interviewing Mr. Angelo, his problem remained a mystery. A second interview revealed that Mr. Angelo's brother had died of a pulmonary embolus secondary to abdominal surgery. However, it was the circumstances that were most germane to Mr. Angelo's present problem. Mr. Angelo's brother had been given a "clean bill of health" by his physician and was encouraged to resume his normal activities and return to work. Mr. Angelo's brother did exactly what his doctor said and "dropped dead" the next day at work. Mr. Angelo had decided for himself that his only chance for survival was to do as little as possible. It became clear that the staff's reassurance was not reassuring at all, but more frightening. Recognizing this and acknowledging it with the patient proved supportive. Using medical psychology—that is, being respectful of the patient's fear and his need to be in control—the intervention was formulated. Mr. Angelo was able to establish an ambulation plan that was acceptable to him and to the staff. The liaison nurse saw the patient daily in attempts to aid him in working through his fear.

As liaison nurses consider therapeutic intervention with hospitalized patients, appreciation of patients' views of their illness and their experience in the hospital is paramount. Appreciation of the medical psychology of patients, an awareness of identification and transference/countertransference issues, and a thorough assessment result in therapeutic intervention. This approach is operationalized on the hospital ward with an individualized nursing care plan, case conferences as needed, and consultation with the psychiatric liaison nurse.

references

1. Florence Nightingale, *Notes on Nursing: What It Is and What It Is Not* (New York: D. Appleton & Co., 1858/1932), pp. 61–62. Reprinted with permission.
2. R. Elms and D. Diers, "The Patient Comes to the Hospital," *Nursing Forum* 2 (1963): 89.
3. Marjorie Kellogg, *Tell Me That You Love Me, Junie Moon* (New York: Popular Library, 1968), p. 61.
4. F. W. Peabody, "The Care of the Patient," *Journal of the American Medical Association* 88:887 (1927): 6–7.
5. Melvin Seeman, "The Hospital," *The Journal of Nursing Education* (November 1971): 24.
6. Lisa Robinson, *Liaison Nursing Psychological Approach to Patient Care* (Philadelphia: F. A. Davis Company, 1974), pp. 31–33.
7. R. K. Zind, "Deterrents to Crisis Intervention in the Hospital Unit," *The Nursing Clinics of North America* 9:1 (March 1974): 30.
8. Carol D. Taylor, "The Hospital Patient's Social Dilemma," *American Journal of Nursing* 65:10 (October 1965): 96.
9. Benita Hall, "Human Relations in the Hospital Setting," *Nursing Outlook* 16:3 (March 1968): 43.
10. T. P. Hackett and N. H. Cassem, eds., *Massachusetts General Hospital Handbook of General Hospital Psychiatry* (St. Louis: The C. V. Mosby Company, 1978).
11. Ralph Kahana and Grete Bibring, "Personality Types in Medical Management," in *Psychiatry and Medical Practice in a General Hospital*, edited by N. E. Zinberg (New York: International Universities Press, Inc., 1964), pp. 108–123.
12. Robert L. Spitzer, *Diagnostic and Statistical Manual of Mental Disorders*, 3rd ed. (New York: American Psychiatric Association, 1980).
13. Joyce Travelbee, *Interpersonal Aspects of Nursing*, 2nd ed. (Philadelphia: F. A. Davis Co., 1971), pp. 59–60.
14. S. V. Kasl and S. Cobb, "Health Behavior, Illness Behavior, and Sick Role Behavior," *Archives of Environmental Health* 12 (February 1966): 531.
15. Joyce Travelbee, *Interpersonal Aspects of Nursing*, 2nd ed. (Philadelphia: F. A. Davis Co., 1971), pp. 59–60. Reprinted with permission.
16. H. Peplau, "Professional Closeness," *Nursing Forum* 8:4 (1969): 345.
17. Zind, p. 29.
18. Z. J. Lipowski, "Psychosocial Aspects of Disease," *Annals of Internal Medicine* 71:6 (December 1969): 1200.
19. I. K. Zola, "Culture and Symptoms—An Analysis of Patients' Presenting Complaints," *American Sociological Review* 31 (1966): 615–630.
20. David Mechanic, "Social Psychologic Factors Affecting the Presentation of Bodily Complaints," *New England Journal of Medicine* 286:21 (May 25, 1977): 1135.
21. Z. J. Lipowski, "Physical Illness, the Individual and the Coping Process," *International Journal of Psychiatry in Medicine* 1:2 (April 1970): 98.

22. Ana-Maria Rizzuto, "The Patient as a Hero," unpublished paper presented at the Tufts Psychiatry Symposium (1978). Reprinted with permission.

23. R. F. Gillum and A. J. Barsky, "Diagnosis and Management of Patient Non-Compliance," *Journal of the American Medical Association* 228:12 (June 1974): 1563–1567.

24. E. H. Erikson, *Childhood and Society* (New York: W. W. Norton & Co., Inc., 1963).

25. J. J. Schwab and W. A. Bradnan, "Life Phases in Health and Illness," *Psychiatric Clinics of North America* 2:2 (August 1979): 278–279.

26. J. Zilbach, "Family Development," in *Modern Psychoanalysis*, edited by Judd Mason (New York: Basic Books, Inc., Publisher, 1968), pp. 355–386.

27. Henry D. Lederer, "How the Sick View Their World," in *Social Interaction and Patient Care*, edited by J. K. Skipper and R. C. Leonard (Philadelphia: J. B. Lippincott Company, 1965), p. 162.

28. Erich Lindeman, "Symptomatology and Management of Acute Grief," *American Journal of Psychiatry* 101 (1944): 141–148.

29. Travelbee, p. 85.

30. J. J. Strain and S. Grossman, *Psychological Care of the Medically Ill: A Primer in Liaison Psychiatry* (New York: Appleton-Century-Crofts, 1975), p. 23.

31. Kristie Gebbie and Mary Ann Levin, "Classifying Nursing Diagnoses," *American Journal of Nursing* 74:2 (1974): 250–253.

32. J. Reynolds and J. Logsdon, "Assessing Your Patients' Mental Status," *Nursing '79* 9:8 (August 1979): 26.

33. Roger MacKinnon and Robert Michels, *The Psychiatric Interview in Clinical Practice* (Philadelphia: W. B. Saunders, 1971).

34. Brian Bird, *Talking with Patients* (Philadelphia: J. B. Lippincott Company, 1973).

35. *Webster's New Collegiate Dictionary* (Springfield, Ill.: G. & C. Merriam Co., 1981), p. 924. Reprinted with permission.

36. Daisy Tagliacozzo, "The Nurse from the Patient's Point of View," in *Social Interaction and Patient Care*, edited by J. K. Skipper and R. C. Leonard (Philadelphia: J. B. Lippincott Company, 1963).

37. Kahana and Bibring, pp. 108–123.

38. G. E. Vaillant, "Theoretical Hierarchy of Adaptive Ego Mechanisms," *Archives of General Psychiatry* 24 (February 1971): 107–118.

39. Lipowski, p. 94.

40. James E. Groves, "Taking Care of the Hateful Patient," *New England Journal of Medicine* (April 20, 1978): 885.

41. Dorothy Gregg, "Reassurance," *American Journal of Nursing* 55:2 (1955): 171–174.

bibliography

books

ALEXANDER, FRANZ. *Psychosomatic Medicine: Its Principles and Applications.* New York: W. W. Norton & Co., Inc., 1950.

BECK, AARON T. *Depression: Clinical, Experimental and Theoretical Aspects*. New York: Harper & Row, Publishers, Inc., 1967.

BELAND, IRENE and PASSOS, JOYCE. *Clinical Nursing Pathophysiological and Psychosocial Approaches*. New York: Macmillan, Inc., 1975.

BIBRING, GRETE and KAHANA, RALPH. *Lectures in Medical Psychology*. New York: International Universities Press, Inc., 1968.

BROWN, M. M. and FOWLER, R. *Psychodynamic Nursing: A Biosocial Orientation*. 2nd ed. Philadelphia: W. B. Saunders Co., 1961.

GARFIELD, C. A., ed. *Stress and Survival: The Emotional Realities of Life-Threatening Illness*. St. Louis: The C. V. Mosby Co., 1979.

HOLLINGSWORTH, C. E. and PASNAU, R. O. *The Family in Mourning: A Guide for Health Professionals*. New York: Grune & Stratton, Inc., 1977.

HOLMES, M. J. and WERNER, J. A. *Psychiatric Nursing in a Therapeutic Community*. New York: Macmillan, Inc., 1966.

JACO, E. G., ed. *Patients, Physicians and Illness*. Glencoe, Ill.: The Free Press, 1958.

JANIS, I. L. *Psychological Stress*. New York: John Wiley & Sons, Inc., 1958.

LAMBERT, V. A. and LAMBERT, C. E. *The Impact of Physical Illness and Related Mental Health Concepts*. Englewood Cliffs, N.J.: Prentice-Hall, 1979.

LAZARUS, R. S. *Psychological Stress and the Coping Process*. New York: McGraw-Hill Book Co., 1966.

LEIGH, H. and REISER, M. *The Patient: Biological, Psychological, and Social Dimensions of Medical Practice*. New York: Plenum Medical Book Co., 1980.

MILLON, T., ed. *Medical Behavioral Science*. Philadelphia: W. B. Saunders Co., 1975.

MOOS, R. H. *Coping with Physical Illness*. New York: Plenum Medical Book Co., 1977.

SCHWAB, J. J. *Handbook of Psychiatric Consultation*. New York: Appleton-Century-Crofts, 1968.

SIMONS, R. C. and PARDES, H., eds. *Understanding Human Behavior in Health and Illness*. Baltimore: Williams and Wilkins, 1977.

SKIPPER, J. K. and LEONARD, R. C. *Social Interaction and Patient Care*. Philadelphia: J. B. Lippincott Company, 1965.

WERNER-BELAND, JEAN. *Grief Responses to Long-Term Illness and Disability*. Reston, Va.: Reston Publishing Co., 1980.

WOLFF, H. G. *Stress and Disease*. Springfield, Ill.: Charles C. Thomas, Publisher, 1953.

ZINBERG, NORMAN, ed. *Psychiatry and Medical Practice in a General Hospital*. New York: International Universities Press, Inc., 1964.

articles

ABDELLAH, F. and LEVINE, E. "What Patients Say About Their Nursing Care," *Hospitals* 23:1 (1957): 44–48.

BADONAILLE, M. L. "Human Relations in the Hospital Setting: A Critical Analysis," *International Nursing Review* 27:5:233 (September–October 1980): 142–143.

BARKER, R. G. et al. "Adjustment to Physical Handicap and Illness," New York: Social Sciences Research Council, 1953, in *Social Interaction and Patient Care*, edited by J. K. Skipper and R. C. Leonard. Philadelphia: J. B. Lippincott Company, 1965.

BERNSTEIN, STEPHEN. "Psychotherapy Consultation in an Inpatient Setting," *Hospital and Community Psychiatry* 31:12 (December 1980): 829–834.

BIBRING, G. L. "Psychiatry and Medical Practice in a General Hospital," *New England Journal of Medicine* 254:366–372 (February 23, 1956): 75–87.

BURGESS, A. and LAZARE, A. "Nursing Management of Feelings, Thoughts and Behavior," *Journal of Psychiatric Nursing and Mental Health Services* (November–December 1972): 7–11.

CASSELL, E. J. "Reactions to Physical Illness and Hospitalization," in *Psychiatry in General Health Practice*, edited by G. Usdin and J. Lewis. New York: McGraw-Hill Book Co., 1979, pp. 103–130.

DROSSMAN, D. A. "The Problem Patient Evaluation and Care of Medical Patients with Psychosocial Disturbances," *Annals of Internal Medicine* 88:3 (March 1978): 366–372.

EISENBERG, LEON. "What Makes Persons 'Patients' and Patients 'Well?'" *American Journal of Medicine* 69 (August 1980): 277–286.

ELLIOTT, S. M. "Denial as an Effective Mechanism to Allay Anxiety Following a Stressful Event," *Journal of Psychiatric Nursing and Mental Health Services* (October 1980): 11–15.

ENGEL, GEORGE. "A Life Setting Conducive to Illness: The Giving-Up/Given-Up Complex," *Annals of Internal Medicine* 69 (1968): 193–200.

———. "Psychogenic Pain and the Pain-Prone Patient," *American Journal of Medicine* (June 1959): 899–917.

———. "The Clinical Application of the Biopsychosocial Model," *American Journal of Psychiatry* 137:5 (May 1980): 535–543.

GROVES, J. E. "Management of the Borderline Patient on a Medical or Surgical Ward: The Psychiatric Consultant's Role," *International Journal of Psychiatry in Medicine* 6:3 (1975): 337–348.

JOHNSON, MARGIE. "Self-Disclosure and Anxiety in Nurses and Patients," *Issues in Mental Health Nursing* 2:1 (1979): 42–56.

KARASU, T. "Psychotherapy of the Medically Ill," *American Journal of Medicine* 136:1 (January 1979): 1–11.

KULP, C. and LEWIS, A. "An Experiential Analysis of the Concept of Separation, A Discussion of the Relational Implications to the Maternal-Child Unit," unpublished clinical thesis, Boston University (1972).

LAWRENCE, S. A. and LAWRENCE, R. M. "A Model of Adaptation to the Stress of Chronic Illness," *Nursing Forum* 28:1 (1979): 33–42.

LAZARUS, R. S. "Psychological Stress and Coping in Adaptation and Illness," *International Journal of Psychiatry in Medicine* 5 (1974): 321–333.

LEHMANN, H. E. "The Emotional Basis of Illness," *Diseases of the Nervous System* 28:7 (July 1967): 12–19.

MULLINS, A. C. and BARSTOW, R. E. "Care for the Caretakers," *American Journal of Nursing* (August 1979): 1425–1427.

NEWLIN, N. J. and WELLISCH, D. K. "The Oncology Nurse: Life on an Emotional Roller Coaster," *Cancer Nursing* 1:6 (December 1978): 447–449.

READING, A. "Illness and Disease," *Medical Clinics of North America* 61:4 (July 1977): 703–710.

REICH, P. and KELLY, N. J. "Suicide Attempts by Hospitalized Medical and Surgical Patients," *New England Journal of Medicine* 294:6 (February 5, 1976): 298–301.

ROBINSON, L. "A Therapeutic Paradox—To Support Intimacy and Regression or Privacy and Autonomy," *Journal of Psychiatric Nursing and Mental Health Services* (October 1979): 14–23.

SAMORA, J.; SAUNDERS, L.; and LARSON, R. F. "Medical Vocabulary Knowledge among Hospitalized Patients," *Journal of Health and Human Behavior* 2 (Summer 1961): 83–92.

SCHMALE, A. H. "Reactions to Illness: Convalescence and Grieving," *Psychiatric Clinics of North America* 2:2 (August 1979): 321–330.

SKIPPER, J. K.; MAUKSCH, H. O.; and TAGLIACOZZO, D. "Some Barriers to Communication Between Patients and Hospital Functionaries," *Nursing Forum* 2:1 (1963): 15–22.

STARKMAN, M. N. and YOUNGS, D. D. "Psychiatric Consultation with Patients Who Refuse Medical Care," *International Journal of Psychiatry in Medicine* 5:2 (1974): 115–123.

STEWARD, M. A.; McWHINNEY, I. R.; and BUCK, C. W. "How Illness Presents: A Study of Patient Behavior," *Journal of Family Practice* 2:6 (1975): 411–414.

STRAIN, J. J. "The Medical Setting: Is It Beyond the Psychiatrist?" *American Journal of Psychiatry* (March 1977): 253–256.

TAGLIACOZZO, D. M. and IRMA, K. "Knowledge of Illness as a Predictor of Patient Behavior," *Journal of Chronic Diseases* 22 (1970): 765–775.

VAILLANT, G. E.; SHAPIRO, L. N.; and SCHMITT, P. P. "Psychological Motives for Medical Hospitalization," *Journal of the American Medical Association* 214:9 (November 30, 1970): 1661–1665.

VERWOERDT, A. "Psychopathological Responses to the Stress of Physical Illness," *Advances in Psychosomatic Medicine* 8 (1972): 119–141.

VOLICER, B. J. "Patients' Perceptions of Stressful Events Associated with Hospitalization," *Nursing Research* 23:3 (May–June 1974): 235–238.

WESSON, A. "Hospital Ideology and Communication between Ward Personnel," in *Medical Care Readings in the Sociology of Medical Institutions*, edited by W. R. Scott and E. H. Volkard. New York: John Wiley & Sons, Inc., 1966, pp. 458–475.

WILLIAMS, F. "The Crisis of Hospitalization," *The Nursing Clinics of North America* 9:1 (March 1974): 37–45.

6

nurses' groups as a consultation modality

*In the relationship between the individual
and the environment, stress occurs when
there is disparity between what an individual
needs and what the environment offers in
the form of gratification and reward. Stress
is exacerbated when the means available to
the individual to reduce the disparity
between need and reward remains outside
one's control.*

ZALEZNIK et al. [1]

section 1   the rationale for a group

The "care-giving" experience is filled with complex expectations, along with identified and unidentified stresses, disappointments, and gratifications. The request for a nurses' group can reflect any of these issues. The expectation on nurses to be patient, nurturing, and supportive is enormous. The very nature of clinical responsibility necessitates that they employ sound judgment while remaining available, objective, and professionally intimate with their patients. Physical symptoms and behavioral responses of patients are observed, understood, and hopefully treated in such a way as to promote the achievement of the highest level of health possible. The practice of nursing, like other disciplines within health care, leaves no margin for error. The unrealistic expectation always to perform to an optimal level and to be consistently therapeutic is prevalent in the nursing profession. The impact of the dichotomy between the real and ideal contributes to the stress. Nurses not only observe, assess, and develop patient/family-centered nursing interventions, but they also benefit from gaining understanding and utilizing their own reactions to the total "care-giving" experience in order to improve the quality of patient care. Sometimes these expectations are unrealistic and cannot be met. This factor alone may validate the need for a group.

Formal education and careful clinical supervision are helpful, but they may not be sufficient for nurses to provide adequate psychological care. Like other health care providers, nurses have strong feelings and reactions to their work and to their patients. They can benefit from an environment in which they explore and understand these reactions. The relationships between health care providers tend to influence the care given to the patient and the professional satisfac-

158

tion of the care givers. Nurses who feel devalued by patients, by other nurses, or by any member of the health care team may respond by not functioning to their potential. Nurses who are baffled by their patient's behavior may be overwhelmed with frustration, anger, or helplessness. This is understandable. They may not be cognizant of the fact that their behavior in response to the patient is less than professional. As a result, they may not be able to provide adequate patient care. The hospital system, with its norms and mores, expects a certain level of behavior on the part of its nursing staff and a certain standard of care for its patients. For the most part, patients expect time, attention, and information, and they believe that care efforts will be curative [2]. Nurses often assume that patients will cooperate with care efforts, that realistic patient care goals can be established and, in most instances, achieved. Obviously, such is not always the case. The complexities of the care-giving experience combine to create a highly charged, emotionally laden atmosphere for patients and for nurses. When "there are some patients who fail to respond to the customary methods of nursing intervention, it becomes evident that nurses are persons at risk for crisis [3]." The value of professional nurses engaged in a group under the leadership of a psychiatric liaison nurse becomes apparent as a vehicle to understanding this ongoing conflict.

The authors' view and experience indicate that nurses' groups are an extremely effective consultation modality, in which nurses can be assisted and supported in their efforts to understand the complexities of the "care-giving" experience. The potential value of the group is multifold. A unique opportunity for nurses to discuss concerns, to validate feelings and reactions, to learn from each other, and to problem solve together may be provided by the group. This opportunity for learning from each other can be both professionally stimulating and satisfying. When there is a high professional morale in a nursing staff, interest and motivation to improve the quality of nursing care is present. This kind of atmosphere also contributes to the interest in nurses' groups. However, morale can be low on a nursing unit, while the need and desire for a group can be very high. It has been our observation that the development of professional cohesion among the members of the group can bring many benefits. We have observed a positive change in the quality of nursing care delivered, personal and professional growth in the group members, and a greater resiliency in terms of weathering actual or fantasized crises inherent in the "care-giving" experience. Regularly scheduled nurses' groups may not only promote cohesion, but they may also serve as a legitimate, structured professional time to discuss, examine, and laugh at, if need be, the potential or actual interpersonal and intrapsychic conflicts that flood the imperfect environment of a hospital.

Liaison nurses are clinically knowledgeable in group theory and in group process, incorporating the group method into their consultation work. The conducting of nurses' groups is an effective means of practicing psychiatric liaison nursing. Where appropriately contracted for, the group is not only a more efficient and cost-effective use of liaison nurses' time, but also another means by which to validate their clinical practice. The opportunity to teach applied psychiatric principles, to role model, to encourage, and to support participation in sharing clinical experiences is dependent on the skill of the liaison nurse. This is also dependent on his or her verbal and behavioral commitment to maintain a patient-centered focus.

"When an emotional reaction of the nurse destroys her objectivity about some aspect of her job, that reaction is a suitable subject for group discussion, but the intrapsychic conflict which may have helped to generate the reaction should not be considered... [4]." For example, in a group meeting, a nurse began talking about a male patient in his late fifties, admitted with acute pancreatitis secondary to a ten-year history of alcohol abuse. The nurse described the patient as intelligent, physically attractive, with a good job and a nice family. "He's the same age as my father, same job too. He's not interested at all in getting help to stop drinking, and he's ruining his family." As the nurse continued, she explained that the patient was "nice enough to take care of, isn't demanding or seductive with me, but it just makes me so angry that he's ruining his family. I'm afraid he'll pick it up and I'll be rejecting him." The liaison nurse asked the group if others were feeling similarly, and some of the nurses nodded their heads in agreement. The liaison nurse then facilitated discussion around alcoholism in general, as well as the anger, frustration, and helplessness that alcoholics often stir up in health care providers. Discussion became focused on problem solving and how to tolerate the angry feelings, while still providing optimal, nonrejecting patient care.

The clues to the psychodynamics of the nurse who initially presented the patient were observed by the liaison nurse. Although it would have been inappropriate to focus on this particular nurse and attempt to explore the comparisons she was drawing between her patient and her father, recognition of their relationship was important. Clearly, the liaison nurse had to acknowledge that it may be more difficult to care objectively for a patient who reminds us of someone in our personal life. It would have been counterproductive to the group and to the care of this patient to dwell on personal issues or to lecture at length on alcoholism or the effects of alcoholism on the family. A specific problem in providing patient care had been identified, and its resolution was the priority. The nurse may or may not have realized how her description of the patient was revealing of her own personal issues. She wanted help so as not to be rejecting of the patient which became the group agenda. The needs of this nurse were also those of the group. A personal issue was refocused as a professional issue. The group provided an opportunity to explore feelings and prejudices. The nurses were supported in that the leader recognized and was empathic to their feelings about this patient. Some teaching about alcoholism was accomplished. Sharing the assignment and keeping expectations of the patient realistic in terms of future alcohol abuse were discussed. The nursing care approach consisted of teaching, as well as support, encouragement, and concern about his health. Hospital and community resources were offered. This intervention provided the nurses with a plan that was potentially helpful and positive, rather than rejecting and angry.

A nurses' group is not a magical modality for providing psychiatric nursing consultation. Not every ward wants, needs, or is ready for a nurses' group. Not every request for a nurses' group is appropriate (Table 6-1). Although there can certainly be exceptions to the rule, the following viewpoint is offered as a basis of understanding the rationale for a nurses' group. Nursing staffs who have not utilized psychiatric nursing consultation and/or who have not found it to be helpful are usually not ready for a group. In such instances, they often do not recognize any need for a group. More importantly, they may interpret such offerings by the liaison nurse as threatening, evaluating, and/or devaluing of them—"You have a problem, so you need a group." The reverse of this situation may also occur, and a professional need for a group may be identified. However, a head nurse or staff who has never utilized the liaison nurse or who has not found psychiatric nursing consultation helpful may request a group whose goals are not appropriate. For example, they may want a therapy group in which the focus is more on their personal issues than on patient care. They may want a group to complain about hospital and/or nursing administrative policies. As a major focus, these kinds of issues are in disharmony with the goals of nurses' groups.

To summarize, nurses' groups are an efficient use of time, and they can be an effective method of providing psychiatric nursing consultation. Through group process, psychological care issues can be

TABLE 6–1 EVALUATING THE REQUESTS FOR A NURSES' GROUP

1. *Clear requests from nurse consultees:*

"We have very difficult patients on this unit and need support in order to take care of them."

"Many of our patients have emotional problems; we aren't sure how to help them."

"Some of our patients are very depressed and we don't know how to talk with them."

"We're really depressed because so many of our patients have died recently."

"The morale is low on this unit, and we want to learn how to support each other."

2. *Unclear requests from nurse consultees:*

"There are some racial problems among the nursing staff members that are interfering with care."

"We need to talk because we're having problems with the doctors. They give lousy care to their patients."

"We're having trouble with the evening nursing supervisor, and she doesn't listen to our problems."

"We don't agree with the new overtime policy and want some help in planning a response to nursing administration."

identified and explored. When issues become problematic, the group can utilize their assessment to formulate a nursing care plan. The "care-giving" experience itself indicates that a period of professional time be designated for members of the nursing staff to engage in this segment of their professional work.

section 2 goals and format

The goals of a nurses' group, which are consistent with the goals of consultation, serve as criteria by which to create, maintain, and evaluate the group. These goals are:

1. To demonstrate and teach mental health concepts and their application to clinical nursing practice.
2. To effect appropriate psychiatric and nursing intervention.

3. To support nurses in continuing to provide quality nursing care.
4. To promote and develop the professional and personal self-esteem of the nurse.
5. To encourage tolerance among the members of the nursing staff of those situations in which immediate and/or effective intervention or resolution is unattainable.

What structured guidelines do liaison nurses utilize in negotiating and contracting for a nurses' group? First, they must very clearly appreciate the goals of such a group. They then proceed to assess the ward, its history, its culture, and its nursing staff. In addition, it is valuable to research carefully the past and present use of groups, along with the group experience in general on the medical-surgical wards. They proceed to carefully consider and evaluate their alliances with the head nurse and the staff. The quality and availability of nursing leadership are other important considerations. Liaison nurses observe the patient care needs and pace of the ward. They assess the head nurse's and the staff's level of concern and interest in psychological care issues and their use of psychiatric nursing consultation in the past. After this assessment is completed, negotiations for creating and conducting a nurses' group begin with the appropriate nursing leadership personnel.

Liaison nurses adopt the process they engaged in when initially negotiating their role. They adopt aspects of it as needed to the process of nurses' group creation. (Chapter 2, Section 2.) During this process, it is useful to restate the patient care focus of a nurses' group and to differentiate it from a psychotherapy group.

Once the head nurse and nursing staff are clear as to the focus and goals of a nurses' group, other elements are understood and agreed on. The membership of the group is an area of concern. It can be very helpful for the liaison nurse to be involved in the decision regarding membership. If the result of this decision is one that is counterproductive to group goals or to the functioning of the liaison nurse, the group will most likely be a failure. It could potentially be a disaster. It has been our experience that, when they are not participants in this process, liaison nurses may learn group membership is to include the ward clerk, intern, ward social worker, psychiatrist, nutritionist, and a variety of other individuals. Although these individuals do make valuable contributions to patient care and may benefit from a group experience, the goals of this group are strictly centered around clinical nursing practice. In some instances, it may be very reasonable to request that a health care provider from another discipline attend a specific group session. It is preferable that this visit occurs with the permission of the group and its leader, the liaison nurse. Also, the liaison nurse is aware that such attendance does, by its very nature, change the group. The session may not be a group at all, but rather a case conference. At these times, specific nursing staff issues are excluded from the discussion unless a group decision is made to the contrary.

The majority of head nurses and nursing staff with whom we have negotiated nurses' groups have agreed that membership should include all members of the nursing staff—RNs, LPNs, nursing technicians, and nurses' aides. In most instances, this membership is profitable and effective. Some head nurses and nursing staffs have requested that group membership include only professional nurses. Others have requested that nursing students and their instructors be included. Again, there can certainly be times when the professional nursing staff needs its own session and times when students should attend the group. LPNs, aides, and technicians may have reactions to being excluded from the group, and these reactions can greatly influence the communication and rapport that they have with the RN staff. Non-nursing staff membership can alter the focus of the group so that a milieu or team meeting, rather than a nurses' group, takes place. It is beneficial when membership rules are clearly understood, as they influence the functioning of the group.

Group consultation, like individual consultation, is a nonevaluative experience. The group does not serve as an opportunity for a head nurse to evaluate the clinical practice of the staff. This is not to say that areas needing input from nursing leadership personnel cannot be identified or attended to, but rather that a nonevaluative stance is attempted by all members of the group, be they staff nurses, nursing leaders, or, of course, the liaison nurse. Presumably, group members will feel reasonably safe with one another while exploring problems, worries, and actions that they may have taken. For example, during a nurses' group, one of the members seemed upset. The group meeting had just begun, and no definite agenda had been decided. The liaison nurse noticed the staff nurse's anxiety and asked her if there was something she might like to bring up in the group. The staff nurse nodded yes. The other group members, including the head nurse, asked how they could help. The staff nurse replied, "I don't know. I accepted money from a patient, and now the patient is very demanding and is driving me crazy. I shouldn't have accepted the money. It was a lot too. But Mrs. Seidler got so upset when I tried to refuse, and she's just recovering from her second MI. I'll probably be written up for this." The staff nurse directed this last comment to her head nurse who in turn responded: "We can discuss the policy about accepting money from patients later. Now, let's just figure out what to do." Through further discussion, similar confessions were made.

Mrs. Seidler was demonstrating a behavior change that was assessed to be based solely on her foiled attempt to "bribe the nurse." Although the staff nurse was anxious and guilt-ridden about accepting money, it was the impact on the patient's behavior that motivated her to bring this matter up in the group. The liaison nurse maintained her nonevaluative stance, but the subtle difficulties in achieving this stance are noted. Obviously, this was most difficult for the head nurse. The staff nurse needed support in talking with this patient. An opportunity for role modeling and teaching was utilized.

The group can be a supportive opportunity for sharing and learning. The life of the group raises the issue of confidentiality. Confidentiality is a necessary aspect of group consultation as it is with individual consultation. The content of group meetings is shared with members of the group who may not have been present at a particular session. Indeed, this is a group expectation. Group content should be shared only with group members. However, if the group feels that another health care team member needs to be made aware of a patient-focused issue that was arrived at in the group, this individual can be contacted by one of the group members or by the liaison nurse.

Finally, the head nurse and the staff identify a day, time, and place for the nurses' group. Most occur once a week and are 45 minutes to an hour long. However, depending on the needs of the nursing staff and the pace of the ward, variations in the frequency, as well as in the length, of sessions are negotiated. Most important is that the group be regularly scheduled and that both the nursing staff and the liaison nurse be committed to meeting. Given the patient care demands, possible short staffing, various crises, and the element of the unknown, the liaison nurse and the group are flexible. Any one of these factors may result in the members feeling that the group has to be cancelled. At the same time, they may experience great conflict and guilt over doing so. The liaison nurse remains attuned to the conflict and assumes responsibility for cancelling and rescheduling the group, when needed. It is quite possible that any of the factors that result in cancellation may necessitate scheduling additional time for the group. Nevertheless, sometimes there is really no other option but cancellation. It is both an indication of flexibility and support to share with the group members the observation that "today" does not appear to be the best day to have the group. Reasonable effort should be made to reschedule. Regardless of whether or not this can be accomplished, the members are informed that the liaison nurse will return for the next regularly scheduled group and remain available until that time. In some instances, cancellation may be an indication of resistance. Experience demonstrates that when a group is cancelled, regardless of the reason, it is helpful for the liaison nurse to remain on the unit, at least for a short time. She may find that although the staff cannot attend the group, some of them may request individual consultation.

Once the goals and format are clearly understood and agreed on by the liaison nurse and consultees, the name of the group is not exceedingly important. A variety of names, as well as no names, have been used. However, there may be hidden meaning in the "misnaming" of the group. Although negotiation has occurred with the discussion of the group goals, the testing of the group and its leader is inevitable. Testing is frequently reflected in the misnaming of the group. Jokes made by the consultee about psychiatry and/or psychiatric nursing may, in some instances, be enjoyed, but they should be taken seriously by the liaison nurse. Any catchy phrases that title the group but inaccurately describe it, or that are devaluing in some way, should be addressed immediately. It is essential that, if the group is titled, the name of the group either accurately reflect its goals or at the very least be benign.

section 3 a theoretical framework

The authors' intent is not to review in depth various theories pertaining to group development and group process, nor to revalidate the use of groups as a therapeutic psychiatric treatment modality. Numerous texts and articles in the literature carefully and thoughtfully examine the pertinent concepts [5]. Therefore, a brief review of certain terms and concepts that are applicable to nurses' groups is provided. It is assumed that the reader is well acquainted both theoretically and clinically with group theory.

To conceptualize and conduct a nurses' group, it aids liaison nurses to be proficient in blending and applying the principles of consultation theory and group theory. According to Labovitz, a "group is something more than collections of individuals. It has a definable membership; its members share a sense of consciousness, or group identity, and they also share a purpose, common goals or ideas [6]." As stated in the previous section, the liaison nurse remains clear as to the goals and format of a nurses' group. Flexibility on the part of the group leader helps to maintain the group's agreed-upon clinical focus and operational guidelines, such as membership, time, day, place, and other terms. "Every group interaction has two levels of function which take place simultaneously: the task level and the process level [7]." The former refers to the manifest work engaged in by the group members to achieve group goals. The group dynamics or process level of the group refers to the interactions and patterns of interactions that occur with the group. The process level also includes the relationships among group members and those between group members and group leader over time. Process is the "constant movement as group members seek to reduce the tension that arises when people attempt to have their individual needs met yet work to help meet group goals [8]." Liaison nurses are aware of the process of the group and respectfully utilize it to promote the group as a modality for psychiatric nursing consultation. Their ability to recognize that they are consultants *first* and group leaders *second* is of prime importance.

Bion's basic assumptions concerning groups reflect major developmental stages and identify themes that are characteristic of each stage. The first assumption concerns dependence on leaders and their role in protecting and conducting the group. The second is focused on the leader's use of power and the fright-or-flight stance of the group members. The third assumption deals with intimacy and hope, and it is characteristic of the stage of pairing [9]. Observing stages and listening for themes can be useful when attempting to understand the group experience for the nurse/consultee. However, unlike a psychotherapy group or a work group, in a nurses' group there is no contract to discuss personal dynamics or to hear psychodynamic interpretations. The achievement of personal insight is neither a group goal nor a group expectation. If nurses gain understanding of *how* they react to specific kinds of patients, this knowledge may be helpful to them. If they gain an understanding of *why* they react to specific kinds of patients, this insight is a bonus. If this knowledge is expressed within the group, the potential exists for all members, including the liaison nurse, to also benefit.

Expectations of the group leader are consistent with expectations of the liaison nurse as a consultant. In this sense, the members, as consultees, can direct the group, while the liaison nurse, as consultant, can operationalize the goals and format of the group. As consultees, the group members can state that there are "no problems" to talk about in the group, that they and the ward are "fine." In essence, they can thank the liaison nurse for coming by, while cancelling a group meeting. Maintaining a consultative stance and not personalizing the rejection can be difficult at these times, but doing so is clearly significant to the achievement of group/consultation goals.

Some of the theoretical principles of task-oriented groups, support groups, psychotherapy groups, and adult learning theory are utilized as a base for conceptualizing the elements of a nurses' group. This combined theoretical application to nurses' groups requires blending with consultation theory (Chapter 2, Section 1). To weave a theoretical model that is applicable to clinical practice, specific factors inherent in the development, as well as in the functioning, of the group necessitate delineation. As a consultation modality, nurses' groups are not curative. It is an expectation and goal that they are supportive and educational. Incorporating some of Yalom's concepts described in his "ten primary categories of curative factors in group psychotherapy [10]," the authors propose nine categories of working factors in nurses' groups.

Working Factors in Nurses' Groups

1. Sharing the "nursing experience,"
2. professional growth,
3. ventilation or "catharsis" [10],
4. identification or "universality" [10],
5. task orientation,
6. support,
7. "instillation of hope" [10],
8. collaboration, and
9. teaching.

Yalom is of the opinion that "the curative factors operate in every type of therapy group, ... they assume a differential importance depending on the goals and composition of the specific group [11]." The working factors in nurses' groups have similar properties. The five basic goals inherent in nurses' groups can be influenced by a variety of factors. The specific ward, the group membership, sophistication and professional development, and the nature of the issues being presented can all influence which goal takes precedence. For example, if the behavior of a patient has severely affected the self-esteem of the nurses in the group so that they cannot function professionally, the nurses' self-esteem becomes the group goal of priority. This further illustrates that not every goal can be reached in every group. Identification and promotion of the working factors aids in making the group a realistic experience.

1. sharing the "nursing experience"

Nurses can become preoccupied with and overwhelmed by the many treatments, procedures, and needs of their patients. Although striving to maintain a holistic approach to patients, to identify and meet their needs, to coordinate and plan their care, nurses appear to be plagued by time constraints and professional demands. In addition to the expectation of clinical competence, a great deal of emphasis in nursing is placed on organizational skills and priority setting. These may be offered as solutions to the problems of insufficient staffing, inadequate communication, and low professional cohesion. With the advent of primary nursing as a method of nursing care delivery, increased emphasis has been placed on responsibility and accountability [12]. Although these two issues have always been present in the nursing profession, there is now increased attention focused on them. These issues account for a large percentage of the anxiety that nurses experience.

Organizational skills and the ability to identify priorities are necessary components of professional nursing practice. In-service educational programs, patient care conferences, and clinical supervision are vehicles by which a nursing department assists its staff in organizational skills and priority setting.

Nevertheless, "nurses are persons at risk for crisis [13]," regardless of the illness and/or age category of the patients. Nurses often feel devalued by patients or their families, by each other, by physicians and other members of the health care team. They often feel impotent in terms of resolving patient care problems, of interacting therapeutically with patients, and of completing their work on time. It is not uncommon for nurses to feel like they are constantly engaged in a game of "beat the Kardex" (getting everything checked off on time)—a game that they rarely win, yet against which they often measure their professional performance.

Nurses need and can benefit from a designated period of time to discuss the experience of being nurses. In addition to reviewing patients and issues regarding the providing of nursing care, the group serves as an opportunity to share the inherent difficulties in being responsible and accountable. It is a place where nursing professionalism can be augmented. The group is a place where intra-nursing staff issues and patient-focused issues can be discussed in hope of promoting professional cohesion and better patient care. The mere existence of the group is a validation that the views, feelings, and reactions of nurses are important. The group has the potential for nurses "to get" something for themselves, to increase their ability "to give" more therapeutically to their patients, and hopefully to perform in a more professional manner in general. The value of the group is not always demonstrated in solving either patient problems or staff problems. Somewhere in between these poles lies the core of the group process. This middle ground deals with the problems, struggles, and responsibilities that face nurses in learning to care for themselves while caring for their patients. To quote a staff nurse, "The group meeting is for us. We share concerns about patients and our feelings as nurses. It's supportive and stimulating. The group is helpful in encouraging us to look at what we do and how we feel about it." The fact that the group is sanctioned by the system, by the department of nursing, and by the head nurse enhances this working factor by acknowledging that nurses need a time to share their professional experiences.

2. professional growth

The nurses' group provides an opportunity for a unique sharing of professional concerns and clinical work. Since there is no fixed format, as there is with case conferences, expectations of members are less clear. Keeping the goals of consultation in mind, each nurse has the potential to develop professionally. Through the group and its process, the nurse is afforded a special opportunity to view and explore the nature of his or her care-giving experience and the experiences of peers. Peer consultation within the group stimulates professional growth by promoting collegiality.

3. ventilation or "catharsis"

Ventilation as a working factor in nurses' groups is basic to the functioning of this type of group, as it is to other groups. The tension-reducing value of catharsis—of expressing powerful, important emotion in psychotherapy—is well commented on in the literature [14]. The application of this concept to the theoretical model of nurses' groups rests in the process and intent of the group itself. Under the supportive direction of the liaison nurse, members are encouraged to identify and openly share feelings regarding patient-care-focused situations. They are encouraged to acknowledge frustrating and

upsetting experiences. This sharing serves to decrease a sense of isolation, to increase motivation for collaboration, and to provide the
benefits of a cathartic experience. Analytic explanation of emotions,
to promote interpersonal learning, is discouraged. Insight-oriented
discussion, concerning the origins of why a nurse feels or reacts to a
patient and/or colleague in a particular fashion, is both inappropriate as well as counterproductive to the purpose of the group. Although
catharsis has a meaningful and significant place in the group, the goal
is to aid the nurse, whenever possible, in therapeutically intervening
with patients.

4. identification or "universality"

Because a nurses' group is not a psychotherapy group, the goals are
not aimed at curing psychopathology. Yet identification or "universality" serves an important function. The therapeutic value of identification is experienced in knowing that other nurses have had similar
feelings or problems and have felt similar emotions. "As patients perceive their similarity to others and share their deepest concerns, they
benefit further from the accompanying catharsis and from the ultimate acceptance ("cohesiveness") by the other members [15]." As
liaison nurses, we have observed this phenomenon in nurses' groups.
The impressive power of identification is demonstrated in the mobili-
zation of the nurses' professional and personal energy. This energy is,
in turn, directed toward the achievement of group goals and toward
the provision of high-quality patient care.

5. task orientation

The major focus of the nurses' group is on the health care needs of the
patient. An attempt is made to direct any topic raised toward this
focus. Questions and concerns about caring for patients, about feelings and reactions to patients/families or to health care providers
from other disciplines, about problems of morale and communication among members of the nursing staff are appropriate areas for
discussion within the group. The liaison nurse is continually processing the discussion, keeping in mind the agreed-upon group focus and
guiding the discussion in an attempt to answer the following questions:

- How does this discussion relate to the delivery and the quality of nursing care?

- How can the quality of nursing care be promoted through this discussion?

Without such guidance, the group content may be in conflict with the established and agreed-upon goals. This working factor validates the purposeful existence of the group and dismisses any fantasy that the liaison nurse may be harboring a hidden agenda, such as psychotherapy for the nurses.

Any attempts at psychotherapy made by the liaison nurse with the nursing staff, either through the group process or individually, are inappropriate in this professional relationship. Such attempts are also contrary to the collaborative relationship that is fundamental to the practice of psychiatric liaison nursing. When psychotherapy is requested or personal problems are identified by the consultee, the liaison nurse can facilitate a referral.

The tasks and responsibilities of the group leader and group members are combined to maintain a patient care focus. Although not task-oriented groups in the traditional sense, nurses' groups do take on some characteristics of this type of group. "The intent of the task-oriented group is to provide a shared working experience wherein the relationship between feeling, thinking and behavior, their impact on others and on task accomplishment and productivity can be viewed and explored ... task accomplishment is not the purpose of the group ... the task provides a frame of reference which helps to keep in focus what is relevant to explore [16]." The intent of the agreement between the group leader and group members to maintain a patient-care-centered group focus is the task orientation of a nurses' group. Foulkes and Anthony refer to this "manifest declared activities of a group as the groups' 'occupation' [17]." The shared work is professional work, the shared experience is professional experience, the shared reactions and feelings are both professional and personal.

The liaison nurse carefully monitors the quality and quantity of self-disclosure during the group. The potential for such exposure to become problematic is very real. For example, it may be demonstrated in work relationships among group members. The nurse who persistently attempts to utilize the group to grieve personal tragedies may be viewed as seeking "special privileges" that are neither realistic nor reasonable. In addition, allowing sharing of this nature to take place within the group may be misinterpreted as encouragement. In this way, an inaccurate expectation may be inadvertently placed on group members.

The task orientation extends a bit further, if we again consider the goals of the group. Many of the same steps that liaison nurses utilize when providing individual consultation can be applied to the group. The problem-identification/problem-resolution approach is utilized, even if after identification, the very nature of the problem limits successful intervention. This is the essence of the group process. Intervention may or may not be developed and implemented. The problem may or may not be resolved. Nevertheless, the key elements are the sharing and learning that occur as the group process continues. The patient-care-centered orientation is a legitimate frame of reference. This orientation is a necessary factor that validates the group's existence and that supports its productivity.

6. support

One of the basic tenets of psychiatric nursing consultation is the provision of support and understanding to the consultee while hopefully assisting in problem solving a specific situation. Within the nurses' group, support is a working factor and a group goal. With the direction of the liaison nurse, members not only receive support from the leader, but they also learn how to support each other through particularly difficult times. It is significant to note, however, that a stressful situation does not have to exist for the group to be experienced as supportive. The authors have received feedback from nurses attributing the supportive value of their respective groups as being purely a function of attending the group, regardless of specific content. The mere fact that a group existed was perceived by many nurses as supportive of their professional practice and of them as individuals. Nevertheless, the format and content, the nature of member participation, and the skills of the leader can influence the supportive experience of the group.

7. "instillation of hope"

Liaison nurses as consultants are recognized sources for information, clarification, and support. Their presence symbolizes the hope and the reality that some problems may be solved, that others may be understood, and that nursing staff may be supported without having their clinical performance evaluated. The very existence of the group provides a sense of hope. The nurses' group is a place in which nurses may conceivably experience these benefits. The benefits become real and are experienced within the process of the group. Again, the skill of the liaison nurse aids this transition from hopeful wanting to experiencing. When new members join the group and learn the group's legacy from the older members, this sense of hope is transmitted.

8. collaboration

In the process of providing consultation and of developing an alliance with the consultee, the value of a collaborative approach cannot be overemphasized. As a working factor within the nurses' group, collaboration tends to dispel the fantasy that the leader is omnipotently knowledgeable. The creation of a climate in which the sharing of thoughts, feelings, and opinions is encouraged and valued is fundamental to a nurses' group, as well as to other types of groups. The methods chosen to achieve this overall purpose, however, depend on the specific goals and type of group being conducted, as well as on the needs and abilities of its members. In this regard, a psychotherapy group differs from a socialization group, a TA group from an educational group. As stated previously, the generalized purpose of a nurses' group is to improve psychological care given to the patient by helping nurses to recognize and work with the complicated issues involved in the "care-giving" experience. In keeping with this purpose, the liaison nurse, as group leader and as consultant, creates a climate in which mutual teaching and learning may occur, and in which members are encouraged and supported in their efforts to help each other. In this sense, collaboration resembles "altruism." "Altruistic acts often set healing forces in motion [18]." When group members share views and information, true collaboration with the liaison nurse and with each other occurs. Through this working factor, the assumption that the members have a great deal to teach the leader and each other is acknowledged. The leader does not merely facilitate discussion, but rather participates with the members in attempting to gain understanding and, if possible, to reach problem resolution.

The encouragement of collaboration within the group supports the reality that this is a professional group in which competition is recognized while respectful appreciation of each other's clinical knowledge is dominant. The shared responsibility of the previously described task is also validated in an atmosphere of collaboration. "When members of the group do not have to spend time defending their ideas or trying to be heard, they tend to use this energy more constructively. They begin to build on the useful components of the thoughts and suggestions of other members. As a result, each (team) member is likely to feel that a portion of his or her idea is a part of the outcome [19]." Collaboration is a vote of confidence in the group members. It can reduce anxiety and confusion. It is a basic element of the nurses' group and tends to potentiate other working factors.

9. teaching

Nurses' groups may provide an opportunity for learning through the identification and clarification of emotional issues. However, as previously illustrated, the intent is neither insight nor a corrective emotional experience for members. "Interpersonal learning is a broad and complex curative factor representing the group therapy analogue of such individual therapy curative factors as insight, working through the transference, the curative emotional experience, as well as processes unique to the group setting [20]." The working factor of teaching most resembles Yalom's curative factor "imparting of information—the didactic instruction about mental health, mental illness, and psychodynamics given by the therapists, as well as advice, suggestions, or direct guidance about life problems offered either by the therapist or other patients [21]." Through this working factor, information is offered and shared by both leader and members. The information may reflect knowledge of mental health, mental illness, and psychodynamics under the general heading of psychological care needs of patients and their families. Personal issues relating to the psychological problems and/or care needs of group members are avoided. At times, it may be very difficult to comfortably avoid these kinds of issues as members may persistently present them. It is important to actively intervene by commenting on the personal quality of the discussion and the original contract of the group. If this interferes with the group process, such comments may be made on an individual basis outside the group.

Nine working factors in nurses' groups have developed as a theoretical model. This model augments the process of conceptualizing and of understanding nurses' groups. Various theories, as well as clinical experience and personal philosophy, have been blended together to illustrate the complicated issues inherent in this consultatively based group. These nine working factors differentiate nurses' groups from other types of groups and necessitate careful consideration by the liaison nurse. In conjunction with the interest, motivation, and degree of sophistication of the group members, the liaison nurse can utilize these factors in making the group a valuable and helpful experience.

section 4   the roles and techniques of the group leader

The techniques utilized by the leader of a nurses' group are varied. The outcome of the group is affected by the implementation of these techniques and the flexibility with which the leader uses them. To effectively apply the theoretical model—that is, the nine working factors of a nurses' group—skill in utilizing specific leadership techniques is required. The liaison nurse as leader assumes several roles. These roles, blended with techniques, result in a nurses' group focused on the goals of psychiatric nursing consultation.

Liaison nurses are knowledgeable by virtue of their theoretical education and clinical experience. Their clinical practice demonstrates their consultative position within the health care milieu. The overall model of leadership used in the groups is similar to a case seminar method of group mental health consultation as described by Altrocchi, et al. [22]. Within the framework of consultation theory applied to group process, issues of power, control, and authority are recognized. The liaison nurse as leader maintains a collaborative stance regarding these issues, to preserve a consistent relationship with the consultees. Mutual performance expectations are not altered.

The medical setting and ward situation dictate immediately the limitations of the group. So that as many staff as possible may attend, it is preferable that group meetings be held on the ward. Interruptions resulting in a continuous flow of traffic characterize the group. At any moment, there may be a medical emergency. In addition, the staff have numerous responsibilities that demand attention and emotional availability. After the group meeting, the consultees return to their patients and provide nursing care. Therefore, a restriction in the full expression of feelings becomes a part of the baseline functioning of the group. The nurses are "on duty," which places a burden of responsibility on the leader to exercise reasonable control. The interweaving of flexibility and expertise in group and consultation theory allows the liaison nurse to persevere in this method of supporting staff and teaching mental health concepts.

roles

The group leader functions in a variety of ways. For purpose of clarity, the roles assumed by the leader will serve as a basis for understanding the techniques utilized. The skill with which the leader assumes roles and utilizes techniques, while maintaining flexibility, influences the group. The roles are:

1. group leader,
2. nurse,
3. teacher, and
4. psychiatric nurse.

1. group leader. The general responsibilities of a group leader include starting and ending the group, utilizing group process, maintaining an appropriate focus, promoting cohesion and safety, and facilitating discussion. In the role of leader, the liaison nurse not only utilizes the group process to augment the professional growth and development of group members, but also continues to promote collaboration and to offer information. The consultee–consultant alliance is strengthened as members experience the group as a supportive and useful consultation modality.

An example of the use of group process in the nurses' group is illustrated by the borderline patient on the medical ward. The patient's pathology may be observed in the group through the process of learning about his or her interactions with the staff. What does it mean when the patient labels some nurses as "efficient" and others as "inefficient"? The problem occurring with the patient may be re-enacted in the group. The nurses may find themselves arguing about whether the patient is "right or wrong." The leader, commenting on the process, aids group members in recognizing their involvement in the split stimulated by the patient. This type of issue requires the expert clinical skill of the group leader.

2. nurse. As a nurse, professional identity with the group members results in a relationship that is fundamental to the group's productivity, not as an experiment or project, but as a cornerstone to nursing care. The liaison nurse does not need to have comparable nursing experience to be effective in the group. However, every common experience does strengthen the professional identity that makes success more likely. A bond, created from their common experiences and their peer relationships as nurses, supports their overall clinical practice. Although other mental health professionals may be skilled in leading groups, the role of the leader as nurse is the unique element that aids in making the group effective and a valuable professional experience. As a nurse, the consultant can offer empathic understanding and clarification of the many complex issues involved in the nursing experience. Clearly the dangers of overidentification exist. However, it is anticipated that the expertise of liaison nurses, coupled with their awareness of the necessity for clinical supervision, would address this potential problem.

3. *teacher.* The theoretical and clinical expertise of liaison nurses, combined with their positions as group leaders, results in the expectation that pertinent information regarding psychological care will be shared and taught. When the need arises, formal presentations are reserved for in-service education programs. Within the group, informal teaching occurs, and it can be meaningful and effective. Topics of particular interest to group members that are within the leader's area of expertise and that pertain to the overall goals of the group are discussed. Continuing to function in the role of consultant, liaison nurses remain acutely aware of the consultation model in this area of their clinical practice. Teaching may occur relevant to the substance of a problem such as anger, depression, lack of motivation, chronic pain, and the like. Teaching and learning are more effective through the subtle and intriguing process of examining the problem and its relationship to the patient. The leader assists the group members in identifying and clarifying their own reactions and feelings to specific patients and to patient care situations. The leader hopes to validate that the group member understands the problem and that learning has occurred. Since the group usually focuses on a particular problem, there is often a sense of anxiety and urgency to achieve problem resolution. When anxiety is reduced, effective teaching and learning are more likely to occur.

Teaching style is based on a synthesis of consultation theory and adult learning theory. In their role as teacher, liaison nurses have goals similar to those in the consultee–consultant relationship. However, superimposed on that relationship is the process of the group. As teachers, leaders are cognizant of the group process. They are also aware and respectful of the varying degrees of internal motivation to learn, learning needs, clinical confidence, the nursing specialty, and level of professional practice among the group members. These issues influence their role as teacher.

4. *psychiatric nurse.* As psychiatric nurses, liaison nurses are striving to "diagnose the total consultation" as issues are discussed within the group. It is important to offer aid and assistance as a psychiatric nurse when situations discussed seem to warrant it. Practical, con-

crete help goes hand-in-hand with "understanding feelings." The consultee's unrealistic expectations of psychiatry and psychiatric nursing may be exposed. Deftly and skillfully, psychiatric nurses acknowledge that, just as medical intervention does not solve all medical problems, neither does psychiatric intervention solve all psychiatric problems. However, in their role as psychiatric nurse, they recognize when there is a need for more active psychiatric involvement for the sake of patient safety or of a potentially unrecognized psychiatric disorder. If they assess that the group is overwhelmed by anger, anxiety, or feelings of inadequacy, they may decide to be more active in presenting a willingness to assist. Psychiatric nurses consider the risks, just as they do in any consultation. These risks may be related to misunderstanding the group process. The role of leader as a psychiatric nurse is fundamental to clinical work. Their knowledge, experience, and clinical skill provide validity to their role as legitimate resources and practitioners.

techniques

The roles assumed by the leader work in concert with the techniques. There are similarities in the techniques utilized in nurses' groups to those utilized in psychotherapy groups. To effectively apply the nine working factors of a nurses' group, the liaison nurse employs specific leadership techniques (Table 6–2). The techniques discussed are consistent with the goals and format of the nurses' group. These techniques are:

1. *direction of affect.*   Liaison nurses are attuned to the affect within the group. Once recognized they attempt to keep the affect within tolerable levels. If more feeling than is workable in the work situation is

TABLE 6–2 LEADERSHIP TECHNIQUES

1. Direction of Affect
2. Promotion of Professional Development
3. Building Group Legacy
4. Recognition of Defense Mechanisms
5. Refocusing of Group Content
6. Incorporation of Milieu Life
7. Support and Catharsis
8. Role Playing

expressed, they attempt to keep it within reasonable limits. Effective direction is accomplished through the accurate recognition of the origin, quality, and intensity of the affect being expressed in the group. The leader may raise or lower anxiety by discussing the concept rather than the affect or by deferring or ignoring interpretations. Referring to "old" patients and using similar situations provide consultees with permission to discuss the affect with more objectivity and distance. Mr. Litke, admitted with Crohn's disease, infuriated the staff with his request for two telephones and the installation of a computer terminal in his room. A major control struggle was beginning as the nurses were joining forces to keep Mr. Litke in line and not violate hospital policy. The liaison nurse reminded the group about Mr. Josh, also suffering from Crohn's disease, who had on admission made unrealistic demands on the staff. They remembered that, as he became less threatened about his illness, his need to be in control diminished, and he became a pleasant, cooperative patient. The use of self to legitimize affect or to illustrate a common emotional reaction is both effective and safe for the group. In a nurses' group, the members presented their helplessness surrounding the case of Mrs. Paul, a patient on bed rest. It was apparent that they tried every possible measure to provide this patient with psychological support. Their efforts proved to be only minimally successful and Mrs. Paul remained critical, demanding, and sarcastic. The nurses were unable to acknowledge the anger that they experienced toward this patient. Therefore, the liaison nurse, using herself, expressed that she would find it very difficult to care for Mrs. Paul and would be angry with the patient. The nurses were then able to recognize and discuss the way they really felt.

2. *promotion of professional development.* Since a major goal of consultation is to aid the professional development of the nurse, it is important as a technique to observe the level of sophistication of the group. Carefully and skillfully, the leader attempts to foster clearer conceptualization of the psychological problems experienced by patients. It is useful to explore the limitations of the group members. Personal motivation, level of education, the milieu, and leadership of the ward affect the professional development of nursing staff. The group leader clarifies the nursing staff's understanding of problems and ascertains the feasibility of their carrying out interventions. It may be possible to initiate only minimal change. This technique is vital to an accurate assessment of the professional level of nurses in integrating psychological concepts into patient care.

3. building group legacy.   The open-ended nature of the group and the changing membership do not always provide the opportunity to learn by repetition. There is very little, if any, carry-over for the group, so there is a sense of repeating the same issues continually. These are later described as "themes." A group with transient membership may develop a legacy. Group norms and group culture get passed on from group session to group session and from generation to generation [23]. In our experience in ongoing groups, active over eight years, there has been continued member turnover. The positive or negative legacy can either sustain a group or impede its progress. The legacy itself may become powerful in validating or in negating the importance of psychological care.

4. recognition of defense mechanisms.   Defense mechanisms may be adaptive not only for patients and staff but within the group itself. Humor and intellectualization, for example, may aid the staff in dealing with unsolvable problems and in accepting their limitations as care providers. These and other defense mechanisms are understood and sometimes encouraged. Only when they are no longer adaptive or helpful are they dealt with directly. An effective technique within the group is to explore and analyze the patient's defense mechanisms and coping strategies. What becomes evident is that many conflicts between the nurse and the patient, as well as between the nurse and coworkers, arise as a result of having minimal understanding of the effects of stress. The technique utilized is demonstrating within the group, most often by case example or by nonthreatening examples within their own lives, how defense mechanisms protect us against more frightening feelings or events. If a group member presents a patient who is nasty and hostile to staff, it is necessary to break the inevitable nonproductive cycle created between the patient and the nurse. This objective may be accomplished by encouraging building an alliance with the patient, identifying the defense mechanisms, understanding their function, identifying the hidden affect, and building empathy.

The following two illustrations are examples that may be employed to demonstrate how anger is expressed when fear is felt:

1. A 2-year-old child runs out into the street where there is a car approaching. With heart pounding and intense fear, the mother races out into the street, swoops up the child, and moves from the path of the car. When she reaches the sidewalk, she finds herself screaming at the child and spanking him. But is she frightened, guilt-ridden, or relieved?

2. You have made arrangements to meet your boyfriend at the movies, and he appears two hours late. While you are waiting, you are frightened and worried that he has been in an accident. When he arrives, you have an argument.

Examples are effective only if they depict situations with which the nurses in the group can identify. Suddenly, they not only understand how they feel, but also how fright may produce another reaction to protect the individual. This reaction serves to normalize the behaviors of the patient, which aids in conceptualizing the function of defense mechanisms.

5. *refocusing group content.* The group leader has the responsibility to remember the goals of the group and to maintain an appropriate focus within the group. In a therapy group, material may be interpreted in terms of the group process. In nurses' groups doing so may be possible, but it is usually more productive to redirect the material to the milieu situation or to the patient interaction. The following example illustrates this point. In the context of a discussion about Mrs. S, a patient with multiple sclerosis, a newly employed nurse began to reveal the feelings she experienced living with her mother who also was afflicted with MS. The group fell silent. In a therapy group, the group's reactions and/or feelings, as well as those of the nurse, might have been explored. In a nurses' group, both would be avoided. The group leader would redirect discussion to maintain an appropriate group focus. This goal may be accomplished by acknowledging the affect through a generalizing statement, which recognizes that patients' emotional and physical problems may touch us all in special ways. By redirecting group content, the leader encourages professionalism, while recognizing the personal feelings of the consultee.

6. *incorporation of milieu life.* The leader can use life events to demonstrate mental health concepts. In the continued attempt to normalize patients' feelings and reactions, drawing on ongoing life stresses—such as separation, termination, and the like—helps to emphasize the normalcy of the patient's behavior. Group members may also discuss ward events that may be influencing patient care. It is possible to involve group members' experiences in an effective way. Nurses usually feel free to express thoughts about their own hospitalization or that of family members. The group leader generalizes these feelings, which may produce more positive group interaction.

In a nurses' group on a medical floor, it was possible to effectively discuss the role of denial in illness through a group member's experience. The group, which had been an active group for over two years, began by expressing concern about the head nurse who had been wearing a neck collar for three days and who was obviously in pain. Her illness was affecting the ward. Permission was obtained from this head nurse to discuss with her in the group the feelings and thoughts she was experiencing with this infirmity. The nurse most effectively unfolded the meaning of the injury to her and how denial was her protection for underlying fears. It was moving for the group to intensely share the power of denial. The group members generalized this information and stated that they now understood the purpose of denial in the patient suffering from a myocardial infarction. The fears that the MI patients were experiencing probably made them increase their activities just to prove to themselves that they were not going to die. Somehow it didn't seem so strange and foreign anymore, but it made some sense. What is most important, however, is that the nurses now knew that just as the head nurse came to work as a form of denial, so did the MI patient ambulate when he was on bed rest as a form of denial. And they also knew that being angry at the head nurse for being so "stupid" was just as ineffective as being angry at the MI patient. With empathic understanding there can be effective intervention.

7. *support and catharsis.*   How is support provided within the nurses' group when the need is recognized? The technique is to explore data about the patient or about the situation, which can possibly provide a basis for support. Generalized statements can be interpreted by staff as patronizing, whereas demonstrating the positive action taken or the impossibility of the situation can offer relief. Although a valuable and necessary technique, providing support and an opportunity for catharsis may not result in problem resolution. However, offering thoughtful and honest support and encouraging group involvement may impressively cause cohesiveness and the "esprit de corps" to emerge from the most complicated of human interactions. The sense of failure and/or frustration that staff may experience around issues needing support may be too powerful or explosive for the group situation on medical wards. It takes restraint, judgment, sensitivity, knowledge of systems, and clinical skill to bridge this gap and to be effective. Adhering to group goals and format, encouraging feedback, asking group members to evaluate the experience of support within the group, and working together to improve the nursing experience can prove to be supportive measures themselves.

8. role playing.   An effective technique, which may demonstrate the experience or feelings of an interaction, is role playing. A modified adaptation is more beneficial in a medical ward setting. It takes time and concentration to become involved in an artificial model. Therefore, role playing has certain limitations. What proves to be more effective and essentially more helpful is to suggest or to encourage the group to state the actual words in an interaction. For example, a group member may discuss feelings about talking with a discouraged patient. She may tell what she actually said to the patient, and the group might think together of what else exactly could be said in that situation (role playing). This type of role playing is concrete, real, action-oriented, and helpful. Knowing the words that can be used is like a tool. It is reminiscent of a young nursing student who wants to learn how to ask a patient about bowel habits or sexual functioning. It does help to practice a few acceptable ways to phrase the question.

The interweaving of roles and techniques is not only flexible, but it is an evolving process. Responding to case material or to specific issues requires spontaneity and creativity on the part of the liaison nurse. This conceptualization of roles and techniques then serves as a guide. The group leader remains cognizant of the goals of the group, which are also the goals of consultation.

section 5   group themes

One of the most striking aspects of nurses' groups is the repetition of themes, which illustrate the life of the group. The reoccurrence of themes is demonstrated in various forms in the context of case material. The themes have been divided into patient issues, professional issues, affectual issues, and illness issues. This list is not intended to be exhaustive but rather a conceptualization of the type of themes that have, in our experience, been dominant in nurses' groups.

patient issues

depressed patients.   The very nature of illness itself, which necessitates hospitalization, can be sufficient to cause depression in patients. Clearly, the most common type of depression experienced in the hospital is reactive depression. Care providers therefore become very accustomed to dealing with depression. The theme of depression in the nurses' group is of a more severe nature. The presentation of the depression may occur in many forms, such as patients' lack of motivation, refusal of care, or lack of acceptance of diagnosis. Clinically significant depression requires assessment, observation, and differentiation from sadness. Patient behaviors, which are actually concealing depression, may be discussed. In extended or prolonged hospitalizations, depression may necessitate intervention. The need for intervention is a paramount consideration.

demanding patients. Patients who express their discontent by behaviors that put unending demands on the nursing staff are frequently presented in the nurses' groups. Rich discussions often develop around this theme because patients who are demanding get everyone's attention, as well as being disruptive to the milieu. As a rule of thumb, if the entire staff is in agreement about the patient's behavior, the problem is more likely the patient's rather than the staff's. If the staff is divided in their tolerance or their opinion, it is more likely the patient's problem combined with the individual staff reaction. The first task is to attempt to discover the reason for the behavior and, through group problem solving, develop some plan of nursing intervention. This aim may involve nonpunitive limit setting and/or behavior modification. There is no formula for demanding patients. Intervention is again based on an individual assessment of the patient and his or her behavior.

For example, nurses in the group may express anger and rage at patients that frequently use their call light for what seem like trivial requests. Through group discussions and interaction, it may be discovered that the patient is frightened and looking for reassurance. The emphasis in the group is on the type of issues that tend to be brought up around demanding patients. Although it is beneficial to express frustrations, the major work of the group is directed toward problem solving and intervention. In addition, continued involvement with the nursing staff is important, given the inherent difficulty, anxiety, and frustration in caring for demanding patients.

At a regular nurses' meeting, Mrs. Wexler was presented as a demanding, irritating, 53-year-old LPN who had suffered her first MI. She was complaining about her care and finding fault with everything. The group members were very annoyed and angry and had not carefully considered the cause or the source of Mrs. Wexler's behavior. Through group discussion the missing pieces of fear, loneliness, and loss of sense of self were revealed. The following day, the liaison nurse was approached by a staff nurse who had been at the group meeting. "We were talking after our nurses' meeting and decided we should all make a real effort to attend the group. Mrs.

Wexler is doing much better. Talking about it helped—what we discussed was common sense, but we all needed to hear it. Sometimes we lose our perspective when we get involved with a patient. It is impressive that this hospital understands these problems of patient care."

unappealing patients. Nurses are often required to have prolonged and rather intimate contact with patients who are not only physically but psychologically unappealing. In addition, the crisis of illness may exaggerate offensive character traits. Nurses often experience an internal struggle between the feeling that they should like their patient and the feeling that they are repulsed by the patient's physical and/or psychological presentation and needs. Within the group, this theme is carefully assessed before the intervention can be considered. Sometimes with discussion, ventilation, and understanding about the patient, the nurses are increasingly able to be tolerant. Other times, the behaviors may be so extreme and/or destructive that the nurses may need assistance in focusing on therapeutic limit setting.

patients receiving placebos. Frequently, patients may not experience pain relief—whether assessed as real or imaginary, organic or functional—through the ministrations of narcotics or analgesics. These patients are often presented for discussion in the nurses' group. The suggestion by nurses or physicians may have been placebo treatment. Patients in the hospital receiving placebos have been described as being generally disliked by the nurses and house officers [24]. Such a reaction has become evident in the nurses' groups when discussions ensue concerning patients having prolonged and unrelieved pain. Relief of pain may be produced temporarily from placebos, but the relief of pain by placebo does not mean that the pain was nonexistent [25]. Group discussions about addiction and/or drug abuse are beneficial in uncovering feelings that affect attitudes toward patient care. Furthermore, encouraging the exploration of the possible origins of pain and the ventilation of concerns regarding placebo administration and the individual patient are useful.

patients who seem bizarre. There is a large classification of patients described as "weird" or "bizarre." When nurses have difficulty understanding behavior and/or when the behavior is exceptionally bizarre, it is common that the patient has been inaccurately assessed. More often than not, these patients or their visitors have major characterological problems or psychiatric illnesses. The group discussion in these cases often begins with joking about the strange behavior and then, hopefully, switches to assessment, understanding, tolerance, and appropriate intervention. These situations require exquisite sensitivity. The liaison nurse can be neither aloof nor involved in the frequent disparaging remarks. Although the tendency of staff to be judgmental may exist, the necessity for them to find safe outlets for tension is clear. In the process of assessment, the patient's behavior may be validated as bizarre and/or psychotic. Such patients understandably engender anxiety and fear in nurses.

prolongation of life.   The feelings surrounding prolonging life, when there is questionable medical viability, is another frequent theme in nurses' groups. The difficult struggle between heroics and humanism is discussed with the hopes of allowing nurses to be more accepting and understanding of themselves and of the medical team, while being sensitive to patients and their families. In this theme, there tends to be more personalization and expression of affect by group members through the sharing of philosophical, religious, and moralistic beliefs.

dying patients.   Patients who are dying have a variety of expectations of the health care delivery system. The expectations on the nurse are a consistent issue discussed within the group. Even with an increased awareness of the psychological impact of death and dying, within the general hospital, there is a strain on the nurse who is required to care simultaneously for patients who are fighting for life and for those who are facing death. Within the nurses' group, the focus of discussions around death and dying are as varied as those dealing with life and living. Sometimes nurses want to explore and better understand patient/family reactions. At other times, they merely want to express their sadness or feelings of helplessness. With this theme, the group leader emphasizes openness, assessment, and individualized interventions. There is no formula for dealing with a dying patient. Remaining aware and respectful of individuality is important. Honesty, availability, support, and involvement are the guidelines for meeting whatever expectations the patient may have for the staff.

anticipatorily grieved.   Patients who have been identified as terminal are usually receiving palliative medical care, as well as nursing care focused toward comfort. If these patients are going to die in the hospital, it is quite common for the nurses, like the patient's family, to assume a type of death watch. In many instances, these particular patients have suffered greatly and their impending death is viewed as a blessing. They have been anticipatorily grieved. When the death watch becomes lengthy, this theme is presented in nurses' groups. By exploring this theme, the group serves as a means of support and reassurance to the nurses as they struggle to live through the watch.

sexuality. With much more frequency, the issues of sexuality are being acknowledged and discussed by staff. Recent publications discuss much of the factual and attitudinal information [26]. However, the group discussions tend to focus on acceptance and integration of deviant sexual styles in the medical-surgical setting. The nursing staff is required to give physical care to homosexuals, prostitutes, and transvestites. The nurses' group becomes a logical place for exploration of feelings of sexuality. The heightened awareness by staff of sexuality as a segment of human relationships can have beneficial effects on the care of all patients. The normalcy of sexual feelings for patients can be emphasized when this theme is introduced. As a teacher, the leader utilizes the opportunity to promote discussion, for example, on illness and sexual health.

patients who are special. Hospitalized patients can acquire the status of being "special" by virtue of who they are, who they know, what they did, or what was done to them. Victims of violent crime, celebrities, relatives, members of the hospital staff, and others may present unique problems to the nursing staff. As these patients are discussed within the group, members explore together the problems presented. The treatment plan is aimed at meeting the needs of each individual "special" patient. Rather consistently, nurses feel like police or maids when they attempt to integrate the special patient into the hospital world. A physician who was hospitalized with thrombosed hemorrhoids illustrates this point. Dr. Morris was in pain and annoyed to be in the hospital. He basically wanted to be left alone, although the "hospital family" paraded into his room all day long. Dr. Morris felt obligated to be the host, yet viewed the visits as intrusive. After discussing within the group her concerns about caring for Dr. Morris, his primary nurse agreed to discuss the treatment plan with the patient. Dr. Morris was enormously relieved to have privacy restored and to be assured of the rest he needed. An envelope was placed on the door asking hospital friends to aid Dr. Morris's recovery and allow him to rest. A request was made to please leave a message for Dr. Morris, which he would have to enjoy reading when he awakened. The result was that the "hospital family" felt involved and not annoyed, and, most important, Dr. Morris was allowed to be a patient and to receive appropriate treatment and care.

Within the group the emphasis moves away from who the special patient is or what happened, and toward what this illness means for this particular patient. When there is fanfare around a patient, it can be difficult to remain focused on the central issues of nursing care. "Special" patients create a myriad of feelings in nurses, which are then discussed within the group. What does it feel like to intimately care for someone who has murdered? What about the rage and horror of caring for a battered woman or an abused child? Patients who are special are appropriately, effectively, and safely discussed in the nurses' group.

professional issues

victimization. Because of the usual stresses of the hospital, nurses may feel unjustifiably victimized or blamed for inadequate patient care. When tension increases on a ward, it is not unusual for professional relationships to become strained. The issue of feeling victimized is presented in various forms in the nurses' groups. For example, the doctor is enraged because the patient who is on forced fluids has only had 200 cc by 3:30 PM. However, the patient was delayed in x-ray until 2:30 PM. The nurse is held responsible. One of the most difficult concepts to convey is the necessity of dealing directly with each other about feelings. The group setting allows for the ventilation and the exploration of possible alternative interactions with other health care providers. The sharing and mutual support allow nurses, most often, to see the conflict in perspective and then to deal with it directly. Since little is accomplished in the heat of anger, discussing in the group a chain of events that resulted in the nurse receiving the "heat" cools the situation. It increases the possibility that the nurse may deal with the situation more rationally and less defensively.

patient advocacy. It is not uncommon for the nursing staff, through the intimate and prolonged contact with patients, to find themselves as the advocate for the patient. A vigorous approach by house staff, resulting in frequent uncomfortable procedures for the patient, may result in confusion and disagreement on the part of the nursing staff. Why subject this elderly gentleman to a diagnostic test, the result of which will not change the course of treatment or prognosis? Through the group discussion, nurses can explore together and gain understanding of the complexity of treatment decisions and responsibilities. With this understanding, communication with the physician staff may improve and reduce feelings of helplessness, frustration, and inadequacy.

nurse–doctor relationship.   Nurses frequently bring up nurse–doctor conflicts, which may serve as a foil for nursing staff conflicts. A common victim may be the new intern or the elderly physician, who are the most defenseless. It is rare and threatening for nurses to discuss the inadequacy of and competition between nurses, but they often have less restraint with other health care providers. On wards where respect between professions is genuine, this sort of conflict is less likely to occur. The approach of the leader is consistent by proposing communication between the nurse and doctor to encourage understanding. Often the nursing staff feel relieved by complaining, and they resist talking to the doctor. However, when they do decide to work at improving the relationship, nurses find that there can be a change in nurse–doctor relationships, especially when they share their anxiety with each other. Communication in conflict situations has been found to be difficult for nurses as a group. Kramer encourages a reorientation of nurses toward conflict, advocating the learning of skills to manage conflict [27].

male–female.   The changing roles of men and women have had their affect on the nurse–doctor relationship. As sex stereotyping changes, especially in the profession of medicine, nurses are confronted with different relationships. The competitiveness between female nurse and female doctor replaces for some the seduction between male doctor and female nurse. The changes in society are reflected in the group issues. Roles may not be perceived as clearly. All this produces anxiety for patients and professionals. This theme is emerging as an important professional issue.

Achilles heel.   The group leader may recognize a sensitive area or an issue for certain staff members in the group, which may or may not be recognized by group members. Sometimes group members volunteer their sensitive and/or personalized area, that is, their "Achilles heel." A medical nurse in the group frequently mentioned being sensitive to patients' auditory systems when they are in a coma, as she had an experience with her brother who had been in a coma for a year. Another nurse focused on diabetic teaching because her father was diabetic. The important point is, more often than not, that the leader is unaware of the nurse's personal life. Therefore paying attention to the probability of sensitive areas may help the nurses to acknowledge these feelings, if they wish, or to silently recognize them. Using a case example from another clinical setting can promote this process in a comfortable way.

competition between nurses.   As professionals, nurses are encouraged
to work together. Among nurses, personal competition is often discouraged and denied, although it is an integral part of human relationships. Issues of competition are masked and are rarely dealt with
openly. Cliques and/or subgroups within the nursing staff are common vehicles for the expression of competition. Barriers are erected
between arbitrary groupings such as between the 3-to-11 and the
11-to-7 shift nurses, between newly employed and more senior
nurses, between the young and the old, or between hospital units. In
one hospital, the competitive spirit erupted in the group meetings
when it became known that several surgeons preferred admitting
their patients to a particular surgical unit because they thought the
nursing care was better. Within the group, competition was acknowledged and a problem-solving approach was utilized.

nurses as martyrs.   Nurses caring for patients in a hospital have, in addition to the stress put on them by the patient's illness, the added burden of stresses within the institution. What becomes apparent in the
groups is the theme of martyrdom. When there is a sick call, a volunteer is needed to work nights. Many times, especially with less experienced nurses, their expectations of themselves may be unrealistic. If
nurses are unable to set limits for themselves, they may feel angry
and unappreciated. This is the precursor to being "burned out." Discussion concerning setting limits and establishing realistic expectations becomes vital.

burn-out.   At least twice a year in each nurses' group, the liaison nurse
finds a staff quiet and lifeless. This phenomenon usually occurs after
a long period of difficult patients, staff resignations, or multiple
patient deaths. The group is unable to focus on any patient issue and
remains listless. When the concept of feeling burned-out is brought
up, the group often quickly identifies with the multiple problems
contributing to their overwhelming feeling of discouragement.
Maslach describes the burn-out syndrome as being characterized by
physical and emotional exhaustion in which the professional person
no longer has any positive feelings, sympathy, or respect for patients
or clients [28]. Ventilation is important with this theme. However,
the priority remains on resolving the present situation, diminishing
the intensity of reoccurrence, and continuing to provide therapeutic
patient care.

rescue fantasy.   On occasion, nurses as a group or as individuals may become so involved with a patient that they believe in some way their interaction will bring a major change to the patient's life. There is some attraction in the patient that precipitates this phenomenon. This tendency is most readily recognized in the nurses' group when a sense of unreality about the patient emerges. The interaction between staff and patient is so intense and powerful that the exposure of the fantasy must be slow, deliberate, and sensitively executed. A young drug-addicted woman from a local prestigious college was admitted for surgery. The patient was not the stereotype drug addict, and the staff was unable to accept her as a drug addict. As a staff, they saw themselves as "understanding" the patient, and they saw previous health care providers as "misunderstanding" the patient. It is very painful for nurses to recognize that they have lost their perspective.

affectual issues

Although many feelings are expressed within the group, the nature of the hospital setting results in a repetition of the following affectual themes.

anger.   Ventilating pent-up feelings of anger and hostility is cathartic. There are few opportunities to react freely to the tension and intensity of ward activities. Many of the cases presented in the group are unsolvable. The patient remains in the hospital, as does the myriad of problems. When the anger at the system, health care providers, patient, family, or anyone can be expressed by the group members, as well as heard and tolerated by the liaison nurse, the consultee feels a sense of relief. As the staff must return to the bedside, it is far better to acknowledge, accept, and diffuse the anger than to deny or ignore it.

frustration.   The goals of aiding the sick and of restoring them to health are frequently interrupted by medical complications and limitations of the hospital system. These interruptions lead to frustration. Short staffing and sick calls place additional burdens on the nurse. Extended hospitalizations, which sap the patients' psychological energy, place an even greater burden on nurses. As patients' illnesses require nurses to assume more of their ego functioning, nurses become tired and depleted. This theme is experienced in the form of general malaise, depression, or displacement. The complexities of the milieu are a consideration in attempting to discover with the group the possible causes of frustration in the staff and to identify possible resolutions.

sadness.   The professional education of nurses tends to discourage the
theme of sadness to emerge with high frequency. If nurses were to
react sadly to the multitude of problems and infirmities observed,
they might become nonfunctional. At times the proximity and/or
rapidity of highly charged situations extinguishes the more acceptable coping mechanisms and results in overt expressions of sadness.
The group can acknowledge, tolerate, and normalize these feelings.

loneliness.   A less obvious, but persistent theme, is that of loneliness.
When patients, most often elderly, are alone without family or
friends, the feelings aroused in nurses are intense and personalized.
Nurses may be struck by the sense of abandonment and isolation of
the patient. Many of the nurses, in their identification with these
issues, feel both frightened and protective for themselves and/or for
their families. This feeling may be expressed obliquely, or it may
result in interactions with the patient anywhere along the spectrum of
empathy to withdrawal. In dealing with this theme, the work of the
group is to assist nurses in identifying ways of being professionally
available to patients.

illness issues

drug/alcohol-addicted patients.   The very nature of patients who are
addicted may make their hospitalization traumatic for them and for
the health care providers. The structure of the hospital and the
restrictions of the ward often precipitate unmanageable behaviors in
the addicted patients. Liaison nurses are frequently involved in the
management of these patients. Their adaptation to the hospital often
results in acting out behavior that requires immediate attention. The
necessity of limit setting is clearly apparent for staff, but achieving it
without being punitive is problematic. Since addicted patients have
usually learned to manipulate many systems to support their addic-
tions, the inevitable clash with the health care system occurs rapidly.
To effectively intervene, it is helpful to become aware of potential
problems early in the hospitalization.

    Addicted patients are commonly presented in the nurses' groups
because they are often disruptive on the ward. The individual needs
of the patient, the anticipated problems associated with addiction,
and the medical illness are explored in the group. There is an opportunity through the group process to develop more effective and realistic interventions. Nurses are also afforded the opportunity to

achieve a professional stance toward addiction rather than assuming a moralistic or judgmental viewpoint.

extended hospitalization. Patients suffering from multiple trauma or fractures that require a prolonged hospitalization in an acute care setting frequently experience psychological difficulties. Characteristically, such illnesses do not affect the mental alertness or acuity of the patient, whereas illnesses that have systemic effect may dull the awareness of the patient. The patient with a fractured femur requiring a six-week hospitalization usually becomes involved, by the nature of his or her confinement, in some degree of self-struggle or struggle with the staff. Within the nurses' group, attempts are made to anticipate problems that may erupt and to engage in preventive care. Patients who are immobilized must be assessed individually and cared for with appropriate treatment plans. Their psychological adaptation is a frequent subject for discussion in nurses' groups.

psychological reactions to specific physical illness. As liaison nurses, we have increasingly observed predictable feelings or stages that patients seem to experience around certain illnesses. Cassem and Hackett have written extensively about the coronary patient [29]. When MI patients display extreme and sometimes bizarre denial, through group discussions nurses can begin to understand the "normalcy" of their behavior. Learning that behaviors can be adaptive helps the nurses to support patients. Learning the usual psychological course of the post-myocardial infarction patient is as helpful as learning the usual medical course. It allows nurses to reassure patients appropriately yet to be consistently aware of individual differences and reactions.

As nurses' groups develop, group members become increasingly interested in learning about predictable psychological stages in certain illnesses. With the MI patient as an example, it becomes clear that this awareness and knowledge by the staff is helpful to patients. A further development of this is the concept of patient-to-patient peer counseling [30]. The assurance that others have felt the same way is potentially helpful.

The list of possible themes is endless. We have chosen to discuss a few of the more common to illustrate the predictable content of the nurses' group. Other themes that have been observed include:

- noncompliant patients,
- patients from different cultures,

- patients suffering from specific illnesses such as cancer, COPD, or mutilating surgery,
- chronically ill patients, and
- patients presenting a diagnostic dilemma.

These categories certainly deserve consideration and, coupled with those not mentioned, may represent an important area for research in psychiatric liaison nursing.

section 6   group resistance and interpretation

Liaison nurses attempt to recognize resistance and its effect on the process of the group. Utilizing consultation theory, they "diagnose the total consultation," while applying their knowledge of groups and their observations of the process within the group. If the group process and the achievement of group goals are being significantly inhibited, as group leaders, they try to intervene. Although continually searching for ways to strengthen their alliances with the consultees, as group leaders, they have certain responsibilities. Sharing observations of repeated examples of resistance in a nonjudgmental, yet supportive and questioning manner may become necessary. (For example, "I have become aware that X keeps happening ... It seems like this is becoming a problem ... I'm confused as to why ... .") The purpose is to clarify the etiology of the resistance and hopefully to resolve it. In doing so, liaison nurses may learn that the consultees are still not clear on the goals and format of the group. They may also learn that a nursing staff that they believed to be ready for a group was really not ready at all.

The success of a nurses' group is dependent, in part, on the clinical skills of the liaison nurse. Nevertheless, there may still be times when the group will be ineffective, just as there are times when individual consultations will be ineffective. The variables that can influence the effectiveness of the group are numerous. Many are beyond the control of the liaison nurse. Most unsuccessful nurses' groups are a result of some kind of internal ward problem, which may never be identified. The success of a group is dependent on staffing, high morale, and effective leadership on the ward [31]. An accurate assessment of the ward prior to group negotiation and creation, combined with an ongoing reassessment, can aid in decreasing possible resistance.

Confrontation on issues that are clearly demonstrative of resistance is more often than not counterproductive. Unless the consultee–consultant alliance is firm, psychodynamic interpretations may promote a very negative reaction in the consultees. This reaction can be either overt or covert. The result can be the termination of the nurses' group and/or a decreased use of the liaison nurse. Confronting resistance can be misunderstood and/or distorted by the consultees.

Clinical example: A nurses' group was conducted on a gyn ward for four and a half years. During that time there had been many different head nurses. The group had been renegotiated with each head nurse so as to avoid the group being unwillingly inherited. The group had occurred with great regularity, and feedback had been quite positive. The nursing staff usually had patients that they wished to discuss, as well as many feelings and reactions to working with gyn patients in general. When the ward was under the direction of one head nurse, there were fewer and fewer meetings. The head nurse frequently cancelled the meetings, stating that the ward had "no problems" to discuss and that everything was "fine."

The liaison nurse overestimated her consultation alliance and underestimated the anxiety of the head nurse. She confronted the head nurse's resistance to the group by sharing with her that the group, until this time, had always been an integral part of the ward's milieu and was not sure as to why it was being cancelled so frequently. The confrontation was personalized by the head nurse. She experienced it as a criticism of her leadership abilities. The liaison nurse failed to first adequately explore with the head nurse her understanding of the purpose of the group. The liaison nurse failed to solicit feedback from the head nurse as to what did and did not make the group valuable for her staff. The head nurse responded that although she had heard that the group had been helpful in the past, talking about sexuality and how patients make nurses feel was, in her opinion, often harmful to nurses because it got them "very upset and stirred up."

At this point, any attempts to reclarify, explain, and/or modify the content of the group was impossible, as the head nurse was clearly angry with and threatened by the liaison nurse. From a psychodynamic standpoint, it was important for the liaison nurse to understand the kind of threat that she and the group posed for the head nurse. However, this knowledge could have been obtained without getting into a control struggle with the head nurse who, by the very nature of her administrative position, could and did terminate the group. Consultations on this ward also decreased in number until such time as the liaison nurse rebuilt her alliance with the head nurse.

In clinical supervision and psychotherapy, that which may be accurately diagnosed as resistance is usually taken up with the client. Reluctance or refusal to meet in the group can be an indication of anxiety. Perhaps the group process has been too hot or too threatening. This is best dealt with by providing clear re-explanation of the group's goals and format and by case illustrations of how the group may be utilized. A reluctance or refusal to meet can also be an indication of negative feedback regarding the value of the group. If this is the case, the etiology of the resistance may be explored with the consultees. The liaison nurse needs to ask the consultees if the group has been helpful. If the response is negative, the liaison nurse explores this with the group members. Hopefully, specific ways in which the group can become a more valuable experience will be identified.

If the consultees feel that the group has been helpful, the liaison nurse continues to attempt to understand, with the group members, the reluctance or refusal to meet. Is this truly resistance or is something else going on? Perhaps the consultees just do not have the energy to participate in a group that day. Perhaps the ward has been unusually chaotic, and the nurses are determined to leave work on time. The group meeting may potentially prevent their doing so. This is not to say that the group is not important. The group is important, but other concerns are important as well. Perhaps the consultees do not believe that it is necessary for the group to meet. The overt expression of not needing to have a group is not always an indication of "ominous latent content." Respectful tolerance of the wishes and views of the group members is important at that time, regardless of whether or not the leader fully agrees. Even if the liaison nurse is aware of a difficult or potentially difficult situation on the ward, if the consultees claim that they are not having any problems, the tenets of consultation theory and not group theory are followed.

Some examples of resistance by group members are:

1. refusing to carry out interventions that are clinically and theoretically sound as well as in the best interest of the patient;
2. presenting patients in the group when the most knowledgeable nurses in terms of these specific patients are not present;
3. consistently attempting to utilize the group for discussion of personal and/or administrative problems;
4. engaging in multiple simultaneous conversations within the group;
5. allowing unnecessary interruptions during the group;
6. refraining from asking nonmembers to leave the room in which the group is being held;
7. making unnecessary phone calls during the group;
8. writing nurses' notes, charting meds, and performing other tasks during the group;
9. cancelling group meetings; and
10. leaving the group early.

Historically, when nurses feel like they are being analyzed, they flee. Simon and Whitely found that when they invited nursing staff to join them in writing about their group experiences, there was resentment and anger [32]. Resistance is observed by the leader in terms of the ongoing integration of group process. However, it is not usually verbally acknowledged.

section 7   evaluation of groups

When evaluating a nurses' group, specific parameters prove useful. The following parameters will be discussed:

1. verbal feedback,
2. behavioral feedback,
3. group legacy,
4. requests for formal psychiatric consultation,
5. utilization of social workers and other mental health professionals,
6. group content,
7. "problemless groups,"
8. peer teaching,
9. group cohesion,
10. hidden agendas,
11. documentation,
12. requests for nurses' groups,
13. patient-care/management crises,
14. preventative consultation, and
15. dependency.

Verbal feedback is a useful criterion for evaluation. Just as asking for feedback on a specific consultation can be helpful to the liaison nurse, so can the same request be made of group members. This is a very direct method of attempting to gather data, while encouraging members to participate in making the group experience valuable.

Behavioral feedback, also an important criterion, can be demonstrated in more therapeutic interventions with patients. In addition, it has been our experience that many members try to schedule their time and come in early or on days off to attend the group.

As the group continues, a *legacy* develops. As older members leave, the legacy is passed on to new members. The liaison nurse may receive direct feedback concerning the nurses' group as an outgrowth of its legacy. New members may ask the liaison nurse about the group and in so doing share the "grapevine version."

Certain parameters appear to be significant in terms of evaluating the utilization of the nurses' group. It has been our experience that, if the group is successful—that is, if it is working toward the achievement of appropriate goals—there is an *increase in the requests for formal consultation* from the psychiatry service. Through the process of the group, members can not only learn to apply mental health principles to general nursing practice, but also to recognize areas in which psychiatric consultation is needed. More specifically, members can demonstrate their ability to *differentiate which mental health professional might be employed* for consultation. Experience in the group aids members in identifying areas in which they are clinically responsible.

Through collaboration, teaching, and support, more sophisticated patient-care issues may be presented and discussed in the group. Hence the *group content* advances. The level and type of consultation requested within the group can dramatically change, as illustrated in the section on themes. Consultation may be requested in the context of a desire either to become more professional or to improve psychiatric assessment and intervention skills. The discussion of issues that are appropriate to group goals is a reasonable criterion to utilize in evaluating the group. Even if the same kinds of issues are repeatedly presented, the group may still be a valuable experience for its members. Liaison nurses review the process over time, the nature and influence of the milieu in which the group exists, and the needs of the group members. They continually consider the group goals and determine which one(s) take precedence, given these other factors. The inherent value of the group is not a function of reaching all the goals within a specific time frame. Each group differs in its ability and readiness to achieve its fullest potential. Therefore, as long as group content is appropriate, professional development is more likely to occur.

It is helpful to understand the *problemless groups* when evaluating nurses' groups. A problemless group is one in which the members do not present a specific patient or patient-care situation for consultation and discussion. The members either directly or indirectly convey that they are not having any problems, while still wanting the group to take place.

At times, problemless groups may be an indication of anxiety and resistance. In these instances, the problemless group may be a result of the members' fear of evaluation and criticism. Liaison nurses assess how clearly and consistently they have demonstrated and promoted safety, confidentiality, and nonevaluation. Frequent problemless groups may be a signal to liaison nurses that they and the group are not trusted. They may also be an indication that the members feel that they have overburdened the leader. The problemless group may be an expression of "pseudo-burn-out." Group members may feel a need to refrain from discussing problematic situations.

However, there may be times when problemless groups are not an indication of anxiety and resistance. They may be an indication of group cohesiveness and of a positive group experience. This group may be motivated by a desire to share with the leader "good things" as opposed to "problems." The problemless group may be a gesture to include the leader in the "more enjoyable" aspects of life on the ward. It may be an attempt to assure the group leader that the members are "OK" despite the difficult problems with which they are often faced. It may be a time for the members and leader to become closer, while expressing genuine interest and enjoyment in spending professional time together. The problemless group may be a time for liaison nurses to identify previously unrecognized needs of the group members, as well as their own learning needs. It can serve as a time to listen for feedback and further evaluation. However, they note the frequency with which problemless groups occur, in order to differentiate possible resistance from a potentially productive use of group time.

Liaison nurses keep in mind that throughout the group, the expectations on them as group leaders and as consultants remain constant. They may find that, as a consequence, the provision of empathy is also expected. This is an ingredient in creating a meaningful group experience. Empathy is the unique expression of warmth and understanding. It is related to the development of a sense of identification within the group. With a sense of commonality in the group, cohesiveness increases, resulting in empathic communication. The problemless group may be an expression of the degree to which empathy has been experienced in the group. If liaison nurses never experience a problemless group on a ward where the nurses' group has been relatively consistently occurring, they may benefit from assessing the quality and quantity of empathy that they are expressing and encouraging within the group.

The frequency and quality of *peer teaching*, along with the degree of *group cohesion*, are useful evaluation criteria. There is value for members in sharing patient care experiences—and not only patient care problems. Peer teaching and learning can occur at these times. In turn, group cohesion is augmented.

Although a professional group where problems and issues concerning clinical nursing practice are explored, the expectation on group members to develop and implement solutions, to always demonstrate and apply learning from previous experiences, is minimal. The expectations on members, which the liaison nurse conveys throughout the group, are syntonic with the principles of consultation theory. The nursing staff does not have to be faced with a specific patient-care problem to have the group. Consequently, group members need not feel that they must work diligently during the group to present the leader with a great nursing care plan or newly attained clinical insight.

As previously mentioned, a nursing staff that is very eager for a group may not be ready for a group. In this situation, the nursing staff is usually not clear as to the goals and format of such a group and are looking for something quite different. The identification of a *hidden agenda* within the process of negotiating for a nurses' group or within the workings of the established group is an appropriate evaluation criterion. A discovery of this nature would indicate poorly understood and/or not agreed-upon group goals.

Although less important, other criteria must be considered in evaluating a nurses' group. *Documentation*, as demonstrated in nurses' progress notes, nursing care plans, Kardex, and retrospective audits, can reflect the effectiveness of the work of the group, as it reflects the bedside care of the patient. *Requests for nurses' groups* from staffs that do not have groups may indicate that the nurses' group is regarded as a meaningful and valuable experience. Liaison nurses may also notice that the number of *patient-care management crises* on a ward that has a nurses' group greatly decrease. In addition, they may observe that the group members request consultation and/or inform the liaison nurses of a specific situation prior to its reaching crisis level—that is, for *preventative consultation*. Also, problems that would normally reach crisis level are safely managed until they can be discussed in the group. Problems that would usually frustrate a nursing staff may no longer be viewed as problems. They may have been mastered and the group members themselves may recognize this.

The quality and expression of *dependency* on the group and on its leader is another evaluation parameter. The group may frequently end with the members "thanking" each other and the leader for the meeting. Liaison nurses may observe that the group assumes that they are knowledgeable of certain patient-care situations. These specific situations are presented in such a way as to imply familiarity on the part of the leader. In making this assumption, the group members demonstrate both their dependency on the leader as well as the degree to which he or she is regarded as a member of the group.

In evaluating a nurses' group, some of the usual parameters prove nonapplicable. For example, group attendance would be a less valid means by which to evaluate the effectiveness of the group experience. The very nature of the hospital milieu and the patient-care demands makes consistent group attendance difficult. The frequency and intensity of emotional reactions shared in the group are not reliable parameters. Nurses' groups differ from each other in terms of the members, their values, their norms, and the patient-care needs of each ward. There is variation in the thematic content of nurses' groups. The group's understanding and expectation that emotions can be shared may be present. Nevertheless, members vary in their ability to identify and to express emotions. There is variation in the level of professional sophistication within any group. Some members are more skilled than others in conceptualizing patient-care issues and in formulating interventions. Nurses vary in their abilities, internal motivations, and degrees of commitment in fulfilling clinical responsibilities and in participating in the group.

summary

As a nurses' group exists and functions over time, the working factors are operationalized. During this process, the group members challenge and validate the goals, format, and the norms of the group. The legacy of the group develops and is passed on to new members. The identification of specific stages of group development, although possible, may not be as helpful in understanding the group process as is the identification of the issues being presented for group consultation. Since the nurses' group is yet another modality for consultation, the emphasis is on the "diagnosis of the total consultation" rather than on the delineation of the developmental stages of the group. This emphasis is paramount to the success or failure of the nurses' group.

All psychiatric nursing consultation has a process level. As previously stated, this level reflects the latent or unconscious content of the consultation, and the nature of the interpersonal relationship between consultant and consultee. The process level includes the identification issues, the manner in which they are expressed and the role these issues play in the success or failure of the consultation. Within the group, the process level of interaction is magnified. Multiple transferences are cognitively acknowledged by the liaison nurse. Similarly, the specific roles that individual group members assume, as well as the relationships between them, are acknowledged.

If goals are to be achieved, liaison nurses attempt to support the group members in their efforts to interact with each other and with the leader. Utilizing their knowledge of group theory, they listen for the latent content but refrain from sharing interpretations. The purpose of formulation, or of recognizing the etiology and degree of anxiety/resistance in groups, are purely for the edification of group leaders. Coupled with their efforts to assist members in accomplishing the task of the group, liaison nurses have demonstrated their clinical skill through their individual consultations prior to the establishment of a nurses' group. Hopefully, the issues of trust, confidentiality, and safety have been addressed. Woven into the consultation alliance, these issues augment the potential for members to productively utilize the group. However, this is by no means an absolute. The development of a nurses' group, as well as its progression and its regression, can be influenced by many variables. Among these are group meeting regularity, attendance, general investment, manifest and latent content, degree of participation, level of trust, the interplay of the working factors, and the skill of the group leader. Regardless of which issue or which working factor takes precedence in influencing the direction of the group, the responsibilities of the leader, the liaison nurse, remain constant. "It is the consultant's role to disentangle the interwoven group factors presented to him and find some clarity and sense in the total picture so that some positive change, however minimal, may be effected [33]."

The value of a nurses' group can be measured through the utilization of the previously described criteria. Any improvement in the quality of nursing care, any indication that professional consciousness regarding the psychological needs of patients and nurses has been raised, indicates, to some degree, the potential benefits of such a group. All the ramifications of nonjudgmentally supporting group members in their efforts to understand the "care-giving" experience is immeasurable. The value of time, specifically designed for the group, regardless of how consistently it is utilized, is also immeasurable. Clearly, nurses' groups are another means of achieving the goals of psychiatric nursing consultation.

references

1. Abraham Zaleznik, Manfred F. Q. Kets de Vries, and John Howard, "Stress Reactions in Organizations: Syndromes, Causes and Consequences," *Behavioral Science* 22:3 (1977): 160. Reprinted with permission by James Grier Miller, M.D., Ph.D., Editor.

2. Anita Lewis and Sue Foster, "An Examination of the Hospitalization Experience and the Role of the Nurse in Patient Advocacy," a research study on Primary Nursing conducted at the New England Medical Center Hospital, Boston, Mass., 1977.

3. Janice K. Janker, "The Nurse in Crisis," *The Nursing Clinics of North America* 9:1 (March 1974): 17.

4. Beulah Parker, "Psychiatric Consultation for Non-Psychiatric Professional Workers," in *Public Health Monograph*, No. 53 (Washington, D.C.: Department of Health, Education and Welfare, 1958), p. 2.

5. The reader is referred to the bibliography at the end of this chapter for a listing on writings of group therapy, group process, technique, and related subjects.

6. George H. Labovitz, "Criteria and Processes of Group Formation, Managing Groups: The Key to Productivity," Individualized Education Services, Modu-Learn Systems, *Motivational Dynamics* (Minneapolis Control Data, 1975), pp. 1–5.

7. Jean A. Werner, "Relating Group Theory to Nursing Practice," *Perspectives in Psychiatric Care* 8:6 (1970): 257.

8. C. Clark, *The Nurse as Group Leader* (New York: Springer Publishing, 1977), p. 172.

9. W. R. Bion, *Experiences in Groups* (New York: Ballantine Books, 1974), pp. 132–151.

10. Irvin D. Yalom, *The Theory and Practice of Group Psychotherapy* (New York: Basic Books, Inc., Publishers, 1975), pp. 3–82. Reprinted with permission.

11. Yalom, p. 5. Reprinted with permission.

12. Karen S. Zander, *Primary Nursing Development and Management* (Germantown, Maryland: Aspen Publication, 1980).

13. Janker, p. 17.

14. The reader is referred to the bibliography at the end of this chapter for a listing on writings of group theory, group process, techniques, and related subjects.

15. Yalom, p. 11. Reprinted with permission.

16. Gail S. Fidler, "The Task-Oriented Group as a Context for Treatment," *Journal of Occupational Therapy* 23:1 (1969): 45.

17. S. H. Foulkes and E. J. Anthony, *Group Psychotherapy: The Psychoanalytic Approach*, 2nd ed. (England: Penguin Books Ltd., 1965), p. 33.

18. Yalom, p. 11. Reprinted with permission.

19. Amargit Chopra, "Motivation in Task-Oriented Groups," *Journal of Nursing Administration* (January–February 1973): 60.

20. Yalom, pp. 16–35. Reprinted with permission.

21. Yalom, p. 6. Reprinted with permission.

22. J. Altrocchi, C. Spielberger, and R. Eisdorfer, "Mental Health Consultation with Groups," *Community Mental Health Journal* 2 (Summer 1965): 127–134.

23. S. Bailis, S. Bernstein, and S. Lambert, "The Legacy of the Group: A Study of Group Therapy with a Transient Membership," *Social Work in Health Care* 3:4 (Summer 1978): 405–418.

24. James Goodwin, Sean Goodwin, and Albert Vogel, "Knowledge and Use of

Placebos by House Officers and Nurses," *Annals of Internal Medicine* 91 (1979): 106–110.

25. Goodwin, Goodwin, and Vogel, pp. 106–110.

26. Robert Kolodny, William Masters, Virginia Johnson, and Mac Biggs, *Textbook of Human Sexuality for Nurses* (Boston: Little, Brown & Co., 1979).

27. M. S. Kramer, "Conflict: The Cutting Edge of Growth," *Journal of Nursing Administration* (October 1976): 10–25.

28. Christina Maslach, "The Burn-Out Syndrome and Patient Care," in *Stress and Survival*, edited by C. Garfield (St. Louis: The C. V. Mosby Company, 1979).

29. N. H. Cassem and T. P. Hackett, "Psychiatric Consultation in a Coronary Care Unit," *Annals of Internal Medicine* 75 (1971): 9–14.

30. F. G. Guggenheim and S. O'Hara, "Peer Counseling in a General Hospital," *American Journal of Psychiatry* 133 (1976): 1197–1199.

31. L. J. Weinstein, M. M. Chapman, and M. A. Stallings, "Organizing Approaches to Psychiatric Nurse Consultation," *Perspectives in Psychiatric Care* 17:2 (1979): 67.

32. N. Simon and S. Whitely, "Psychiatric Consultation with MICU Nurses: The Consultation Conference as a Working Group," *Heart and Lung* 6:3 (May–June 1977): 497–504.

33. A. Issacharoff, R. Redinger, and D. Schneider, "The Psychiatric Consultation as an Experience in Group Process," *Contemporary Psychoanalysis* 8 (1972): 261.

bibliography

books

COHEN, R. G. and LIPKIN, G. B. *Therapeutic Group Work for Health Professionals.* New York: Springer Publishing Company, 1979.

GLASER, B. G. and STRAUSS, A. L. *Awareness of Dying.* Chicago: Aldine Publishing Co., 1965.

GRAY, W.; DUHL, R. J.; and RIZZO, N. D., eds. *General Systems Theory and Psychiatry.* Boston: Little, Brown & Co., 1969.

KAPLAN, H. I. and SADOCK, R. J., eds. *Comprehensive Group Psychotherapy.* Baltimore: The Williams and Wilkins Co., 1971.

KUBLER–ROSS, E. *On Death and Dying.* New York: Macmillan, Inc., 1969.

LIFF, Z. A., ed. *The Leader in the Group.* New York: Jason Aronson, Inc., 1975.

LOOMIS, M. E. *Group Process for Nurses.* St. Louis: The C. V. Mosby Company, 1979.

OLMSTED, M. S. *The Small Group.* New York: Random House, Inc., 1960.

SLAVSON, S. R. *An Introduction to Group Therapy.* New York: International Universities Press, Inc., 1970.

SKINNER, B. F. *Science and Human Behavior.* New York: The Free Press, 1953.

YALOM, IRVIN D. *The Theory and Practice of Group Psychotherapy.* New York: Basic Books, Inc., Publishers, 1975.

articles

BERMAN, L. "Countertransference and Attitudes of the Analyst in the Therapeutic Process," *Psychiatry* 12 (1949).

BILODEAU, C. and O'CONNOR, S. "Role of Nurse Clinicians in Liaison Psychiatry," in *Massachusetts General Hospital Handbook of General Hospital Psychiatry*, edited by T. P. Hackett and N. H. Cassem. St. Louis: The C. V. Mosby Company, 1978, pp. 508–523.

CASSEM, N. H. and HACKETT, T. P. "Psychiatric Consultation in a Coronary Care Unit," *Annals of Internal Medicine* 75 (1971): 9–14.

CLARK, C. "Burnout: Assessment and Intervention," *Journal of Nursing Administration* 10:9 (September 1980): 39–43.

GLADSTONE, T. U. and McKEGNEY, F. P. "Relationship Between Patient Behaviors and Nursing Staff Attitudes," *Supervisor Nurse* (June 1980): 32–35.

GLASER, INA and HORVATH, KATHY. "A Tool for Dealing with Nursing Problems," *Supervisor Nurse* (April 1979): 46–52.

IVANCEVICH, JOHN and MATTESON, MICHAEL. "Nurses and Stress: Time to Examine the Potential Problem," *Supervisor Nurse* (June 1980): 17–22.

LARKIN, B. and CROWDES, N. "Nurse Consultation: The Instilling of Hope," *Supervisor Nurse* 7:11 (November 1976): 54–58.

LARSON, MARGARET L. and WILLIAMS, R. A. "How to Become a Better Group Leader," *Nursing '78* (August): 65–72.

LEWIS, A. and ANTOS, P. "Psychological Care of the Patient and the Self-Esteem Needs of the Nurse." Unpublished Survey. Boston, Mass.: New England Medical Center, 1981.

MENDELSON, M. and MEYER, EUGENE. "Countertransference Problems of the Liaison Psychiatrist," *Psychosomatic Medicine* 23:2 (1961): 115–121.

MENIKHEIM, MARIE. "Communication Patterns of Women and Nurses," in *Women in Stress: A Nursing Perspective*, edited by D. Kjervik and I. Martinson. New York: Appleton-Century-Crofts, 1979.

MOHL, P. C. "A Review of Systems Approaches to Consultation—Liaison Psychiatry," *General Hospital Psychiatry* 3:2 (June 1981): 103–110.

———. "A Systems Approach to Liaison Psychiatry," *Psychosomatics* 21:6 (June 1980): 457–461.

———. "Group Process Interpretations in Liaison Psychiatry Nurse Groups," *General Hospital Psychiatry* (1980): 104–111.

NETZER, ROSEANN E. "Nursing Management of the Chronic Pain Patient." An unpublished clinical paper, Boston University (May, 1980).

PALERMO, ELEANOR. "Mental Health Consultation in a Home Care Agency," *Journal of Psychiatric Nursing and Mental Health Services* (September 1978): 21–23.

PARKER, BEULAH. "Psychiatric Consultation for Non-Psychiatric Professional Workers," in *Public Health Monograph*, No. 53. Washington, D.C.: Department of Health, Education and Welfare, 1958.

RANDOLPH, B. M. and BERNAM, K. "Dealing with Resistance in the Nursing Care Conference," *American Journal of Nursing* (December 1977): 1955–1958.

REIMAN, D. W. "Group Mental Health Consultation with Public Health Nurses," in *Consultation in Social Work Practice*, edited by L. Rapaport. New York: National Association of Social Workers, 1963, pp. 85–98.

SCHEIDLINGER, SAUL. "The Concept of Empathy in Group Psychotherapy," *International Journal of Group Psychotherapy* 16 (1966): 413–424.

SCHNEIDER, I. "The Use of Patients to Act Out Professional Conflicts," *Psychiatry* 26 (1963): 88–94.

SCHULDT, SALLY. "Supervision and the Informal Organization," *Journal of Nursing Administration* (July 1978): 21–25.

SCHULMAN, BRIAN M. "Group Process: An Adjunct in Liaison Consultation Psychiatry," *International Journal of Psychiatry in Medicine* 6:4 (1975): 489–499.

SEDGWICK, RAE. "The Role of the Process Consultant," *Nursing Outlook* 21:12 (December 1973): 773–775.

SHUBIN, S. "Rx for Stress—Your Stress," *Nursing '79* (January 1979): 53–55.

VITALE, JOHN; PRESTON, LUELLA; MARKFELD, JAN; and MULLIN, SANDRA. "Small Group Method on a General Hospital Unit," *Journal of Psychiatric Nursing and Mental Health Services* (May–June 1973): 9–12.

WILLIAMS, MEYER. "Limitations, Fantasies and Security Operations of Beginning Group Psychotherapists," *International Journal of Group Psychotherapy* 16 (1966): 150–162.

7
the professional
process

The scientist's prime aim is the description
of the social world; the practioner's prime
aim is the control of that world.

GREENWOOD [1]

section 1 transference and countertransference

The medical ward was buzzing with the morning news. Mr. Roberts, an attractive, 32-year-old drug-abusing and alcoholic patient, recently discharged after a bout with pancreatitis, had appeared the previous night at the apartment of Ms. Powers, a staff nurse. He claimed that he had nowhere to stay and after negotiating with Ms. Powers to spend the night, robbed her and locked her in a room. How did this happen? What effect did the patient's issues have on this nurse? Was her relationship with him while he was hospitalized therapeutic? Why did she entice him by providing her address to him? Was she acting out a rescue fantasy? Was she not knowledgeable about "professional relationships" and simply did not understand the potential dangers? Or did this patient arouse conflictual issues that are not resolved for the nurse? Is it transference, countertransference, or simply identification?

This example raises many issues for the liaison nurse. Mr. Roberts had been hospitalized for many weeks, and as his physical condition improved he became the attractive, pleasant, misunderstood special patient. Ms. Powers spent much time talking with Mr. Roberts. Should the liaison nurse, having observed this, mention the problems of dealing with manipulative and physically attractive patients? Although not being asked to consult, would it seem intrusive to discuss this with the nurse? Once the incident occurred in the nurse's apartment, how would the liaison nurse have a role? How would it differ from the role of the head nurse?

The nurse–patient relationship may be understood on various levels, ranging from a superficial involvement to one that may be representative of intrapsychic conflicts. This relationship may precipitate transference and countertransference issues. Peplau defines the appropriate nurse–patient relationship as professional closeness, which is focused exclusively on the interests, concern, and needs of the patient [2]. Human behavior tends to repeat itself and occurs in situations where there are unresolved and unconscious conflicts [3]. Strong identification of nurses to patients has been defined as their inability to separate themselves and their problems from those of their patients. They do not perceive the uniqueness of individual patients and respond accordingly, but instead they respond to "themselves" in the patients [4]. Nurses may be viewed as comforting mothers, convenient and common love objects for frightened, ill, and frustrated patients. They may also be viewed as hated objects, representing other figures in the patients' lives: a nurturing grandfather, a despised older sister, an unfaithful friend, or the like may be bound up in patients' perceptions of nurses. These responses warrant attention as they may be reflective of transference/countertransference issues.

The psychological regression (Chapter 5), which accompanies illness and hospitalization, is a precursor to transference, just as regression precedes transference in psychotherapy. The experience of being a patient, as discussed previously, is rich with possibilities of identification and transference. Closeness with patients may stimulate a variety of fantasies and responses for both patients and nurses. For example, the intimacy of physical contact may produce sexual fantasies or anxious withdrawal. When overwhelmed psychologically, patients, in their more child-like state, may confide in nurses in a manner uncharacteristic to them. As they recover, they may feel angry toward the nurses who were with them when they were exposed either physically or psychologically. For some patients this exposure would make visiting the ward staff after discharge painful and embarrassing. Yet some patients, affected differently by this exposure, continue to return for months. Obviously, other factors influence visiting after discharge. The liaison nurse observes, thinks about, speculates, but does not interpret the relationship between nurses and patients. The hallmarks of liaison practice are navigating without adequate information and being aware of the frequent and likely possibility of error in understanding the transference.

Transference between patients and their nurses and countertransference between nurses and their patients can have both positive and negative elements. These issues can enhance or detract from the nurse–patient relationship. *Transference*, in its purest form, refers to the unconscious identities of the past ascribed to a new person. Transference also refers to unconscious emotional feelings, responses, and expectations of oneself and a person in the past, ascribed to a new relationship. Although the term transference was originally used to describe the process in psychoanalysis (Freud), manifestations of transference have been described in other professional relationships including those between nurses and patients. *Countertransference* also refers to unconscious identities, emotional feelings, responses, and expectations that are based on past relationships and ascribed to a new person. These reactions are valuable to notice yet almost never discussed with patients or nurses by the liaison nurse. A care provider's unresolved problems, displaced onto task situations, has been described as theme interference. A conflict based on real or fantasized experiences may preconsciously or unconsciously persist as a theme [5]. For this discussion, "transference/countertransference" will be applied to unconscious processes, and "identification" will be applied to conscious processes.

Identification issues also characterize the nurse–patient relationship. They are usually obvious to the liaison nurse and to the consultee. Common examples of identification issues, as experienced by nurses in regard to their patients, are stimulated by patients of the same age and sex, patients who are nurses, patients whose illness is age-related to them or to a significant person in their life, and the like. Patients may identify with nurses around issues of age, associations with other care providers, physical appearance, social interests, and so on. These identification issues may or may not indicate underlying transference/countertransference issues.

Patients may revive unresolved conflicts in the health care provider [6]. An unmotivated patient may make the provider feel unsuccessful. New patients may revive in the health care provider anxiety about strangers or change. Patients undergoing mutilating procedures may evoke fear and terror in the provider. Unless there is some understanding of this process, nurses may become too involved with patients or too remote. Nurses can usually recognize when they feel especially angry, sympathetic to suffering, emotionally drained by patient's demands, or very saddened by the ravages of illness. The responsibility rests with professional nurses to deal with conflicts in their own lives. The priority and goal are their emotional and professional availability to patients. Nurses remain responsible for their own behavior as it has the potential to influence the response from patients. Nurses struggling with their own conflicts remain unavailable to patients. In some instances these personal struggles may be so intense for them that their actions may become destructive to patients. At these times psychotherapy for nurses may be indicated.

Mr. Howard, a 62-year-old retired construction supervisor, was hospitalized for the fourth time in two months with end-stage pulmonary disease. An alcoholic most of his life, he had been estranged from his family and was experiencing difficulty living alone. Like many chronic lung patients, he clung to his cigarettes. A struggle raged with Ms. Roy, his nurse, around the safety, location, and frequency of his smoking. The covert struggle raged around control. The patient saw his nurse as a controlling female figure. Mr. Howard raised issues for Ms. Roy, the source of which remained unclear. She was unable to explore his need for control without becoming angry and feeling personally attacked. It was virtually impossible for Ms. Roy to have therapeutic interaction with Mr. Howard. The liaison nurse encouraged increased nursing staff involvement to diffuse the intensity in this clinical situation. In addition to practical suggestions, like allowing Mr. Howard to make some decisions, the liaison psychiatrist continued to work with the patient, and the liaison nurse continued to work with the staff. Their availability allowed both the staff and patient to express their rage, frustration, fear, and helplessness. In this situation, the possible transference/countertransference issues were too hot to explore. The ultimate goal of the consultation was to ensure safe and effective care for Mr. Howard, while providing Ms. Roy with permission to distance herself.

Issues of identification are usually less dangerous to the consultation alliance, generally understandable, and easier to discuss than unconscious processes. There are situations, however, when acknowledgement of the possible transference/countertranference issues by the liaison nurse prove necessary and potentially helpful. These interpretations/discussions are based on a sound alliance with the consultee, and they may be generated by the question, "What is this patient doing to you?" The decision to pursue this avenue in the consultation is based on:

1. potential or actual harm to the patient,
2. the consultee is anxious and is seeking help in understanding why, and/or
3. the consultee is visibly suffering.

Certainly not all emotional difficulties with patients are based on critical conflictual areas, but they may also be based on inexperience. The identification that occurs between the novice therapist and the patient has been noted [7]. The novice therapist feels vulnerable and anxious while the patient feels anxious and helpless. When a hospitalized patient is emotionally distressed, the inexperienced nurse feels pressured for immediate action. This pressure may emanate from a wish to be therapeutic, a fear of failure, peer pressure, supervisory pressure, and/or a wish for emotional relief. When the nurse is unable to create or implement an appropriate "treatment plan," the increase of the patient's frustration leads to an intensification of unrealistic demands. As nurses begin to feel more vulnerable, they may identify the patient as the aggressor and not solely as a possible countertransference object in their lives.

Mr. Adam, a 42-year-old patient who had cellulitis of both legs, had an uncomplicated hospital course. Initially he had resisted admission but finally did agree to hospitalization. At first, Mr. Adam's response to his illness did not interfere with his overall compliance. A close examination of the situation prior to his barricading his room and acting "psychotic" revealed a series of events that continued to escalate. The inexperienced young nurse did not recognize the significance of these events. What did it mean when Mr. Adam started refusing to swallow his pills or objected to having his blood pressure taken? When he threatened to get dressed and leave the hospital at 2:00 AM, the nurse was more frightened and overwhelmed than conflicted. Unable to recognize that Mr. Adam's behavior was based on his fear, which supported his denial of his medical needs, the nurse ineffectively tried to scare him more by explaining each medication and treatment as life saving. The young nurse did not conceptualize Mr. Adam's behavior as his response to his illness. He was viewed as uncooperative and crazy.

Relationships between nurses and patients are continually changing. As the health of patients progresses or regresses, there are different expectations in the relationship. The feelings that nurses have about themselves are subjected to judgment, threat, or stimulation. They are vulnerable to patients' suffering massive psychological trauma (Mr. Adam, in the previous example) with a resulting disorganization of their ego functions. They may also be vulnerable to patients who, during their recuperation, fight like adolescents to shed their dependence in a provocative way. At each stage, and with each patient, there may be a stimulus to a sensitive part of the nurse's own psychological makeup. The expectation on nurses by the liaison nurse is to remain aware of their feelings and reactions but not necessarily to explore the origins.

The manifestations of transference/countertransference may be

noted by liaison nurses and nurse consultees in their individual interactions with patients. Menninger and Holzman describe some of the
common cognitive, affective, and behavioral ways in which countertransference may be identified [8]. Just as this awareness is necessary
in a psychotherapy relationship, it can be an aid in therapeutic
interaction with the medically ill. Some manifestations of
transference/countertransference have been altered, applied to the
nurse–patient relationship, and listed as follows:

- repeatedly experiencing affectionate feelings toward a patient, [8]
- depressed or uneasy feelings during or after interactions with a
  patient, [8]
- permitting and even encouraging resistance in the form of acting out,
  [8]
- persistently attempting to impress the patient, [8]
- cultivating the patient's continued dependence in various ways,
  especially by unnecessary reassurances, [8]
- sadistic, unnecessary sharpness in interactions, [8]
- experiencing a strong need to care for the patient,
- experiencing conscious satisfaction from the patient's praise, appreciation, and evidence of affection, [8]
- continually arguing with the patient, [8]
- sudden increase or decrease in interest in a patient, [8]
- trying to help the patient in "extra" ways, such as financially or
  socially, [8]
- having an instant like or dislike to the patient,
- not trusting anyone else to care for the patient,
- worrying/dreaming about the patient, or
- feel intimidated by or angry with a patient.

How do transference and countertransference affect liaison
nurses? In direct encounters with hospitalized patients, the ramifications of these issues are similar to the nurse–patient interaction.
Liaison nurses are vulnerable to the same pitfalls. Presumably, their
psychiatric education and experience help them to interact in a
manner that is therapeutic for patients. Clinical supervision, a recognized adjunct to quality professional practice, assists liaison nurses in
maintaining a constant vigilance on the quality of their practice
(Chapter 3, Section 4).

There is, however, a paucity of literature on the transference/
countertransference issues specifically in liaison nursing practice.
Mendelson and Meyer's experiences as liaison psychiatrists [9] revealed that what seemed initially to be realistic pessimism or despair
in their assessment of patients was not always predictive of their

eventual value to the patient and physician. Instead their counter-transference caused them to underestimate the potential for effective intervention. For liaison nurses a similar phenomenon exists.

Mr. Green, a 34-year-old drug addict and pusher, was admitted with multiple abscesses covering his extremities. His social history was rampant with societal failures, marital discord, and inter-personal deficits. The staff nurse expressed her disgust regarding both the physical appearance of the patient and her disapproval of drug addicts and especially pushers. The liaison nurse found herself feeling the same way. When the staff nurse suggested that the patient might benefit with "help" from the liaison nurse, the latter felt helpless, hopeless, and disinterested. Previous unsuccessful attempts at in-tervention with other drug addicts had left the liaison nurse frustrated and feeling that drug addicts were very difficult to engage. Attempting to overcome her countertransference issues, the liaison nurse interviewed the patient, became engaged with him, and was able to outline and implement interventions. Some of the interven-tions included a referral to the drug treatment specialist, group meetings and daily contact with the nursing staff, a referral to social service, and collaboration with the psychiatrist and surgeons re-garding pain management and detoxification during Mr. Green's hospitalization. Only when the liaison nurse observed the nurses' change in attitude regarding Mr. Green did she understand how an inability to recognize her manifestations of countertransference might have affected care.

The liaison nurse may symbolize a variety of people, issues, and conflicts for the consultee. The reverse of this may also occur. It is possible that the liaison nurse may represent the all-knowing, protec-tive parent whose approval is sought by her/his children, the con-sultees. Liaison nurses may represent the accomplished older sibling, and the consultees may identify with them as such. Depending on how they feel about their "older sibling," the consultees may respond with feelings of pride, admiration, emulation, or unhealthy competi-tion and aggression. As an example in contrast, the consultees may represent the immature teenager or the autocratic grandparent. Is there a difference between a young, inexperienced, attractive nurse presenting the impossible patient and a middle-aged, unattractive, experienced nurse presenting the same patient?

An exploration of the triadic system of nurse–patient–liaison nurse warrants attention. Parallel processes have been identified in psychoanalytic supervision when supervisees re-enact with super-visors their interactions with patients [10]. Parallel process in the continuous case conference between the therapist/presenter, the patient, and the seminar members has also been noted [11]. Parallel processes may be observed in families when issues or conflicts are re-enacted with the family system. Parents re-enact with their children their interactions with each other or their past. A similar parallel process exists between the nurse, the patient, and the liaison nurse. Consideration is given, when a consultation is presented, to the identification between the nurse and the patient (Chapter 5). A parallel process may occur and also warrants attention when the conflicts in this relationship are re-enacted in the relationship with the liaison nurse.

Miss Paul, a 78-year-old active and independent woman who had never been hospitalized, was recovering after numerous medical complications from multiple surgical procedures for terminal cancer. She was presented as quiet, depressed, and uninvolved in her care. The nurse felt she was unresponsive to her. As the liaison nurse collected her data, prior to interviewing the patient, she felt helpless and wondered how it would be possible to get this case moving. She also thought that it might be better for the patient to give up her fight for life than prolong an inevitable downhill course. Clearly the staff nurse had re-enacted with the liaison nurse her own issues with the patient. This illustrates parallel process. The liaison nurse began to experience the same feelings as the staff nurse, as if they were contagious. If this process goes unrecognized, the liaison nurse may approach the patient with a mind set that has implications for the care of the patient and for the learning of the consultee. Counter-transference issues for the liaison nurse may or may not be related.

It is important for liaison nurses to maintain a balance between observing, experiencing, and acting on feelings, thoughts, and behaviors. Their ability to experience the intensity of the relationship with the patient through the nurse is invaluable. An appropriate level of identification with the consultee makes liaison nurses effective. Sharing the same profession, liaison nurses and staff nurses share similar experiences. The quality of the identification warrants attention. It is important to first recognize the identification and subsequent parallel process in the hope of using it to better understand the clinical problem.

Mrs. Berg, a 62-year-old widowed woman recovering from vascular surgery, was an unusually demanding patient. When her needs were not immediately satisfied, she screamed for the nurse. The liaison nurse, after interviewing Mrs. Berg, assessed that her fear of the hospital, of the surgical procedure, and of abandonment was superimposed on her personality, making the patient a complicated management problem. Carefully negotiated care plans were sabotaged by the patient. The nurses felt enraged and helpless. They persistently and frequently requested that the liaison nurse do something just as the patient demanded that the nurses do something. Recognizing the parallel phenomenon, the liaison nurse remained involved and responded to the consultees' need not to be abandoned. Furthermore, this illustrates one of the goals of consultation: to encourage tolerance among members of the nursing staff of those situations in which immediate and/or effective intervention or resolution is unattainable.

In the process of gathering data regarding a formal or an informal consultation, liaison nurses consider the transference/countertransference phenomenon. The distinctions among considering, recognizing, understanding, interpreting, suggesting, and discussing are recognized. Timing and tact are significant factors in human relationships, psychotherapy, and consultation. Consider the perspective and goal from which liaison nurses would approach the following similar problems:

1. a personal friend in conflict with her controlling mother-in-law,
2. a patient in psychotherapy having conflicts with her boss, or
3. a nurse consultee in conflict with a demanding and controlling middle-aged male patient.

The personal friend is seeking help and advice with her problem. Within the boundaries of friendship, such aid can be appropriately provided. A patient in psychotherapy may also be seeking advice. The liaison nurse as therapist would examine the conflicted areas around control and authority, which would probably be reenacted in the transference and thus become an integral part of the therapy. The nurse consultee may be seeking advice as well. The liaison nurse remains aware of possible transference/countertransference issues between the demanding, controlling patient and the consultee, but refrains from comment. The goal of the interaction with the consultee is to improve the psychological care given to the patient, if at all possible. At the very minimum, the liaison nurse endeavors to aid the consultee in providing psychologically safe care. Insight into the etiology of the consultee's conflict is not a goal.

In the first example, when Ms. Powers was locked in her room by the drug-abusing patient, the role of the liaison nurse can be further explored. The liaison nurse and Ms. Powers had an alliance that facilitated their interaction. If the liaison nurse did not have a prior alliance with Ms. Powers, the sensitivity and delicacy of this problem would have made involvement difficult. Ms. Powers approached the liaison nurse and told her about her experience with Mr. Roberts. Ms. Powers said that she realized that the consequences of her behavior were serious. She chose to view the incident as a mistake in judgment rather than as a clinical error. However, her professional behavior after the incident indicated that Ms. Powers did have some degree of insight into the nature of her error. Rescue fantasy as postulated by Freud [12] is an independent derivative of the parental complex. The child, in struggling with both tenderness and independence, lives in fantasy a wish to rescue the parent of the opposite sex. All of the child's instincts are bound to the single wish of replacing and being his own father or her own mother. Rescue fantasy is bound up in the ambivalence of hate-love relationships. In all health professionals, edges of rescue fantasy operate in a variety of ways. Perhaps Ms. Powers was motivated out of hate rather than love.

As liaison nurses, we endeavor to consistently question what motivates behavior. Is it love or hate that stimulates the rescue fantasy for the nurse? Which patient stimulates which side of the ambivalence for the individual nurse?

The goals of consultation do not include the psychotherapy of the nurse consultee. As a psychiatric nurse, the liaison nurse is sensitive to the possible issues of transferance and countertransference. Aside from professional considerations, contrary to the openness, assertiveness, and confronting style presently in vogue, some things are simply better left unsaid.

section 2   documentation

the patient's medical record and nursing care plan

The documentation process in psychiatric liaison nursing is an important aspect of clinical practice. Documentation, a basic responsibility in all areas of nursing practice, has been viewed by some nurses as burdensome and time-consuming. Although not always the first priority of patient care, documentation is vital to accurate and safe care. Nurses attempt, to the best of their ability, to write assessments, medication sheets, treatment sheets, transfer notes, and the like, even though these may seem at times to be an annoyance. Recently, nursing has focused energy on identifying clear, concise documentation of nursing observations and care as a professional priority and an indication of clinical accountability [13].

From a legal perspective, professional nurses are held accountable for their clinical practice. Documentation is one vehicle through which legal accountability is exercised. If patient care is not documented, it is assumed that it has not been delivered. In most medical-surgical hospitals, nurses' notes are now part of the patient's permanent record. In some institutions, the word "progress" has been added to the phrase "nurses' notes" changing it to "nurses' progress notes." Many hospitals have combined professional documentation by physicians and nurses into a section of the patient's recorded labeled "patient progress notes."

Documentation validates clinical practice. It illustrates much more than the status of the patient and the plan of care. It also illustrates theoretical and clinical knowledge, as well as the ability to conceptualize critically, empathically, and creatively. Documentation in patients' medical records by psychiatric liaison nurses validates the existence of their role by describing their contribution to the care of the patients. It promotes communication and can serve as a vehicle for teaching. It also provides liaison nurses with an opportunity to carefully review their work so as to share it in a jargon-free, helpful way with the health care team.

Rigid policies for documentation in the patient's medical record would be unrealistic. There is tremendous variation among hospitals regarding the method of charting and the organization of the patient's record. It would behoove liaison nurses to become familiar with the policies of the departments of nursing and psychiatry in terms of the prescribed formats for nurses' notes and psychiatric consultation notes. However, while utilizing hospital-sanctioned forms and formats, certain guidelines for psychiatric liaison nursing documentation can be identified.

guidelines for documentation

1. A psychiatric nursing consultation note is placed in the patient's record only when there has been a direct intervention. If the liaison nurse has provided indirect consultation—that is, if the patient was presented to the liaison nurse but was not interviewed—it is the consultees' responsibility to include in their nurses' notes that such a discussion took place.
2. It is strongly suggested that liaison nurses refrain from writing in the patient's Kardex. The long established expectation—and one that is best not altered—is that nurses who are familiar or responsible for a patient's nursing care also remain responsible for writing the patient's nursing care

plan. The involvement of liaison nurses in writing care plans may be viewed as intrusive or controlling, and it may serve as a misrepresentation of their responsibilities. This is certainly not to say that the psychiatric liaison nurse should also refrain from assisting with the development of a nursing care plan. It can be profitable in terms of teaching, role modeling, and strengthening consultation alliances to collaborate with nurse consultees in formulating a nursing care plan.

3. It is most appropriate for liaison nurses to write their consultation notes in the section of the patient's record where other nurses write their notes. The exceptions to this would include the following:

   a. The liaison nurse, hired by the department of psychiatry, is mandated to write notes in the same section of the medical record as the psychiatrists write their notes.

   b. The liaison nurse is requested by a physician to provide consultation for his or her patient and the expectation is that she or he document the work in the doctor's progress notes.

   c. Nurses' notes are not part of the patient's permanent medical record, but are discarded. If liaison nurses feel that it is important that their assessment of the patient remain in the permanent medical record, they may choose to write their notes in the doctors' progress notes. Situations in which this may be an appropriate decision include threat of law suit, serious psychopathology, or refusal of psychiatric treatment.

4. Liaison nurses write a note in the patient's medical record each time they interview the patient/family.

5. Liaison nurses clarify with the appropriate department(s) whether or not their formal consultations need to be cosigned by a psychiatrist. Hospital policies vary widely and are acknowledged.

6. Regardless of who requested psychiatric nursing consultation, liaison nurses may be mandated by hospital policy to document their work in the nurses' notes section of the medical record. However, it can be quite helpful in terms of illustrating both the role and clinical involvement, to place a brief note in the physicians' progress notes. Example: 4/12/81 Psychiatric Nursing Consultation (See Nurses' Notes), name, title, phone extension, and/or page number.

The content of documentation in the patient's medical record by liaison nurses remains consistent regardless of the hospital's policy for charting. Documentation in the medical record is dated and titled "Psychiatric Nursing Consultation." It is recommended that it begin with a statement, which includes the source of the consultation request and the purpose of the consultation. If for any reason the consultation is delayed, a note to that effect is written. Stating when the patient will be seen avoids miscommunication, misunderstanding, and unnecessary confusion. If traditional narrative format is being utilized, a brief summary of medical and social history followed by a description of the interview is written. Data gathered from other members of the health care team or family is included as appropriate. Clinical impressions—a general assessment of the patient utilizing nursing diagnosis and treatment recommendations or suggestions—are included. Liaison nurses indicate in the note what their role will be in effecting their recommendations, as well as the extent of their availability. The note is then signed with their title, phone extension, and/or page number. If medical records are organized in a problem-oriented format with SOAP notes [14–16], this same information can still be included, although the history is usually briefer.

examples of documentation in the patient's medical record

1/2/81 psychiatric nursing consultation

Ellen is a 13-year-old white female with anorexia nervosa admitted to medical pediatrics by the child psychiatry service. Per request of this service and the nursing staff, I interviewed the patient and will be involved in her treatment, specifically the ward management and behavior modification program. Ellen is the fourth of five children—three older sisters and one younger brother. The patient has lost 38 pounds over the course of two months. Intensive medical evaluation has been negative. She is in the seventh grade and is an excellent student. Parents and siblings are without psychiatric history and are in good health. With the daily collaboration of the psychiatric, dietary, nursing, and pediatric teams, I will be formulating the behavior modification program. The patient's daily weight and medical status will serve as the basis for program development. I will communicate the program daily to the patient. I will also introduce myself to her parents who with Ellen will be in psychotherapy with members of the child psychiatry service. The nursing staff has been encouraged to assume a supportive stance with patient and family while directing questions regarding the behavior modification program to me. Presently, the patient weighs 30.4 kg.

S: "I just want to get out of here as fast as I can. I don't want to weigh any more than 80 pounds, but I think I'm OK now. I was just too fat."

O: Extremely thin, pale, boyish preadolescent, lying on bed and dressed in pajamas and heavy robe, TV on; smiled initially at interviewer, but eye contact poor.

A: Superficially cooperative, very angry about hospitalization, denies feeling ill, although vital signs are reported as low. Medical status reported as stable. Denies thinness and hunger, appears to understand purpose of hospitalization and dangers of severe weight loss but does not share our concerns. Specific psychiatric etiology of anorexia not clear at this time.

P: 1. Daily meetings with treatment team.
2. Daily meetings with patient.
3. Observe patient/family behavior.
4. Daily weights in AM after voiding; patient to wear johnny only.
5. Regular diet.
6. No restrictions in terms of activity, visitors, and other privileges at this time.
7. Behavior modification program to begin in two days if patient fails to gain weight on her own.

Will follow daily—Anita Lewis, RN, MS (Psychiatric Nurse Consultant), Page 334 or extension 5576.

7/21/81 psychiatric nursing consultation

At the request of Dr. Joshua, Mrs. Evans was interviewed in the presence of her primary nurse. The patient is a frail, 83-year-old devout Catholic Italian white widow whose husband died from an MI 16 years ago. Mrs. Evans was admitted 10/1 via the ER with question of head trauma secondary to fall at home. She was brought in by her youngest daughter. Gastric cancer has been diagnosed during this admission. The patient is felt to be increasingly withdrawn, noncommunicative, and anorexic. She has been told her diagnosis and is presently awaiting nursing home placement. Mrs. Evans has been told that her medical condition necessitates that she not return home.

Mrs. Evans appears quite depressed; affect generally flat, eye contact poor. On mental status exam she is unable to do proverbs or serial sevens. She is not oriented to time, date, month, stating that it is "1956." She knows that she is 83, but is unable to remember her birthday or her home address. Mrs. Evans does remember her arrival at the hospital. "I fell, and my daughter came and brought me here." Mrs. Evans does not remember how long she has been in the hospital, but states that she is "very ill." She is not able to describe her illness. Mrs. Evans appears frightened at times and agreed that she is "very sad." She also said that she "just wants to die." Appetite poor and not sleeping well. Mrs. Evans has no complaints of physical pain.

Mrs. Evans has two married daughters and five grandchildren. According to the nursing staff, daughters describe their mother as "very independent." Mrs. Evans states that she sees her daughters frequently, and this has been validated by them. The patient states that she is visited by her husband who "talks with her and wants her to come home." Mrs. Evans does not appear to be aware of her confusion.

Impression: Vegetative signs present in this elderly woman who has never been ill or in a hospital until this time; mental status deteriorating; auditory and visual hallucinations present.

Formulation: Probable psychotic depression secondary to loss of health, home, and familiar environment, some organicity present.

Plan: I will discuss this patient with Dr. Gottlieb from the psychiatric liaison service and would suggest:

1. formal psychiatric consultation for differential diagnosis of functional versus organic components of depression and psychotropic medication evaluation;
2. consultation with hospital chaplain, since patient is very religious;
3. familiar objects from home to be brought in, i.e., bible, pictures;
4. as consistent nurses as possible, and frequent orientation to time and place, night light;
5. daily contact with liaison nurse.

> Joyce Sasson, RN, MS
> (Psychiatric Liaison Nurse)
> page or extension 1164

consultation records

Each request for psychiatric nursing consultation requires documentation in private consultation records. If liaison nurses practice in collaboration with the consultation-liaison service of a psychiatry department, they may find that this service uses a variety of forms on which to record requests for psychiatric consultation and completed consultations. There may be instances when it is both useful and appropriate for liaison nurses to employ these same forms. For example, if they are clinically responsible for providing formal psychiatric consultation, they may also be required to document, in a prescribed fashion, for the department of psychiatry. It may also be common practice in the hospital for all "consultants," be they representatives of psychiatry or some medical-surgical specialty, to document in the patient's medical record on carbonized paper, retaining a copy of the consultation note for their own records. Liaison nurses may choose to do the same and proceed to maintain some kind of consultation note-filing system, perhaps by unit or by diagnostic category. The recordkeeping system is effective only if it is clear, concise, useful over time, and efficient.

A variety of tools and methodologies may be adapted to meet the needs of liaison nurses and to reflect the psychiatric consultation needs of the hospital. Our experience has been that, when carefully and consistently accomplished, brief documentation of the "total consultation" serves as invaluable data from which to extract and evaluate not only clinical practice and impact, or the lack thereof, but also the learning needs, problems, and repetitive difficulties encountered by the consultee(s). It can serve as a basis for formulating research hypotheses, as well as for illustrating the breadth of the liaison nurse's practice. Again, this information can be further categorized in terms of specific wards, diagnostic categories, "types" of consultation questions, or direct versus indirect intervention. Documentation tools that may be employed are included. Some of these may also be reduced to index cards (Tables 7–1 through 7–5).

Private documentation on nurses' groups is also worthy of mention. If liaison nurses are to process these groups over time, record-keeping is essential. A process recording format is useful, one in which group attendance is noted, the group theme and consultation questions (overt and covert) are identified, as well as the roles assumed by members.

section 3 evaluation

Psychiatric liaison nurses are accountable to their patients, themselves, their profession, and their employers. As previously discussed, they are accountable for "diagnosing the total consultation," for their recommendations, and for the interventions that they directly institute with patients. They are also responsible for any clinical teaching that they provide for consultees. Responsibility, as a precursor to accountability, is founded in intellectual honesty, maturity, a desire to be recognized as a professional, and the motivation to identify and learn from mistakes. "Accountability involves disclosure; its purpose is evaluation and decision making, and its method is open communication [17]."

There are three aspects of evaluation: the formal process, the informal process, and the identification and role of the evaluator(s). Each is considered separately, and each is of significance in the achievement of a comprehensive evaluation of the practice of the psychiatric liaison nurse. The achievement of absolute objectivity in the total evaluation process constitutes a goal rarely met.

TABLE 7–1 EXAMPLE OF DOCUMENTATION OF CONSULTATION

Patient # _____   Date of Admission _____

Date of Referral _____

Date of Discharge _____

Medical Diagnosis _____

Psychiatric Diagnosis _____

Source of Referral _____

Formal Consult   yes _____ no _____

(Addressograph)   Clinician _____

Age _____ Race _____ Marital Status _____ Floor _____

Nature of Concern Presented	Further Definition of Problem

INTERVENTIONS (Date & Time)

1. Patient Interview
2. Nurses
3. Staff Conference
4. Physicians
5. Significant Others
6. Other Care Givers
7. Psychiatric Collaboration

RECOMMENDATIONS

1. Psychotropic Medication _____
2. Change in Staff Approach _____
3. Therapeutic Relationship with Liaison Nurse for Patient _____ for Family _____
4. Team Involvement _____
   a. Formal Psychiatric Consult Collaboration _____
   b. Social Worker _____
   c. Others (Specify) _____
   _____
5. Environmental Change _____

Documentation Form, Psychiatric — Mental Health Nursing Program, Yale University School of Nursing, New Haven, Conn., Jill Nelson, RN, MS, and Dianne Schilke Davis, RN, MS. Reprinted with permission.

TABLE 7–2 EXAMPLE OF DOCUMENTATION OF CONSULTATION

REQUEST FOR PSYCHIATRIC NURSE CONSULTATION

Routine _____ Emergency _____ Date _____

I. Reason for request. Please check appropriate response(s).

    _____ Difficult patient to care for.

    _____ Unsure of how to effectively care for the emotional needs of the patient.

    _____ Patient needs supportive counseling.

    _____ Patient and family having difficulty coping with illness or resulting disabilities.

    _____ Family interfering with nursing care of patient.

    _____ Nursing staff needs support in taking care of this patient.

    _____ Other.

        Any additional comments on above?

II. Has the patient received the services of any of the following:

    _____ Social Services

    _____ Rehabilitation Counselor

    _____ Psychiatrist

    _____ Alcoholism Counselor

    _____ Continuing Care

III. Is the patient aware of the request for this consultation?

IV. Is the doctor aware of the request for this consultation?

V. What do you hope will be accomplished through this consultation?

_____
                        Consulting Nurse

Documentation Form, Lemuel Shattuck Hospital, Jamaica Plain, Mass., Department of Nursing, Mildred Davis, Director of Nursing. Reprinted with permission.

TABLE 7–3 EXAMPLE OF DOCUMENTATION OF CONSULTATION

| DATE: _____

| TO: _____

(TO BE FILLED OUT BY PERSON MAKING REFERRAL)

Diagnosis: _____

Referred by: _____

Primary Nurse: _____ Primary Physician: _____

Reason for Referral: _____

(TO BE FILLED OUT BY CONSULTANT)

ASSESSMENT: _____

PLANS/GOALS: _____

INTERVENTION: _____

EVALUATION: _____

CONSULTATION MADE BY: _____

DATED: _____

Documentation Form, Rush University College of Nursing, Chicago, Ill., Luther B. Christman, RN, Ph. D, Dean. Reprinted with permission.

TABLE 7–4 EXAMPLE OF DOCUMENTATION OF CONSULTATION

C/L SERVICE	Pt:
Pt. Stamp	Psych. Diagnosis Past Psych. Diagnosis and Therapy
Initial Consult Date: _____ Length: _____	Mental Status:
F/U VISITS: Date | Length | Date | Length	Psychiatric Formulation: ppt. to symptoms, to hospitalization, character style, occupation, level of function, defenses:
CONSULTING PSYCHIATRIST: Consult Initiated by: RN SW MD Referring MD/Service: _____	
Reason Referred: Overt: _____ _____ _____ Covert: _____ _____ _____	INTERVENTION Individual _____ Family/Couples _____ Drugs/Medical Psychiatric _____ Dose: _____
MEDICAL DIAGNOSIS	OUTCOME: Subjective: _____ _____
Milieu response to pt:	Objective: _____ _____ Disposition: _____ _____

Documentation Form, Adult Psychiatry Consultation/Liaison Service, New England Medical Center, Boston, Mass., Myrna Weiss, M.D., Chief Consultation/Liaison Service. Reprinted with permission.

TABLE 7–5 CONSULTATION—NURSES' GROUP

Nurses' Group		
Ward		
Attendance		
Theme		
Group Member	Dialogue	Process and Affect

Overt Consultation Question(s)

Covert Consultation Question(s)

Recommendations and Interactions

Follow-up

formal evaluation

It is not unusual for liaison nurses to find that they must develop role-appropriate evaluation criteria. It is helpful to review the evaluation tools presently being utilized by the nursing department. Perhaps one of them is appropriate or can be modified to achieve applicability. It is possible that the expectation for evaluation may be a narrative with no specific guidelines.

The basis for evaluation is in accord with the specific tasks and responsibilities discussed in the liaison nurse's job description (see Chapter 2, Section 2, "A Model Job Description"). In light of the job description and tenets of practice, basic areas to consider in evaluating performance emerge. These are:

1. consultations, direct and indirect,
2. interpersonal skills,
3. leadership/professionalism,
4. teaching skills, and
5. academic advancements.

With these areas as a guideline, liaison nurses identify specific evaluation criteria and proceed to document their professional activities.

Regardless of the clinical setting, certain evaluation criteria can be identified and are applicable in most general hospitals. Liaison nurses can tabulate, on the basis of their consultation records, the number and types of consultations received. The "numbers" of consultations as an evaluation criterion can be deceptive. This information can be broken down further in terms of consultation theme, the specific ward, the identification of the consultee requesting the consultation, and relationship/utilization of the liaison nurse over time. As the legacy of the role develops, liaison nurses may receive both consultation requests and recognition from both physician staff and various departments within the hospital. They may receive more requests for in-service education programs. Resistant wards may become more open to them. New nursing orientees and physicians may have learned of their existence and seek their advice. As a result, the level of consultation may become increasingly sophisticated. Maintaining documentation that reflects all these areas constitutes the basis for formal and objective evaluation.

The "Consultation Evaluation Guide" (Table 7–6) is included to assist liaison nurses in their efforts to obtain objective data regarding the consultation. They may also use this guideline to enhance and

TABLE 7–6 CONSULTATION EVALUATION GUIDE

The Consultee's Responsibilities:

1. Gathering and reviewing data pertinent to the problem situation *prior* to the consultation using:
   a. nursing assessment,
   b. past and present medical records,
   c. observation/interaction with patient, and
   d. a formulated master problem list, nursing index, and nursing care plan.

2. Formulating the problem to the best of your ability:
   a. Describe the problem.
   b. Clearly state "what you need help with."
   c. Clearly state short- and long-term goals.
   d. Describe previously proposed and/or tried solution.

3. Making your needs known:
   a. Share your previous experience (if any) in dealing with similar problems.
   b. Ask for clarification of the consultant's suggestions.
   c. Ask for direct support in carrying out interventions if necessary.

4. Giving feedback to the consultant.

---

focus their dialog with consultees, to implement a collaborative approach to problem solving, and to gather feedback from the consultee.

In addition, liaison nurses may request that consultees complete a "Consultation Evaluation Questionnaire" (Table 7–7), as a further method of obtaining objective data for evaluation.

Feedback from consultees provides liaison nurses with valuable information concerning the consultees' understanding of the consultation, their understanding of the situation necessitating the consultation, as well as their expectations of and reactions to liaison nurses.

informal evaluation

This process refers to subjective evaluation that is based on thoughts, feelings, or personal perceptions of liaison nurses.

The problems and situations that come to the attention of liai-

TABLE 7–7 CONSULTATION EVALUATION QUESTIONNAIRE

1. Did the consultant appear interested and concerned about the problem?

2. Did the consultant take into account your previous experience (if any) with similar problem situations when offering you solutions?

3. Was the consultant interested in your formulation of the problem?

4. Did the consultant allow sufficient time to discuss the problem and possible solutions with you?

5. Did the consultant understand the problem?

6. Did you find the consultant supportive, critical, attentive?

7. Did the consultant offer to see the patient with you? To implement the proposed interventions with you? If no, why? If yes, was this helpful?

8. Did the consultant's suggestions make sense to you?

9. Did you implement the consultant's suggestions? If no, why? If yes, what was the effect of these interventions?

10. Were your needs for consultation met? If yes, how? If no, why?

11. Did you fulfill your responsibilities as the consultee?

12. Would you call the consultant again? Why?

son nurses are not only complex, but they are often personalized by the consultee. The success or failure of a clinical consultation often depends on much more than accurate patient assessment and sound clinical application of theory. Data obtained through "diagnosing the total consultation," the quality of the consultation alliance, and the transference issues between consultant and consultee all combine to influence the effectiveness of a consultation. In addition, facets of ward life, as well as specific information regarding members of the health care team that the liaison nurse may never be knowledgeable about, can impede or enhance the usefulness of psychiatric nursing consultation. Finally, changes in patients' medical status, regardless of whether or not they are coupled with changes in their psychological status, influence their response to psychological intervention. Utilizing "successful consultations" as an evaluation criterion may be misleading. Sometimes problems presented for consultation are resolved before or in spite of the consultation. Certainly, successful consultations can be tabulated and may validate clinical skill. A successful consultation is defined as one in which recommendations and

TABLE 7–8 A MODEL FOR QUARTERLY EVALUATION

Three-Month Objectives:

1. To continue professional writing and research.

2. To assist in the organization and to provide supervision/consultation for a patient support group on the medical oncology ward, to be conducted by two members of the nursing staff.

3. To conduct the "Group Dynamics and Leadership" course for nurses who were unable to attend last month's course.

4. To participate in the planning and presentation of educational programs (Renal and Family Workshop).

5. To develop alliances with the general surgical service via teaching conferences and increased availability.

6. To set aside two additional hours per week for clinical follow-up.

Evaluation Tools, New England Medical Center, Department of Nursing, Sandra Twyon, Chairperson. Reprinted with permission.

interventions suggested to the consultee are implemented. The outcome of this action is either resolution of the problem, a decrease in its severity, and/or the achievement of any of the goals of consultation. A successful consultation is also characterized by a strengthening of the consultant–consultee alliance. Therefore, "successful," as well as "unsuccessful," consultations can be reviewed with clinical supervisors as a part of the evaluation process.

Other tools for informal evaluation include documentation in the patient's medical record and/or Kardex by the consultee concerning the psychiatric nursing consultation and subsequent recommendations/outcomes. These notes are valuable to review. Peer audit and peer review are other methods of evaluating practice. If the liaison nurse is receiving clinical supervision from a qualified individual, evaluation criteria may be identified within the supervision.

In the majority of settings, the most difficult aspect of the total evaluation process is the identification of an appropriate evaluator(s). The liaison nurse's performance may be evaluated, to varying degrees, by a "nontrained" evaluator, that is, by someone who has not practiced psychiatric liaison nursing or liaison psychiatry. When hired by a department of nursing, it is not uncommon to find that the director of nursing or a delegate is the liaison nurse's evaluator. It is not uncommon for the evaluator to be unable to formally assess the liaison nurse's performance. The evaluation may become nonreflective of the actual knowledge and clinical practice of the liaison nurse. Part of the responsibility for appropriate evaluation always rests with the liaison nurse. This responsibility may mean requesting evaluation or, in some cases, designing evaluative tools.

Tables 7–8 and 7–9 are included as further illustrations of evaluation methods and tools.

Professional practice is founded on autonomy, accountability, maturity, and intellectual honesty. Defining practice goals ... formulating and revising behavioral objectives ... sharing and evaluating clinical practice ... these constitute but an illustration of liaison nurses' awareness of their responsibility. The ideal situation for evaluation is accomplished with input from a clinically skilled supervisor, from peers, and with consultee feedback. Although comprehensive evaluation may be stressful, it is a basis for professional and personal growth.

TABLE 7–9 A MODEL FOR ANNUAL EVALUATION

Consultations:

1. Understanding the psychodynamics involved.

2. Assessing the appropriateness of a referral.

3. Utilization of head nurse and/or nurse supervisor channels.

4. Assessing the need for direct versus indirect intervention and using appropriate channels.

5. Decisions and judgments concerning consultations reflect:
   a. professionalism,
   b. current nursing practice,
   c. policies and practices of the department of nursing,
   d. appropriate collaboration with other members of the health care team,
   e. comprehensive assessment of the milieu,
   f. appropriate utilization of available nursing and psychiatric supervision,
   g. documentation, and
   h. teaching.

6. Formulating appropriate nursing care interventions to promote high-quality nursing care.

7. Evaluation and assessment of each consultation and encouragement to the consultee for feedback.

TABLE 7–9 *(continued)*

Interpersonal Skills:

1. Maintaining communication with members of the nursing staff, with nursing leadership personnel, and with other hospital departments, community agencies, and so on.

2. Maintaining appropriate communication with the nursing supervisory group and with the department of nursing, to keep these individuals informed of specific issues, patient care problems, and other matters.

3. Demonstrating awareness of self and its effects on others, along with attempts to control reactions that would be directly or indirectly detrimental to patient care.

4. Maintaining a consultative and nonevaluative role with members of the nursing staff.

5. Maintaining a professional relationship with nursing staff, leadership personnel, patients, and other members of the health care team.

Leadership/Professionalism:

1. Presenting self as a professional.

2. Interpreting psychological goals, policies, and decisions of the department of nursing to nursing staff and other hospital personnel in a clear, supportive manner.

3. Participating actively on various committees, often taking a leadership position, as well as reporting back to appropriate supervisory personnel.

4. Demonstrating responsibility for personal and professional growth.

5. Demonstrating ability to provide effective and creative communications.

Teaching Skills:

1. Seeking opportunities for discussion with nursing leadership personnel of the psychological care given on their units, the needs of their staffs, in order to identify strengths, weaknesses, and other areas of interest.

2. Identifying the learning needs of the nursing staff and providing psychiatric in-service.

3. Planning appropriate conferences and workshops for the nursing staff.

4. Developing and implementing teaching plans for conferences.

TABLE 7–9 (continued)

Academic Advancements:

1. Collaboration with peers and/or colleagues in the identification of areas for the enhancement of patient care.

2. Participating in and conducting nursing research.

3. Attending academic programs, conferences, and workshops to further develop level of practice.

Evaluation Tools, New England Medical Center, Department of Nursing, Sandra Twyon, Chairperson. Reprinted with permission.

references

1. Ernest Greenwood, "The Practice of Science and the Science of Practice," in *Planning For Change*, edited by Warren E. Bennis et al. (New York: Holt, Rinehart and Winston, 1951), p. 74, a Brandeis University Paper, published by The Florence Heller Graduate School of Advanced Studies in Social Welfare, 1960. Reprinted with permission.

2. Hildegard Peplau, "Professional Closeness," *Nursing Forum* 13:4 (1969): 345.

3. Lawrence Swartz and Jane Schwartz, *The Psychodynamics of Patient Care* (Englewood Cliffs, N.J.: Prentice-Hall, Inc., 1972), p. 10.

4. Joyce Travelbee, *Interpersonal Aspects of Nursing* (Philadelphia: F. A. Davis Company, 1971), p. 133.

5. Gerald Caplan, *The Theory and Practice of Mental Health Consultation* (New York: Basic Books, Inc., Publishers, 1970), pp. 32–35.

6. James Strain and Stanley Grossman, *Psychological Care of the Medically Ill: A Primer in Liaison Psychiatry* (New York: Appleton-Century-Crofts, 1975).

7. David Sachs and Stanley Shapiro, "On Parallel Processes in Therapy and Teaching," *Psychoanalytic Quarterly* 45 (1976): 403.

8. Adapted from Karl A. Menninger and Philip S. Holzman, *Theory of Psychoanalytic Technique*, 2nd ed. (New York: Basic Books, Inc., Publishers, 1973), pp. 91–93. Used by permission.

9. Myer Mendelson and Eugene Meyer, "Countertransference Problems of the Liaison Psychiatrist," *Psychosomatic Medicine* 23:2 (1961): 121.

10. Helen Gediman and Fred Wolkenfeld, "The Parallel Phenomenon in Psychoanalysis and Supervision: Its Reconsideration as a Triadic System," *Psychoanalytic Quarterly* XLIX (1980): 234.

11. Sachs and Shapiro, p. 394.

12. Sigmund Freud, "A Special Type of Choice of Object Made by Men," in Vol. XI, *The Standard Edition of the Complete Psychological Works of Sigmund Freud* (London: The Hogarth Press and the Institute of Psycho Analysis, 1955), p. 172.

13. G. Marram, M. Schlegel, and E. Bevis, *Primary Nursing: A Model for Individual Care* (St. Louis: The C. V. Mosby Company, 1974).

14. V. K. Carrieri and J. Sitzman, "Components of the Nursing Process," *The Nursing Clinics of North America* 6 (March 1971): 115–124.
15. P. L. Schell and A. T. Campbell, "Problem-Oriented Medical Records POMR— Not Just Another Way to Chart," *Nursing Outlook* 20 (August 1972): 510–514.
16. M. Woody and M. Malleson, "Problem-Oriented System for Patient-Centered Care," *American Journal of Nursing* 73 (July 1973): 1168–1175.
17. S. Matik, "Accountability: Its Meaning and Its Relevance to the Health Care Field," *HEW Publication* No. (HRA) 77–72, HRP–0500101 (September 1977): 21.

bibliography

books

BINSTOCK, WILLIAM. "The Psychodynamic Approach in Outpatient Psychiatry," in *Psychiatry Diagnosis and Treatment*, edited by Aaron Lazare. Baltimore: Williams and Wilkins, 1979.

Documenting Patient Care Responsibly, A Nursing Skillbook Series. Pennsylvania: Nursing '78 Books, Horsham Publishing, Intermed Communications, Inc., Eugene W. Jackson, Publisher, 1978.

FREUD, SIGMUND. *The Standard Edition of the Complete Psychological Works of Sigmund Freud*, Vol. XI. London: The Hogarth Press and the Institute of Psycho Analysis, 1910.

GRISSUM, M. and SPENGLER, C. *Womanpower and Health Care*. Boston: Little, Brown & Company, 1976.

MAYERS, M. *A Systematic Approach to the Nursing Care Plan*. New York: Meredith Corp., 1972.

SOURS, J. A. *Starving to Death in a Sea of Objects*. New York: Jason Aronson, Inc., 1980.

ZANDER, K. S. *Primary Nursing Development and Management*. Germantown, Maryland: Aspen Publications, 1980.

articles

AMERICAN NURSES ASSOCIATION. "Statements of Psychiatric and Mental Health Nursing Practice," Division on Psychiatric and Mental Health Nursing, American Nurses Association, 1976.

BLAKE, A. E. "Accountability in Mental Hospitals," *Free Association* 6:3 (May–June 1979).

BLOCH, D. "Some Crucial Terms in Nursing—What Do They Really Mean?" *Nursing Outlook* 22:11 (November 1974): 689–694.

CISKE, K. L. "Primary Nursing: An Organization That Promotes Professional Practice," *Journal of Nursing Administration* 4:1 (January–February 1974): 28–31.

DIERS, D. and EVANS, D. L. "Excellence in Nursing," *Image* 12:2 (June 1980): 27–30.

GROVES, JAMES. "Taking Care of the Hateful Patient," *New England Journal of Medicine* (April 20, 1978): 883–887.

GUNTHER, MEYER. "The Threatened Staff: A Psychoanalytic Contribution to Medical Psychology," *Comprehensive Psychiatry* 18:4 (July–August 1977): 385–396.

KERR, A. H. "Nurses Notes, That's Where the Goodies Are!" *Nursing '75* (February 1975): 34–41.

Lewis, Emanuel. "Counter-transference Problems in Hospital Practice," *British Journal of Medical Psychology* 52 (1979): 37–42.

Luborsky, L.; Graff, H.; Pulver, S.; and Curtis, H. "A Clinical-Quantitative Examination of Consensus on the Concept of Transference," *Archives General Psychiatry* 29 (July 1973): 67–75.

McClosky, J. C. "Nurses' Orders: The Next Professional Breakthrough," *RN* 431:2 (February 1980): 99–113.

Malloy, J. L. "Taking Exception to Problem-Oriented Nursing Care," *American Journal of Nursing* 22:11 (November 1974): 582–583.

Meyer, Eugene and Mendelson, Myer. "Psychiatric Consultations on Medical and Surgical Wards," *Psychiatry* 27 (1961): 197–220.

Mundinger, M. O. and Jawron, G. D. "Developing a Nursing Diagnosis," *Nursing Outlook* 23:2 (February 1975): 94–98.

Peplau, H. E. "The Psychiatric Nurse—Accountable? To Whom? For What?" *Perspectives in Psychiatric Care* 18:3 (May–June 1980): 128–134.

Rosenberg, M. L. and Brody, R. "The Threat or Challenge of Accountability," *Social Work* 19:3 (May 1974): 344–350.

Rutledge, K. A. "The Professional Nurse as Primary Therapist: Background, Perspective, and Opinion," *Journal of Operational Psychiatry* 5:2 (Spring–Summer 1974): 76–81.

Ryan, L. J.; Gearhart, M.; and Simmons, S. "From Personal Responsibility to Professional Accountability in Psychiatric Nursing," *Journal of Psychiatric Nursing and Mental Health Services* 15:6 (June 1977): 19–24.

Smith, D. M. "Writing Objectives as a Nursing Practice Skill," *American Journal of Nursing* 71:2 (February 1971): 319–320.

Weed, L. L. "Medical Records That Guide and Teach," *New England Journal of Medicine* 278 (March 14–21, 1968): 593–599, 652–657.

part three
appendices:
clinical papers, standards, and epilogue

appendix a
psychiatric liaison nursing in graduate education

NANCY NEBLE
JANICE RUNZHEIMER

Psychiatric liaison nursing is a rapidly growing area of interest. Beginning in the early 1960s, this type of practice developed from a need and demand for nursing expertise in the management of difficult patients on general hospital units. At that time very few opportunities for preparatory clinical work in consultation were available to nurses, and many psychiatric nurses created their own roles as liaison specialists based on past experiences and ingenuity. While programs specific in liaison nursing were developed at the University of Maryland and at Yale University, at present the path into psychiatric liaison nursing remains in transition. Many nurses still begin consultation roles and learn in practice, while others are obtaining formal education in this specialty prior to assuming the job role. Today many psychiatric nurses with graduate training and/or many years of experience are practicing consultation [1,2]. Graduate nursing students can learn of the rewards, pitfalls, cautions, and practical models of liaison nursing from these practicing specialists before they contract for a job experience.

A clinical rotation in psychiatric liaison nursing can provide a unique graduate experience. Several factors should be considered in choosing such a placement. Supervision as well as one's supervisor contribute strategically to the outcome of the placement. Little, if any, previous experience will substitute equally for first-hand knowledge of consultation liaison theory and process. A broad theoretical base of psychiatric nursing and consultation, coupled with clinical observation, is essential. However, a liaison nurse finds that past working knowledge in many subspecialty areas is a valuable asset. Many of the problems and crises encountered by a practicing nurse consultant also surface during a student practicum. The diversity of the student's experience in consultation depends on the clinical setting, the time available, the goals set by the student, and his or her own skills as a beginning consultant. These and other components of a preceptorship will be discussed more fully.

There is a paucity of information in the literature concerning student experience and education in psychiatric nursing consultation. An article by Jansson describes one such experience provided to undergraduate nursing students as an elective option within their psychiatric nursing rotation [3]. These students had several brief encounters in consultation with their peers in other areas during the semester. Their goal was to provide suggestions for dealing more effectively with patients presenting difficult behaviors. The article identifies three phases—initial, working, and termination—of the consultation process. Another study cites the experiences of undergraduate nurses who again were utilized in follow-up consultation to parents of problem children. Holland et al. point out the role of the students as therapeutic consultants to the parents who had been taught alternative parenting techniques initially [4]. The students made some home visits and were found to have a 60-percent success rate as measured by parental effectiveness and the degree of future problems with the child. Neither of these articles described clearly the process of educating the students in consultation.

Robinson has outlined a graduate program in psychiatric liaison nursing [5]. She points out the need for previous psychiatric nursing experience, courses in brief therapy, much first-hand clinical consultation, and ongoing supervision as essential elements in a nursing consultation program. Nelson and Davis have also outlined a graduate curriculum in liaison nursing [6]. They emphasize a threefold approach to the education of nursing consultants, which includes theory, research, and clinical practice. The program's objectives are to prepare students who can: (1) provide appropriate psychological care to physically ill patients and their families, which considers biopsychosocial factors and capitalizes on opportunities for prevention; (2) serve as consultants to nonpsychiatric nurses to increase their knowledge and skills in dealing with the psychosocial needs of their patients; and (3) plan and implement clinical nursing research. Although these articles address some of the issues in educating the nurse consultant, neither describe the learning experience of the student.

choosing a placement

Clinical work assumes an important position in the graduate student's educational experience. Often the experiential component determines the difference between the mediocrity and the excellence of one's educational preparation. A clinical placement should be chosen with care. The student makes this choice usually through negotiation with the potential clinical preceptor and with the help of a faculty advisor. That choice is based on numerous factors about the placement itself. In addition, the student needs to identify his or her own expectations for the preceptorship.

There are several factors to consider in selecting a clinical placement in liaison nursing. Of primary concern is the quality and variety of experience and learning opportunities available at the agency. The amount of time that the student has to devote to clinical work is limited. Therefore, the most benefit is to be gained from practicing in a hospital that is familiar with the liaison nurse's role and that can ensure the use of the liaison nursing student. The freedom to work with patients, families, and nursing staff enriches the student experience and contributes to professional growth. Excessive amounts of time devoted to gaining acceptance into an institution and creation of the role may deprive the student of the opportunity to put into practice basic consultation concepts. For this reason, a student may find it more satisfying and beneficial to study and practice consultation with a liaison nurse already successful in practice. The availability of an experienced liaison nurse as a supervisor is an important factor when choosing a placement. The need for detailed examination of clinical experiences makes adequate supervision in the placement a high priority. A graduate student should seek an experienced liaison nurse for a supervisor with whom he or she can develop a working relationship.

The agency itself may be large or small, in-patient, out-patient, community, or a multiservice institution. The consultation process may reflect similarities in each setting, but for this discussion the focus will be on a student in the general hospital. The history and philosophy regarding consultation in a hospital may contribute to a decision about a placement. In some hospitals the liaison nurse is required to obtain the physician's approval prior to seeing a patient presented by the nursing staff. This design distinctly impedes the nursing consultation process. Nursing consultants may collaborate with psychiatric residents freely, or the two may provide completely separate services. The model to which we were exposed was one that demonstrated a strong working relationship between the liaison nurse and the psychiatric consultation service. Such a relationship affords the liaison nurse the opportunity to exchange important information with colleagues, to receive support and to insure a more stimulating working environment.

We believe that the optimal method for practicing nursing consultation in a system places the nurse in a staff position accountable to the director of nursing and in collaboration with the psychiatric consultation-liaison service, if it exists. Furthermore, the nurse consultant should have free access to patients. This model provides the necessary freedom, raises fewer questions of authority and responsibility, and is less likely to confuse the liaison nurse role with any other nursing position or function.

These factors are among those that contribute to an enriching educational experience for the graduate student. They are not intended as an exhaustive list of considerations in choosing a placement, but rather as a guide.

preparation and goals

Any graduate student considering a consultation-liaison rotation should be an experienced nurse who may possess both psychiatric and medical-surgical nursing expertise. Many combinations of knowledge and skill can serve the student well. For example, a student may have several years of medical-surgical experience and a year of psychiatric nursing, or much more work in psychiatric nursing and minimal experience in other specialties prior to the graduate rotation. Certain psychiatric nursing expertise is necessary. Without a basic understanding of psychodynamics and group management skills, it is difficult to practice psychiatric liaison nursing. Knowledge and skill in family dynamics is also important. However, these ideas need not be considered absolute, but they do affect the students' goals for the graduate rotation. Thus a graduate placement in consultation may vary both quantitatively and qualitatively according to the student's preparation and goals.

A graduate student must establish goals for the experience. These goals depend on several factors:

1. the ability and experience of the student,
2. the availability of the supervisor,
3. the interests of the student,
4. what is realistic for the student's available time, and
5. what is acceptable within the institution.

One student may hope to gain a basic idea of psychiatric liaison nursing and thus choose to observe the liaison nurse in action. Alternatively, a student may have the interest and ability to function independently of the liaison nurse for a portion of the rotation. Despite the variability of student experience, some basic goals apply to any graduate rotation. The following are common objectives:

1. To identify the roles that the liaison nurse enacts within the institution.
2. To identify areas that are appropriate for the liaison nurse's involvement and intervention, and also those that are inappropriate.
3. To understand consultation-liaison concepts in dynamic situations encountered by the student.
4. To begin to generalize these concepts to meet new situations.
5. To apply previously acquired knowledge, skills, and nursing interventions to consultation-liaison situations.
6. To learn to translate psychiatric terminology into language that is appropriate and meaningful to nonpsychiatric professionals.

These objectives may be attained through observation and more independent functioning by the student.

Prior to beginning the graduate experience a student may expect to feel a high level of anxiety. Anxiety often persists throughout the first several weeks of the experience. The graduate student should understand that these feelings are normal and eventually diminish. This is often a time when exposure to basic consultation-liaison literature may be helpful and increase the student's knowledge base. Information about organizations and the placement agency, in particular, allay anxiety by giving the student some realistic expectations. The quantity of this information should be limited so as not to overwhelm the student. Meetings with the faculty and/or preceptor in the beginning further decrease anxiety. These meetings focus on the learning needs and goals of the student. They may also help to clarify the support system available to the student during the rotation. Appropriate supports become important when problems or questions arise, and when these key people are identified at the outset it proves invaluable. Future meetings can be scheduled during the academic year to review the student's experience and goals in the placement, to vary or reaffirm them accordingly, and to monitor his or her level of anxiety.

Before the student arrives, the psychiatric liaison nurse can alert the nursing staff to the student's coming. Together they plan an appropriate orientation. Initially, the student will benefit from accompanying the liaison nurse on all the requested consultations. Such activity allows the student to observe various means by which the staff utilizes the consultant. It also provides an opportunity for the introduction of the student into the liaison role. The nursing staff become accustomed to a "new" liaison nurse and develop some expectations about his or her role. A collegial representation of the experienced consultant with the student helps the staff to transfer their trust to the graduate student and to develop a working relationship. This exposure to the student may alleviate staff concern about their responsibility to train the newcomer. These beginning activities assist the student consultant in gaining acceptance with the staff.

The liaison nurse may have identified units appropriate for student involvement, and the student may express certain interests. The reception of the consultant by the staff is a consideration in selecting areas for student experience. Some staff groups provide a warm welcome and already understand how to utilize the student effectively. However, staff who are less experienced in using consultation-liaison nursing can also supply the student liaison nurse with a rich, interesting rotation. If the student consultant has sufficient time and investment and the staff, a desire and interest, then this experience may prove ultimately fruitful. A resistant staff may be set up for failure if the student has an inadequate time in which to develop the relationship. When the units have been identified, the student and the supervisor can meet with the head nurse and staff to define the parameters of the student's involvement and to assess their needs and concerns. After this preparation the experienced consultant may slowly withdraw or remain highly involved depending upon the student's needs and goals. Whatever work the student may take on independently, observation and participation with the liaison nurse make for an excellent learning experience, and they should be continued to some degree throughout the duration of the student's rotation.

During the early phase of consultation to a staff the primary work of the student is to build trust and rapport with the staff. This task becomes an ongoing part of consultation work. Certain activities and behavior will promote success in this endeavor.

1. Provide the staff with a clear explanation of one's role and abilities to be helpful.
2. State one's involvement and availability, so the staff know what to expect.
3. Demonstrate a genuine interest in their problems.

4. Maintain visibility with the staff between consultations.
5. Be aware of one's own limitations and avoid acting on the urgency to respond and provide solutions.
6. Work through collaborative relationships and encourage staff nurses to pursue their own ideas, whenever productive.
7. Maintain the relationship between the staff and the liaison nurse or ensure its continuance by utilizing the liaison nurse when appropriate.

These types of behaviors help develop student–staff rapport and increase the acceptance of the student consultant by the staff.

The liaison nurse may provide the student with additional opportunities to facilitate his or her entry into the system. Participation in the hospital's nursing education programs and nursing seminars increases the student's exposure to the staff. At times, other health care providers affect the work of the consultant and the nursing staff. These include the psychiatry department staff, the liaison residents, social workers, other clinical specialists, and nursing administrators. An introduction to many of those colleagues early in the student's rotation will often facilitate a working relationship necessary to the student consultant's later work. These early experiences in the system also increase awareness of available resources, enhance entry into the system, and make the role satisfying.

Obviously, a graduate nursing experience in consultation liaison can be arranged in many different ways. Once the student has found a suitable agency and a practitioner, then a contract or framework can be constructed to meet the learning needs of the student. One method is to define a time-limited and structured experience. Our own practicum was designed similarly.

One clinical rotation lasted a full school year; the other, only one semester. One semester is a minimum unless one's goal is set strictly as an observational experience. Our placement was in a general hospital setting. However, as previously stated, psychiatric liaison nursing can be learned in a variety of settings. At the outset the greatest benefits came through the opportunity for observation. Spending time in the shadow of a successful practitioner, a student can absorb much significant information. The following case illustration clarifies this point:

> Several nurses from the heme-oncology unit presented a 30-year-old man with melanoma for consultation. His disease was progressive, and he had lost control of his bladder function. The nurses said that he remained very quiet and isolated in his room and

talked only about the activities he would pursue at home. He was described further as intelligent, optimistic, and ashamed about current dependency needs. The staff worried about him because it was doubtful that his bladder control would return despite medication and treatment. They also feared that the patient would continue to refuse to accept his loss and to master self-catheterization before he went home. If forced to face reality, the staff thought the patient would become hopeless and desperate. One of the nurses verbalized the thought that the patient was young enough to be her brother. The patient's wife was very supportive, but also very stressed herself with the care of a new baby. The task was to help this patient gain some adaptive skills that would make him more independent at discharge. However, he refused to believe his potential need for such skills as self-catheterization, as he believed strongly that he would regain this function before his discharge. The staff was helped to see that their availability was most important to the patient. The liaison nurse also devised a time-limited schedule for awaiting the patient's return function. The patient was told that at the end of this period he would be instructed in those skills necessary for his discharge since no one could predict future developments and he could not remain in the hospital forever, nor did he want to do so. His doctor's assistance was elicited. This plan was successful, and yet allowed the patient to save face and retain hope. In this brief consultation the liaison nurse had ascertained the patient's areas of conflict, some of his defenses, especially his level of denial, his family support and stress level, and the staff relationship with the patient through skillful questioning and observation. This information was all important in formulating the plan of intervention with the staff.

During our placement some days reverberated with a sense of crisis and pressure, while others moved more slowly and smoothly from one staff group to the next. Many clinical presentations by nursing staff focused on patient problems and problem patients. From time to time, staff raised interdisciplinary conflicts or administrative dilemmas that they felt affected patient care. Frequently, we moved from a discussion about an infant in the ICU to an elderly patient who was CVA-impaired, to a discussion with a head nurse, to a suicidal patient, for example, within two hours. Sometimes, as students, the mass of clinical data became overwhelming. Once a mental framework for categorizing data is developed, the student's anxiety will decrease (Table A-1). Fortunately, this beginning stage of consultation work is normal and does not reflect the entire experience.

As the practicum continues, most graduate students provide

TABLE A–1 A CONSULTATION FRAMEWORK [7]

  I. Identifying Data: Floor, Unit, Date, and Attendance
  II. Requested by Whom and Why
  III. Key Consultation Question
  IV. Case Description: Patient—Problems and Behaviors
                      Staff—Ideas, Opinions, Previous Interventions
                      Whose Side Is Staff On?
                      Others—Physicians, Family, Friends, Auxilliary
                      Personnel
  V. Issues Addressed and Unaddressed: By Whom, When, How, and Why
  VI. Role of the Consultant: Thoughts, Feelings, and Suggestions
  VII. Outcome and Follow-up

consultations and follow-ups on their own. To choose several units or groups of staff from within the agency helps to focus time and energy. It is preferable when these choices are made according to the student's interests and areas of comfort versus discomfort. Areas of discomfort need not be excluded from the experience, for these units may prove excellent sources from which to expand knowledge and skill. However, some nursing units have the potential to present problems that may be too difficult for the student. In our experience, units such as the ICU, dialysis unit, and emergency unit were difficult areas in which to make inroads. This may differ in other hospitals. As a student, there are many anxiety-provoking thoughts and feelings when learning to do consultation. Focusing efforts helps to diminish these feelings somewhat, as do the support and guidance offered by a supervisor.

During the early stages of the consultation process a student or beginning practitioner seeks to develop rapport with the staff and to support their caring for difficult patients. We found that these early solo consults required, on our part, an holistic understanding of the patient, his or her problems, the others involved, and the concurrent group process among the staff. Many times it was difficult to synthesize these numerous factors and to respond to the key questions asked by the staff. However, doing some actual consultations is an integral part of learning the process, as the example below illustrates. Over time, the student begins to tune into all the factors contributing to the key question of the staff. Slowly the skill of suggesting successful intervention develops.

As student consultants we heard about some difficult cases. One of the earliest still stands out clearly. A group of nurses were especially distraught over a 19-year-old male patient who was transferred from a distant community hospital after an automobile accident left him a paraplegic.

> Jim was still living with his family prior to hospitalization and worked outdoors with heavy machinery. He had completed high school the spring before the accident. After being transferred, this patient found himself on a 36-bed unit primarily for infectious disease patients. Most of the other patients could look forward to getting well and resuming their normal activities. It was a busy floor with a moderate amount of nursing staff. At the time of the consultation, Jim had become very withdrawn and belligerently refused nearly all physical care from the staff. Although the staff recognized his anger as legitimate and his withdrawal as a normal grief reaction, they had many distressing and uneasy feelings about the patient and their own abilities to help him. Among the feelings they expressed were guilt, anger, helplessness, sorrow, concern, affection, and frustration.

When we first heard this story, we too felt somewhat devastated by its impact. We experienced sadness and helplessness, which created an urgency to support and assist the staff. However, no words or ideas seemed to provide a solution to the problem: how to help the staff care for this young man and deal with their feelings. With the assistance of our supervisor, we were able to identify many of the dynamics. We understood how our identification with the staff had been immobilizing. As we discussed the patient's needs for trust and support, we grew more capable of helping the staff. Recognizing the limitations to our intervention allowed us, and eventually the staff, to be more effective. Before successful intervention came the acknowledgement that none of us could return to Jim the function of his legs. What slowly helped the staff was their increasing ability to talk honestly with him and to accept his negative feelings, while building rapport and trust in the relationship.

a consultation framework

A consultation framework provides a quick and easy way of organizing the mass of material presented to the liaison nurse (Table A–1). It can be used as a mental outline during an actual case consultation.

Students can also employ this outline for doing process recordings of their experiences. The record later furnishes material for discussion in supervision. In some ways, the format resembles that often used to construct an individual psychiatric evaluation and history. The key question usually reflects the staff's chief concern. The case description includes present as well as past behavior of the patient, if known. The consultant also gains information about various opinions and views of the staff and possibly of the family or significant others. The viewpoints of others may equate with those of the patient, or they may differ. What is not said may be just as important as what is said. The consultant should also heed his or her own nonverbal reactions to the case presentation.

The format of a consultation framework helps decrease stress. If the consultant recognizes his or her own thoughts and feelings evoked by the consultation data, then he or she can often pinpoint the key issues quickly. It is important to acknowledge for oneself and often for the staff, the strong feelings created by the patient's situation. Intense feelings such as helplessness, hopelessness, rage, and anger can be recognized and given some expression during the case presentation. Following this expression by the staff, the consultant may help them redirect their goals and intervention with the patient to decrease the anger-provoking stimuli. Ultimately, the staff will return to care for the patient, while the consultant can leave the situation freely. By adhering to this mental format, the consultant can better manage intense emotions and traumatic data presented by the staff.

The use of this framework provides an organized data base from which to formulate nursing intervention. When suggesting solutions, the consultant often validates them as plausible with the staff. If the staff does not understand or agree with the suggested interventions, they usually refuse to implement them. Such a refusal does not mean that the suggestion will not work. However, the staff may require more support and explanation from the consultant to implement the plan, or it may represent an unrealistic expectation of the staff by the consultant.

For example, a depressed patient was transferred from the psychiatric unit to a general floor. On the psychiatric unit she had been very regressed initially. Through progressive structured activity she had improved and was able to leave the unit on short passes. With the onset of symptoms of gall stones, the patient was transferred. She again grew more depressed, and the staff feared that she might regress. This patient's response to physical illness was typical.

To encourage her to exercise as much independence on the general unit as she was able to assume on the psychiatric unit would not have been feasible. Such intervention might precipitate a tenuous situation if the patient felt unsupported. Therefore, the nurses provided her with support while insisting that she continue assuming responsibility for her daily personal care. They also helped her to structure her time with alternative activities on the unit. In this example the consultation framework helped the consultant to suggest specific intervention in light of the patient's changed situation.

stressors for the student consultant

Some of the significant stressors that are experienced by students include: (1) the varying pace, (2) the element of unpredictability, (3) the monumental amount of information assimilated during one day, and (4) the isolation of the experience. By the very design of the position, the consultant moves quickly from one ward to the next, focusing on one or more new problems and cases in each meeting. Developing the ability to refocus attention quickly and to resist distraction is dependent upon the pace. In managing the case information usually given to the liaison nurse, the student learns to screen for what is meaningful. As the student gains knowledge and skill, he or she can attend to the consultation framework and process mentally during a group meeting. The experienced liaison nurse has usually developed such guidelines for her practice. Guidelines aid the consultant in asking further questions about the case. The student does not yet think routinely about each consultation and often experiences each new situation as scary and alien. His or her response also reflects the volume of information in addition to the pace. It seems that past experiences have not prepared the student for the diversification of problems presented. This stress and anxiety may cause the student to feel that he or she must always have an answer and must act rather than respond. In acting, one may offer premature suggestions or several alternatives that confuse consultees. Realizing that one may not always have a solution or suggestion is important. Learning how to process information and give clear, direct feedback is the key to managing and minimizing stress and anxiety. As a student achieves some skill in the consultation process, he or she incorporates a structure or framework for the organization of much data.

The role of the liaison nurse is isolated by definition. Most agencies employ few, if more than one, such specialists. A student faces similar isolation in this placement. Some support and collegiality can be obtained from the preceptor and university advisor. However, these relationships do not replace the need for peer support. The opportunity to share responses and experiences with a fellow student decreases the feeling of isolation. It increases understanding of consultation work and of the unique system of the agency as well.

a difficult case

Mrs. R is a 72-year-old lady who is a widow with three daughters. Hospitalized on a neurology unit, she recently suffered a CVA (cerebrovascular accident) and has expressive and receptive aphasia. In her history it was noted that the patient was depressed prior to her hospitalization. Naturally, it was difficult for the staff to fully assess her responsive capacity. However, the nurses thought that she understood some of what they said to her. The problem faced by the staff was how to teach Mrs. R about her gangrenous right toe and prepare her for surgery. Since her lower limb circulation was very poor, the surgeons expected to do a below-the-knee amputation to ensure proper healing. At the time that the nurses presented this patient to us, Mrs. R would not even look at her foot. The situation seemed hopeless to the staff. They feared the patient's response after surgery.

From the patient's perspective, the whole hospital experience was probably strange and foreign. The eventual amputation might have been sufficient trauma to cause a total and severe withdrawal, along with increased depression, for this patient. From the nurses' point of view they were faced with a perplexing task—to teach a patient with severe communication difficulty about upcoming surgery and an eventual insult to her body image. Initially our own thoughts and feelings reflected doubt and some helplessness. As we thought further, we realized that the task of teaching this patient was not unlike that of teaching a very young child about surgery.

Together with our supervisor, we developed a teaching plan, using a doll to teach Mrs. R about her upcoming surgery. We blackened the doll's toe and put on a dressing. Each time the nurses changed her dressing they showed her by changing the doll's dressing. After several days the nurses were to amputate the doll's foot and wrap the stump. It was to be shown to Mrs. R the day before surgery. The patient initially cried when shown the doll, which was very moving to the staff and made them feel that she understood what they were trying to tell her. The staff felt that they were making progress with the teaching. They also involved the family in the routine explanations. The stress of the staff and the patient decreased and, the plan succeeded in preparing the patient for surgery.

the intrapsychic experience

The thoughts and feelings experienced by a student in the liaison role represent significant hurdles in the learning process. Despite past experience in psychiatric nursing and other specialty areas, the student role evokes a change in self-opinions. At times graduate students relive the feelings of being "just a student" as if they lack the knowledge and expertise that they had as practicing nurses. Such feelings do not represent reality and will eventually disappear, but they can influence graduate students in doing consultation. They compound or intensify other concerns of the student, which are important considerations and hurdles in this work.

One of the common feelings of graduate nurses is being overwhelmed by the consultation process. Feeling overwhelmed can cause increased anxiety and temporary immobilization. Immobilization often stems from helplessness, the wealth of information shared by the staff, and fear of the unknown. At times the dynamics of the case presentation or of the group process may affect the student's responses during the consultation. There may be a sense of urgency to provide answers, explanations, suggestions, or something helpful to the staff. This feeling can serve to exaggerate the awareness of inadequacies as a consultant. Slowly and painfully students learn to recognize their limitations and reactions and share them with the staff appropriately.

Another important issue for a student arises from the fear of destroying the rapport previously attained with the staff by the liaison nurse. Sometimes damage to or loss of rapport can lead to a decrease or loss of invitation to consult. Although the need for rapport is realistic, its loss need not result in cessation of liaison work. This fear comes from fantasy, as most mistakes are not irreparable. However, in trying to help the staff with a patient, a liaison nurse is cautious not to set the staff up to fail, by providing suggestions that they do not understand or cannot carry out. This hazard can befall students or practitioners who fail to validate whether their proposals seem realistic to the staff nurses. Consultation suggestions reflect available resources. If suggestions are realistic and interventions by the staff successful, the alliance with the liaison nurse will be strengthened. This will increase the use of the consultant by the staff.

Coupled with concern over rapport and the invitation to consult is often the felt need to be successful in consultation practice. Success is directly related to self-esteem. Neither the student nor the practitioner should rely totally on staff for feedback although this sometimes can be a source of validation and support. The major sources of such support, however, are in supervisory and peer relationships.

One of the greatest pitfalls of graduate students learning consultation is related to the achievement of the appropriate level of identification with the staff and the patient. Overidentification with the staff or the patient can cause the consultant to lose sight of the comprehensive picture of the problem and to be at a loss for suggesting helpful alternatives to the staff. Similarly, lack of identification can create difficulty in considering the importance of various aspects of the problem and in providing support through empathy. Lack of identification may stem from horror, disgust, anger, or fright as a response to the problem presented to the consultant. For example, it is not uncommon for a staff member to vividly describe a patient's condition or even show the consultant what the staff nurses are confronted with, such as mutilating surgery. This can cause the student to temporarily feel unable to empathize with the nurse and that he or she has little to offer. In cases of overidentification, the student may react from sadness, desperation, helplessness, or the recollection of a similar past experience. Striving for awareness of personal reactions to various elements of the consultation, a student slowly gains expertise and greater capability of avoiding identification problems.

The most important factor in relation to all these thoughts and feelings about consultation rests on recognizing them as normal. Students and practitioners alike experience these difficulties. Early recognition of personal responses helps to solve these problems. A colleague or supervisor plays a vital role in assisting the graduate student to identify these thoughts and feelings. Recognition may not always effect a change in responses. However, once recognition occurs, the student may manage identification problems more successfully.

problems and obstacles

Many problems encountered by the student providing nursing consultation resemble those experienced by practicing clinicians. These problems are inherent in the role itself. Other obstacles occur that are more unique and isolated to the student role. It is important to differentiate the two types of difficulties.

The student may experience the same uncertainty and resistance with staff in establishing the role, as does the practicing liaison nurse. The staff frequently have questions about the role and the student's purpose. When the role is not established, the staff commonly question its purpose and misunderstand the relationship for many months. If it is not continually explained, the staff may withdraw and cease to utilize the liaison nurse. Where an established practice of nursing consultation exists, the student will find it easier to assume the role. Once the student lays the initial groundwork, these difficulties decrease.

Any liaison nurse or student needs to develop the ability to synthesize an enormous amount of data quickly and attain an understanding of the key consultation questions and the psychodynamics. The next step is to suggest plausible intervention. To suppose that general hospital staff nurses can implement complex "psychiatric" nursing interventions in nonpsychiatric settings is to set the staff up to fail. The task requires the translation of psychiatric interventions into realistic action for many different specialty nurses. This problem does not prove insurmountable. If the student exercises patience and a willingness to examine previous mistakes, he or she can overcome this obstacle with time, practice, and increasing skill.

The title of "student" may represent an obstacle in itself. Most nurses are accustomed to a continual barrage of new students, which can mean an extra burden to the staff. If the staff's perception reflects the idea that students are inexperienced, the student nurse consultant may be unwelcome. A student's availability may also influence the reception that he or she receives. Increased student availability allows the staff to experience greater support and benefit from the relationship. Limited contact can decrease the possibility of effective utilization.

The student remains outside the institution, and this position, one step removed from the system, can create an obstacle. It requires time to understand a system, its politics and policies, and the many interrelationships of the staff. Certain situations may arise that are difficult for the student to fully grasp. Many staff may resist the intrusion of an outsider. The student should clarify with staff the fact that he or she functions under the same rules, limitations, and regulations of the system despite the lack of employee status. Such clarification may reinforce the consultation relationship of the student with the staff.

Needless to say, many of these situations place the student and the consultant under considerable stress. However, with time and practice such obstacles can be mastered.

enhancement of student consultation

The student role in nursing consultation may also promote successful experiences. Many times the staff view students as welcome additions to the team. They bring objectivity, new ideas, and extra time and energy to the health care team. A liaison student can often focus some energy on support for the staff who then benefit from the student's work. The patients also benefit. Ongoing support lessens the daily stress felt by the staff. Being a student and perhaps identified as more neutral, the staff may discuss their concerns and feelings more freely with the student. Such willingness provides the student an opportunity to build greater trust and rapport with the staff, which leads to an increased use of nursing consultation services.

The actions of the perceptor* enhance the student consultation experience. Introduction of the student as a colleague will encourage the staff to accept the student's help. The staff will grow accustomed to working with the student, as he or she participates in group meetings and does follow-ups alone. The preceptor can also encourage the student to work with others on the team, such as residents or social workers. Helpful tips about the system and the agency's internal politics may alert the student to important considerations in providing consultation. These various factors will influence the student's experience positively.

peer support

Peer support is a significant enhancement of the student consultation-liaison experience. The practitioner also derives much support and

---

*It should be noted that the word "preceptor" is used here interchangeably with that of "supervisor" since in our experience, the roles were performed by the same person. In another system, the roles may be performed by two different people.

benefit from a peer group. This relationship decreases the isolation inherent in the consultation role. Students, in particular, who are distressed at times with many thoughts and feelings evoked by their work, benefit from sharing their experience with a fellow student. This opportunity may arise through peer contacts at the university, or several students may share the same placement. The supportive network is often informal, but it may develop in clinical placement groups led by faculty. Whatever the format, peer support groups serve as an arena for the consultant to discuss distressing feelings and difficult case presentations.

Since we shared the placement, the two of us developed a mutual support system rather easily. This relationship provided us with an excellent mechanism for managing the stress of student consultation experiences. From time to time, we met to discuss our thoughts, feelings, and reactions to difficult situations at the agency. Informal opportunities in class or telephone conversations allowed us to share with each other freely and frequently. One significant factor in our development of this open supportive interaction was our previous year's experience on the same unit. There we had learned to respect our similarities and differences as individuals and as clinicians. This mutual respect and friendship fortified our interaction within and outside the clinical setting. We were also able to relate some data about important clinical case presentations to one another, as we did not share the same days in the agency routinely. Sharing clinical information helped each of us to maintain continuity over many case conferences. This meant that our preceptor need not spend extra time in keeping us informed on ongoing events as often. Most important was the opportunity to recognize our responses as normal because we could easily validate them with each other. Exchanging ideas about cases, discussing possible interventions, and validating one another's responses improved our understanding as students and our ability to function in this isolated role.

role of a supervisor

A supervisor fulfills an essential role in the graduate placement in consultation-liaison nursing. Supervision is a forum in which the student can share case material with another skilled, experienced practitioner. The student's supervisor provides support, assistance in problem solving, and constructive criticism to the student concerning consultations that he or she has done alone. It is also possible for the student to gain insight and understanding of the process by discussing consultations done jointly with the supervisor. By inviting the student to observe an experienced liaison nurse in practice, the supervisor serves as a role model. It is advantageous to utilize the preceptor at the agency for supervision, since he or she has greater familiarity with the nursing staff, other health team members, hospital policies, and the milieu of each unit. Without adequate supervision the student cannot derive optimal benefits from the experience.

The experienced liaison nurse has several role functions as supervisor. Specific time should be allocated for the presentation of clinical case material. The supervisor may suggest areas in which the student needs to increase knowledge. Various consultation techniques are discussed to help the student improve skills for use during case presentations. How and why specific intervention succeeds with the staff and the patient is better understood through examination of the consultation content and process in supervision. It is especially important to encourage the student to recognize his or her own intrapsychic responses as useful in doing consultations. They may represent keys to understanding the staff and/or the patient. Such an awareness is also helpful in achieving an appropriate level of identification with the consultee. Supervision will assist the student in identifying significant data, as well as in processing dynamics, strengths, and weaknesses in clinical work.

The data presented and the consultation process are both important to examine in supervision. The first step is that the student learns to organize and process case material. The next step focuses on the identification of the key question asked by the consultee. When the student can correctly isolate the question, the response given to the staff will more closely address the important issues. The next level of supervision helps the student to examine the dynamics of the consultation process. These are relevant to the intervention that will succeed. At this point, the student consultant needs to determine possible techniques and suggestions that will work and examine those that will not be successful. This step in supervision helps the student identify the rationale for intervention. The final step for consideration in supervision is the need for follow-up.

We have tried to include the many aspects of nursing consultation that make it enriching and rewarding for graduate students. There are a number of factors to consider in designing a consultation placement. The experience will allow the student to explore the issues and dynamics inherent in psychiatric liaison nursing, both its content and process. Ultimately, such a preceptorship will better prepare nurse clinicians to assume this role of expanded clinical practice.

references

1. Jill K. Nelson and Dianne A. Schilke, "The Evolution of Psychiatric Liaison Nursing," *Perspectives in Psychiatric Care* 14 (1976): 61–65.

2. Marie Berarducci, Kathleen Blanford, and Carol A. Garant, "The Psychiatric Liaison Nursing in the General Hospital," *General Hospital Psychiatry* 1:1 (April 1979): 66–72.

3. Diane P. Jansson, "Student Consultation: A Liaison Psychiatric Experience for Nursing Students," *Perspectives in Psychiatric Care* (March–April 1979): 77–82.

4. Cornelius Holland, Raymond Daly, and Charles Caparizano, "The Student Nurse as Therapeutic Consultant," *International Journal of Nursing Studies* 15:3 (1978): 153.

5. Lisa Robinson, "A Psychiatric Nursing Liaison Program," *Nursing Outlook* 20 (1972): 454–457.

6. Jill Nelson and Dianne Davis, "Educating the Psychiatric Liaison Nurse," *Journal of Nursing Education* 18:8 (October 1979): 14–20.

7. Anita Lewis, "A Consultation Framework," unpublished material.

appendix b
a clinical entry strategy in the pediatric setting

KATHLEEN O'MEARA

The method that a mental health liaison nurse chooses for entering a system is crucial to his or her overall functioning and subsequent effectiveness in the job. Eventual use of this nurse in a consultation-liaison role is related directly to the degree to which he or she has gained acceptance by other nurses in the system [1,2]. Acceptance cannot be expected automatically. Position and title do not guarantee and, in fact, can inhibit use of the liaison nurse by the staff. What can the liaison nurse do, therefore, to ensure acceptance in the system?

Visibility is essential. The staff have to know the liaison nurse is there; she or he has to be seen and become familiar. *Credibility* is necessary, too. The staff need to see the liaison nurse as someone who will make a difference in their practice. They should perceive him or her as having skills that could help them improve patient care, and the liaison nurse must establish *reliability* for assisting them with these skills. The liaison nurse employs strategies that will give nurses a chance to observe his or her clinical skills.

The opportunities for gaining visibility and credibility in a system are numerous. Some entry strategies to consider are assuming administrative accountability for a broadly based program, participating in rounds on units, attending orientations, and conducting workshops. The following presents a strategy successfully used for system entry in a pediatric care environment. This particular approach can be adapted to a variety of institutional settings.

As the only mental health liaison nurse in a 340-bed pediatric, tertiary care hospital (with extensive teaching and research affiliations), the need to provide an opportunity for broad system exposure was acute. Physically, the facilities are spread throughout several buildings, about the distance of a city block. The potential number of consumers is approximately 600 nurses, who provide a range of services that includes oncology, intensive care, dialysis, medical, surgical, psychosomatics, and ambulatory care.

Coincident with the beginning of this position, there was an organizational realignment of programs. The department of nursing became responsible for conducting programs to prepare children for hospitalization. This seemed a good chance for broad system exposure for the mental health liaison nurse, who could request administrative accountability for preadmission programming. Although the staff position of the liaison nurse may appear to be in conflict, the responsibility for program administration is similar to program consultation. Recommendations and interventions are made to a program. The programs would require involvement from the nursing staff throughout the institution. It would be the responsibility of the liaison nurse to develop and implement the plans, as well as to recruit nurses to staff the program. If all went well, the needed credibility would develop.

description of programs

Hospitals provide preadmission programs to prepare patients and their families for hospitalization. The hospitalization of a child, especially, is a stressful event for the whole family, and thoughtful preparation can help a child adapt well to this stress [3]. The type of preparation chosen is based on knowledge of the stressors, a realistic assessment of what needs can be met on a preadmission basis, and the developmental level of the child. The major developmental tasks that the child is dealing with impact on how he or she will experience hospitalization [4,5]. Also, children learn differently at different ages. Modalities chosen for the preadmission programs differ based on age groups, and they take the above points into consideration.

There is a script to accompany each of our programs. For the preschool group (under 7 years old) we use puppets; for school-aged children (7–12 years old), we have slides and a tour; and we have a combination of tools based on individual patients' requests for our adolescents and young adults (12 and up). We try to be sensitive to adolescents' strivings to be independent and their need to have control over their situation. The message from the beginning is one that includes the adolescent in the planning of his or her preparation.

Scripts cover events common to the day of admission through the day of discharge, and include the perioperative experience. There is a table at each program for displaying hospital equipment—operating room hats, masks, and gloves, stethoscopes, syringes, stuffed dolls, bedpans, urinals, thermometers, and the like. The staff encourage the children to play with what they see and ask questions about them. Children like to "give dolls injections" or "take their temperatures," and often they will play out their concerns about coming to the hospital. This helps a child gain control and a sense of mastery over the stresses of the hospital experience. Staff who take part in the programs are nurses and activity therapists from a variety of areas, including the operating rooms, surgical divisions, and x-ray. Staff were selected who could provide familiarity and concrete information about their particular areas and roles. There is an expectation that the primary nurse relationship will begin preadmission.

Each family is interviewed individually, but informally. The program's staff under the supervision and support of the liaison nurse, attempts to establish a rapport with parents and children that facilitates information gathering about specific fears or fantasies concerning the upcoming hospitalization. It is difficult, if not impossible, for a child to hear the preparatory information if his or her anxiety has not been decreased by clarification and reassurance. For example, one 11-year-old told the nurse who was encouraging him to try on an identification bracelet, that he knew what it was for: "My grandfather told me that it is so they can identify your body when they take you to the morgue." After the initial shock of this comment, the nurse, with the assistance of the liaison nurse, explored with the child the reason for his hospitalization and his own fears. It was then possible for the nurse to offer appropriate and realistic reassurance.

Latency-aged children commonly have a fear of death. We try to explore what they say to us, and use their capacity to reason. It is important to acknowledge similarities in children's stories. One must also separate what is unique about each illness and hospitalization [6]. We emphasize confidence in the expertise of the doctors and the nurses. Our rapport and the leverage of our "experience working with children" are used to reassure a child, to use this child's language that he "will not go to the morgue."

In the script, the fear of death and its equally common converse, which is that the child will wake up during surgery, is addressed during slides of the operating room area: "Children are always asleep during their surgery and always awaken when it is over." Since you can awaken while asleep at night, the sleep for surgery is differentiated for them from going to sleep at night. Nursing staff take this language and use it in their interactions with children on the units.

Nursing interventions that successfully abate a child's anxieties are positive experiences for nurses and can increase their sense of worth and value. The liaison nurse in recognizing their interventions supports the nurses' self-esteem, and offers collaboration in further challenges to their skills. For example, in exploring with staff what information is most pertinent to gather on a preadmission basis, the staff develop skills in eliciting data that is useful to the planning of nursing care. They try to learn the history, not only of a patient, but of the whole family. Factors that are considered are: previous or recent hospitalizations, illnesses or losses and how these were experienced and dealt with, and the history of separations for the child. They seek a developmental overview described physically, cognitively, and psychosocially. They study the family's perception of the reason for or meaning of the illness and hospitalization, how the family has prepared to cope with the disruption of the hospitalization (including expectations about parent/family involvement and participation in the hospital), and any changes they have noticed in the child or the siblings' behavior since knowledge of the hospitalization (sleep disturbances, aggression, bed-wetting, and so on). Interviewers try to learn about the child's fears, such as concerns regarding anesthesia, injections, abandonment (by family as well as by peers), pain, mutilation, and death.

Directing the preadmission programs can benefit the mental health liaison nurse in many ways: system-wide exposure, credibility, alliance building, assessment of needs of nurses, formal and informal teaching, and an opportunity for staff to experience the impact of the liaison role on their practice.

Preadmission programs need total system involvement in order to be effective. They need to be integrated as part of the total hospital experience so the child and the family have a place to discuss their concerns and raise questions before the hospital stay. The information we gather about individual children is communicated to the nurse who will plan the child's care in the hospital. The mental health liaison nurse assists the staff in understanding the significance of their observations. Children tell us through their play, their interactions with their parents, their brothers and sisters, the staff, and other children at the program what their needs are.

Toby, a 5-year old, who was to be admitted for a tonsillectomy, used the syringe to jab vigorously at the genital area of the doll. The liaison nurse encouraged him to talk about what he was doing, and when the boy explained the doll was "getting an operation," she rein-forced that "only his tonsils will be taken out; no other part of him will be touched."

For a boy this age, it is probable that this behavior represents a displacement of the genitals for the body part that was going to be operated on [7]. Through his play, he was expressing his fears of castration made even more poignant as he was facing an operation. This child needed continual reassurance that everything would be the same and work properly after his operation.

Several days after this program, one of the in-patient staff nurses demonstrated how she had benefited from this child's example and the intervention of the liaison nurse, when she observed a preschool-aged child who was clutching at his underwear as he was being prepared for surgery. She remembered the incident above and realized that this child should be allowed to keep his underwear on.

There has been multiple evidence of nurses' taking what they were able to learn at the preadmission programs and incorporating it into their practice, reflecting how much they have grown through this new dimension. All children are striving to grow up, to know themselves as separate persons, to know and control their bodies and functions, and to learn to relate to and communicate with others. Children expend a great deal of energy moving through their developmental stages. As nurses, our task is to maintain and facilitate the developmental strivings of the child who is faced with the enormous stress of hospitalization. The mental health liaison nurse tries to assist nurses in this task.

On another occasion a nurse reported her frustration with the way Judy, a 15-year-old, was treating her mother during an adoles-cent preadmission program. Judy had wanted her mother to come, but ignored her rudely once they arrived.

Later, the liaison nurse discussed with the staff what Judy might have been saying through this behavior. A patient this age wants to make decisions about the things that will happen to her. She has a need to be in control and assert her independence. Much of her self-esteem will come from behaving in more adult ways. However, at this stressful time, she also needs to know it is OK to want her parents with her. Subsequently, the nurse was also able to talk with Judy's mother, who was confused by this adolescent's message. The nurse helped her to understand Judy's needs developmentally as well as her occasional need to regress.

Preadmission programs identify liaison nurses and their work for the nursing staff so they will be utilized in other clinical settings. Also, patients identified at the programs as having outstanding needs can receive follow-up when admitted. The liaison nurse is available to consult to the primary nurse around the plan of care.

credibility

Before introducing the new programs to our institutions, it was important to know what had been going on previously and what staff would identify with this program. History influences how people perceive what is now being offered. Indeed, attitudes regarding the "preadmission parties," as they had been called, were not favorable. Difficulties seemed to stem from the lack of one coordinating person, who was responsible for the overall functioning of the program, and from the absence of a core group of staff committed to participation in the parties. Apparently, nurses were selected randomly and assigned to staff the parties. Often they felt coerced, rather than actively choosing to participate. They could not see the sense in being removed from caring for sick patients in order to attend a "party." They didn't understand the value of preadmission preparation and its effect on a child's hospitalization, and they had not experienced the benefits for the patients and for themselves.

It was vital to the effectiveness of the programs that these concerns be addressed. Most germane to the role of liaison nurses at this time is, first, the staff's perception of them as credible individuals and, second, the opportunity to offer nurses information and skills useful to their practice. The nurses were sought out, and their concerns were listened to carefully. Changes in the program relative to concerns expressed by the nurses were instituted. Collaboration with staff helped them accept liaison nurses as reliable persons. The liaison nurse emphasized that the terms "parties" would not be used. This is an incorrect and unclear message to children, because entering the hospital is not a party. It can be pleasant but certainly not fun. Sometimes health care providers use words that are not accurate in terms of what a child actually experiences in an effort to desensitize the child. If children see discrepancies between what we tell them and what they actually experience, they will be less able to trust us. The establishment of a trusting relationship between a child and a nurse is basic to effective care. To be able to trust restores some of the confidence the child has lost when facing the unknowns of the hospitalization.

The concept of establishing a trusting relationship is basic in addressing the emotional needs of the pediatric patient. Presentation of the preadmission programs provides liaison nurses with a forum for reinforcing with nursing staff this need for trust in the nurse–patient relationship. In addition to the presentation of useful information, exploring with staff the history of the programs, and making plans that include their ideas, liaison nurses can enhance the professional development of staff by using clinical situations that nurses can relate to their everyday practice. For example, one young nurse frequently looked distraught and worried when she was listening to a child talk about his reason (which was serious) for hospitalization. She would tell him not to worry, saying "everything will work out." The liaison nurse pointed out to her the discrepancy between what she was saying and how she looked. This could be confusing to the child, and result in his not being reassured by the interaction.

alliance building

The system-wide visibility attained from developing and implementing these programs created opportunities for the liaison nurse to build alliances. In presenting the programs to the staff, as well as in presenting the role of the mental health liaison nurse, relationships were built with key people in the institution.

In the department of nursing, head nurses are the area gatekeepers [8]. They have the authority to support staff in those activities that affect quality patient care. If they are aware of the purpose of the preadmission programs and believe in their helpfulness to the soon-to-be hospitalized child, they have an opportunity to enhance the quality of patient care by sanctioning staff involvement in the programs. The head nurse can provide for the liaison nurse access to staff for assessing skills they need to develop in order to effectively address patient and family needs. The head nurse is eager to develop staff, and sharing examples like the following from the programs increases the head nurse's support:

Many parents reveal their concerns in the comfortable atmosphere of the program. One mother talked about forgetting to administer medication to her son, as she and her husband were involved in a separation. She sighed, "Now he [her son] has to have an operation." She sat and watched her son, but did not respond as he ran around the room, grabbed things away from other children, and hoarded cookies. Her behavior indicated that she was probably overwhelmed. Her child's nurse tried to reassure her that everything would be fine.

After the program the liaison nurse assisted the staff in understanding this mother's cues, and acknowledging their own reactions to them. The mother's inability to set limits on her child had left many of the staff angry. In the author's opinion, this mother's behavior was reflecting her guilt about her child's hospitalization. Parents are sometimes overindulgent, pampering, or unable to set limits on their hospitalized child as a way to assuage the guilt they feel.

The staff nurse who had talked with the mother was able to acknowledge her feelings of being overwhelmed by this mother's problems and sadness. She had wanted to reassure the mother rather than explore feelings that would be difficult to talk about or situations that she felt helpless to do anything about. Sometimes, nurses bring premature closure to an interaction with parents because the topic is painful. However, when nurses receive validation for their feelings in these situations and learn more therapeutic responses, they are far more likely to explore feelings with parents when appropriate.

Post-program discussion between staff and the liaison nurse provides an opportunity to clarify the meaning of the clinical situation and discuss interventions. An alliance is established around the mutual goal of providing quality patient care, and plans can be formulated to help patients in the impending hospital stay.

teaching opportunities

The educational value of the programs is a major benefit to the liaison nurse in the opportunities they provide to teach staff. The teaching and learning experiences at the programs are numerous, and they offer a uniqueness due to their setting, presence of the family, and the direct patient care involvement of the liaison nurse. The programs provide a forum for reinforcing with nurses how children respond to their environment. The unknowns of the hospital, which may include the people, uniforms, machines, rooms, odors, equipment, procedures, and the like, can all be extremely frightening to children for whom a sense of mastery and control over their world is essential to their sense of well-being. These fears influence how children behave in the hospital.

At the preadmission program, children know they are going

back home that day. They have on their own clothes. They are not sick. Usually they have their families along and they are given a light snack. All these things make them feel more comfortable, more secure. They are allowed to explore the environment at their own pace, to talk to the staff, and to play with hospital equipment when they are ready. Many nurses observe that "the children seem less anxious than in the hospital." They are more engaging and free in expressing their concerns.

Also, the family is encouraged to attend the program, and this provides another valuable teaching opportunity for the liaison nurse. In a pediatric setting, it is not always possible to see a whole family together. Nurses can observe the family interacting at the program, which reinforces the fact that the hospitalization of a child is a stressful event that affects the whole family. The teaching of this concept by the liaison nurse is strengthened by this clinical experience.

The more predictable nature of the preadmission program gives the liaison nurse a chance to work with staff and patients in a different environment. Staff, patients, and their families often feel less overwhelmed than on the day of admission. Staff usually report that the day of admission is hectic, and the child and parents are anxious. There are so many "things" to get done, and nursing care is directed at "getting everything under control." Control often becomes the focus of the interaction between parent and nurse. Establishing a collaborative relationship by giving the parent the feeling that the nurse and the parent are there to work together in the care of the child is optimum. The parent may feel excluded, which increases the sense of helplessness and guilt that parents often feel around the hospitalization of their child.

At the preadmission program, time is more structured and organized. The program climate facilitates staff learning, since there is no pressure to "get everything under control." Liaison nurses are in a "hands-on" position to work with staff in developing their skills and to demonstrate their own.

Gradually nurses increase their interviewing skills, build confidence in their capacity to interview parents, and feel less of a need to dominate or control in the parent–nurse relationship. Nurses experience the parents as collaborators in the care of the child. One nurse reflected: "This head start is great. I guess I always knew, but could never really appreciate, that, in fact, the parents know more about their child than anyone else."

The mental health liaison nurse is knowledgeable about the

developmental strivings of the child. There is an expectation that the programs will be based on an awareness of the developmental concerns of the various age groups. This knowledge is crucial to the effective care of the children. Staff nurses spend much time in close contact with the child. They are in a key position to assess and plan the care that will preserve and promote the child's development. Seeing the children in groups divided by age, as they are at the weekly program, reinforces the nurses' awareness of developmental concerns.

The preschool program uses animal puppets for the delivery of a script that addresses, among other issues, the major issue of separation. Many children feel that the separation due to hospitalization is retribution for the rivalrous feelings so common at this age [9]. The child might believe he or she deserves to be punished and therefore abandoned.

Our preschool script clarifies fantasies about the reason for hospitalization. One puppet says that he is "worried about something." He is worried that he has come to the hospital because he "was bad and hit his brother." The puppeteer asks if people come to the hospital because they are bad [10]. Children in our audiences have responded "yes." There follows clarification that, "coming to the hospital has nothing to do with being bad or being good; it has to do with being sick." Children are assured that no one is to blame for their hospitalization. They also hear that their need to have parents with them is respected and carefully considered.

At the program for our school-age children, staff nurses observe and hear the importance of peers to this age group. Their development is moving these children from a parent/family orientation to an emphasis on relationships with peers. These children commonly have fears of mutilation and of death [11]. Nurses incorporate this understanding of the patient's needs in their interventions.

The staff encourage the participation of in-patients. The soon-to-be-admitted child is reassured by the presence of in-patients who have survived this ordeal and who are responding quite competently to questions. Nurses communicate to a child that they will try to put him in a room with boys his own age. They bring an awareness of the child's growing need for independence from his or her parents and attempt to integrate this with the parents' wishes and needs to participate in their child's hospitalization.

The liaison nurse works with nurses in the program and uses

these real clinical situations to make the learning experience more valuable for each nurse.

value of the liaison role

Staff who participate in the programs experience the value of the liaison role to their practice when they observe alterations in the family's adaptations. Nursing interventions made as a result of work with the liaison nurse validate the usefulness of the role for quality patient care. The following example illustrates this:

> We learned during one program that a 6-year-old sister showed a marked change in behavior when she heard about her 7-year-old brother's impending hospitalization for cardiac surgery. She was seen for hyperactivity by a psychologist at her school. Previously, she had been a quiet and passive child. The children's father had died two years before of a heart attack. He had been taken to the hospital while the children were sleeping, and he died that night.
>
> The liaison nurse suggested that the threat of the brother's hospitalization could have precipitated the behavior changes in the sister, and that she might be thinking that her brother would go to the hospital and never come back (as her father had done).
>
> Exploring this with her mother, we learned that an inaccurate understanding of the visiting policy was making the situation worse. The little sister was under 12 years old so she did not think she would be able to visit her brother. The visiting policy, which attempts to be flexible for siblings, was clarified. A primary nurse telephoned the family before admission to reinforce the message that she wanted the patient's sister to come and visit.
>
> The patient, at 7 years old, was the only male in the family and had assumed a father role toward his younger sister. After admission he was able to talk with the nurse about his fears regarding his open heart surgery. At the preadmission program he had maintained a bravado that there was nothing he was worried about.
>
> The nurse was not a familiar person but was seen as an ally in the care of his sister. The knowledge that the nurse could do some of the father surrogating freed this boy to focus his energy on adapting to the hospitalization. The boy told the nurse, after a visit from his sister, "Can you believe it, she thought she wasn't going to be able to come see me?"

This nurse had made a significant intervention in this family for whom going to the hospital had come to mean not ever coming home.

potential problems

As in any system entry strategy, there are potential risks in this choice to the successful entry of the liaison nurse. Although assuming administrative accountability for the preadmission programs was extremely useful, it also involved problems that need to be considered. Overall responsibility for system-wide programs is time-consuming. Once nurses have initiated the liaison role successfully in the institution, to continue to administrate the programs may not be the best use of their time. However, support from a nursing department to relinquish the director's role may not be readily available. It can be useful, therefore, for liaison nurses to document the amount of time they spend in administering the programs.

The other potential problem is the possibility that staff will be confused by the liaison nurse's position in the organization. Liaison nurses in a staff position who assume responsibility for program administration may need to clarify what seems to be a shift in status. They can be attentive and address any misperceptions directly, reinforcing their staff position as mental health liaison nurses. The staffs' concurrently evolving experience of them in the liaison role will hopefully eliminate any confusion regarding their position organizationally.

Finally, liaison nurses must understand their commitment to the programs as they influence the liaison role. Failure to take seriously the responsibility for directing the programs could result in the programs failing. This could compromise liaison nurses' reliability and credibility severely and would counteract their acceptance by the nursing staff.

Assuming administrative accountability for a hospital-wide program as an early responsibility in the liaison role is a useful strategy for entering the system. Directing programs provides visibility. Implementing them well gives credibility to liaison nurses responsible for these programs. The nurses carry out the function of their liaison role—that is, to assist nurses in developing their skills in addressing the psychosocial needs of the patient—within the concrete structure of the program. Staff experiencing the effectiveness of the programs, both for their own learning and for the quality of patient care, move toward acceptance of mental health liaison nurses and their role.

references

1. Maxine E. Loomis, "The Clinical Specialist as a Change Agent," *Nursing Forum* (1968): 137–145.
2. A Peer Group of Liaison Nurses, "Role Creation: A Challenge to the Psychiatric Liaison Nurse and the Nursing Administrator," to be published.
3. Elizabeth Crocker, "Preparation for Elective Surgery: Does It Make a Difference," *Journal of the Association of Care of Children in Hospitals* (Summer 1980): 3–11.
4. Humberto Nagera, "Children's Reaction to Hospitalization and Illness," *Child Psychiatry and Human Development* (Fall 1978): 3–19.
5. Norine J. Kerr, "The Effect of Hospitalization on the Developmental Tasks of Childhood," *Nursing Forum* (1979): 108–129.
6. Madeline Petrillo and Sergay Sanger, *Emotional Care of Hospitalized Children: An Environmental Approach* (Philadelphia: J. B. Lippincott Company, 1980), pp. 225–228.
7. Anna Freud, "The Role of Bodily Illness in the Mental Life of Children," in *The Psychoanalytic Study of the Child*, edited by R. Eissler et al. (New York: International Universities Press, Inc., 1952), pp. 74–75.
8. Sally Everson, "Staff Development Model of Consultation—Liaison for the Integration of the Role of Clinical Nurse Specialist," *Journal of Continuing Education in Nursing* 12:1 (March–April 1981): 18.
9. Petrillo and Sanger, pp. 42–45.
10. Susan Linn, M., ed., Puppet Therapist, puppet show script.
11. Petrillo and Sanger, pp. 46–48.

bibliography

books

Bowlby, J. *Attachment and Loss: Volume II—Separation*. New York: Basic Books, Inc., Publishers, 1973.
Dawson, R. and Hardgrove, C. *Parents and Children in the Hospital*. Boston: Little, Brown & Company, 1972.
Eggert, L. "Family Subsystem: The Therapeutic Process with Adolescents Experiencing Psychosocial Stress," in *Clinical Practice in Psychosocial Nursing: Assessment and Intervention*, edited by Diane Luongo and Reg Arthur Williams. New York: Appleton-Century-Crofts, 1978, pp. 257–288.
Erikson, E. *Childhood and Society*. New York: W. W. Norton & Company, Inc., 1963.

VERNON, D.; FOLEY, J.; SIPOWICZ, R.; and SCHULMAN, J. *The Psychological Response of Children to Hospitalization and Illness*. Springfield, Ill.: Charles C. Thomas, Publisher, 1965.

WHALEY, L. and WONG, D. *Nursing Care of Infants and Children*. St. Louis: The C. V. Mosby Company, 1979.

articles

FERGUSON, B. F., "Preparing Young Children for Hospitalization: A Comparison of Two Methods," *Pediatrics* 64 (November 1979): 656–664.

GEIST, R. "Consultation on a Pediatric Surgical Ward: Creating an Empathic Climate," *American Journal of Orthopsychiatry* (July 1977): 432–444.

GOLDSTEIN, S. "The Psychiatric Clinical Specialist in the General Hospital," *Journal of Nursing Administration* (March 1979): 34–37.

HEDLUND, N. "Mental Health Nursing Consultation in the General Hospital," *Patient Counselling and Health Education* (Fall 1978): 85–88.

KLEIN, C. and SATTERTHWAITE, M. "Preparation and the Hospitalized Child," *Journal of the Association for Care of Children in Hospitals* (Winter 1980): 60–63.

McGRATH, M. "Group Preparation of Pediatric Surgical Patients," *Image* (June 1979): 52–62.

MELAMUD, B. and SIEGEL, L. "Reduction of Anxiety in Children Facing Hospitalization and Surgery by Use of Filmed Modeling," *Journal of Consulting and Clinical Psychology* (1975): 511–531.

MENG, A. "Parents' and Children's Reactions Toward Impending Hospitalization for Surgery," *Maternal-Child Nursing Journal* (Summer 1980): 83–98.

SIEMON, M. "Family Subsystem: Working with School-Age Children Experiencing Psychosocial Stress," in *Clinical Practice in Psychosocial Nursing: Assessment and Intervention*, edited by Diane Luongo and Reg Arthur Williams. New York: Appleton-Century-Crofts, 1978, pp. 289–318.

VISINTAINER, M. and WOLFER, J. "Pediatric Surgical Patients' and Parents' Stress Responses and Adjustment as a Function of Psychologic Preparation and Stress-Point Nursing Care," *Nursing Research* (July 1975): 244–255.

WEINSTEIN, L. J.; CHAPMAN, N. N.; and STALLINGS, M. A. "Organizing Approaches to Psychiatric Nurse Consultation," *Perspectives in Psychiatric Care* (March 1979): 66–71.

appendix c
a family systems model in the long-term care facility

MARILYN ROSSIER

Psychiatric liaison nurses have repeatedly to decide when, where, and how to relate to patients and staff within an institution. Family systems theory is a valuable framework within which liaison nurses can understand the family-like system that develops on a patient care unit, as well as identify some of the dynamics in operation there. This understanding is helpful in evaluating the readiness and potential response to mental health involvement, and it is a useful tool when planning intervention. Such a system is present in any patient care facility, but it is particularly evident in long-term care (chronic disease hospitals and nursing homes) where relationships develop over a longer time and where patients have given up other homes to live out their lives in an institution.

Statistics gathered in 1979 indicate that 40 percent of all patients in nursing homes in the United States have no immediate family, and that 60 percent have no visitors [1]. It is not surprising that many patients look to the institution to replace their families of origin. They seek a sense of security and belongingness from other patients and staff. It is from the reactions of those around them that they attempt to gain or maintain a sense of dignity and self-worth.

Perhaps less apparent is the attempt of staff to achieve this same kind of support from the patient care system. Staff depend upon reactions from supervisors, peers, and patients to support their own sense of self-worth and to provide a feeling of belonging. Although this is true to some extent in many places of employment, the intimate relations that develop in long-term care facilities seem to foster such attitudes.

Although this mutual dependence can produce positive relationships, living and working in a long-term care facility can also produce an overwhelming sense that there is no escape. Patients come to chronic disease hospitals and nursing homes because they have medical and nursing care needs that are likely to remain for the rest of their lives, and because the care they need cannot be provided at home or by out-patient facilities. They cannot sign out against medical advice because they physically cannot manage to get out the door, and, even if they could, they have no home to flee to. For staff members the fact that the patient population remains relatively constant means that feelings of closeness and attachment develop, and leaving to seek other employment is a wrenching experience, not unlike breaking family ties when one leaves home. Resignation can feel like abandonment to both staff and patients.

Consider the atmosphere on a unit in a chronic disease hospital or nursing home. Patients are likely to be dressed in their own clothing, not hospital gowns and robes. Many are out of bed in wheelchairs or geriatric chairs. Meals are sometimes eaten together in a dining room. There are pictures of loved ones on the bedside table, a special music box on the dresser or art object on the wall. When someone has a birthday, staff member or patient, there are cakes and cards, and everyone celebrates. There is an effort to make the surroundings home-like.

Care patterns become orderly and routine. Sally M always has a cup of coffee before the nurses hear the morning report. John W has his turn in the tub on Tuesday. Friday is the day Mildred F goes to the hairdresser. This is not a temporary stopping place but a place where people live.

Time is available to build healthy relationships, to resolve issues, and to see growth take place. Psychiatric liaison nurses can help achieve and maintain the dynamic homeostatis necessary for such a nurturing climate. They are "friendly outsiders," part of the system because they are part of the health care staff, but not members of the individual unit family. Because they are nurses, they are allies of the nursing staff who can be trusted to understand their frustration and problems. Also because they are nurses, they can help staff keep their focus on the patient and on the goal of ever improving psychological care.

An evaluation of the functioning of a patient care unit as a family-like system and identification of the roles played by various members will aid liaison nurses at the time a unit requests help. Such an evaluation should begin as soon as possible after the nurse is employed, and it is an ongoing process. Liaison nurses can observe staff and patients during the change-of-shift report, the team meeting, and the daily care times to gather data to determine how a unit is functioning. It is important to note here that the role of liaison nurses is not that of therapists to the staff; so such an evaluation is generally not shared with the staff or patients directly but used to help plan an intervention on each unit and to evaluate its effectiveness.

Family-member-like roles taken by people who comprise the patient care unit are not always the same. However, since the doctor is usually male and the nurses female, they most often become father and mother to the patient/children. The role parallels follow when one notes that the doctor is only on the unit briefly each day, while the nurse has the all-day care of the patients, just as a traditional father is usually away from home most of the time, and it is usually the mother who stays home with the children, providing various forms of physical care and feeding. Just as siblings sometimes take on parenting roles for each other in families, patients will sometimes take care of one another in nurturing ways. The system is more like the American family of several generations ago when grandparents, aunts, uncles, and cousins were a close part of the family living under the same roof or in close proximity. If occupational and physical therapy personnel and social workers are part of the care team on the unit, they assume roles similar to these aunts and uncles, sometimes taking on part of the care-giving and disciplinary functions. If the patient leaves the unit to travel to separate departments for treatment, to physical therapy for example, the relationship becomes more like the relationship between the family and school. The patient may say that her therapist wants her to transfer from bed to chair in a particular way and that the nurse is "doing it wrong," just as the child reports at home, "but my teacher said. . . ."

Family systems can be placed on a continuum of health that ranges from the most disorganized and chaotic with little energy coming in from the outside, through those that are less chaotic but quite rigid, to those that are most organized yet are flexible [2]. Various characteristics of attitude, communication, and behavior give clues to the observer as to the relative overall health of family functioning (Table C–1).

Patient care units, functioning like family systems, exhibit similar characteristics that indicate how well they function. Levels of functioning will change from unit to unit in any hospital or nursing home, as well as from time to time.

In most impaired families there is a lack of individual boundaries. Members are usually unaware of how much "group speak" they do and how little attention is paid to individual perceptions and feelings. There are often family members totally ignored by others. Planning in such a family group is almost impossible, since no individual is free to voice an opinion that may be different from the others. For example, the question of how to spend a vacation becomes difficult to answer. Shall the family go to the mountains, the beach, or travel across the country? No on speaks up to voice a preference, fearing it might be different from the others. To be different is to be excluded from the family. If one person does all the speaking for the family, the decision will be made by that one with no disagreement from the others. With no outlet for disagreement or anger, feeling tones become apathetic, empty, and sometimes cynical.

> A patient was transferred from a rehabilitation unit to a long-term unit that displayed some of the above characteristics. On this unit patients were all put to bed at the same hour. The head nurse made all the decisions and told them to her staff, whom she called "my kids." Every television set on the ward was tuned to the same channel, since staff said that everyone liked watching the same programs. Patients sat in their chairs with heads down. As the liaison nurse walked down the corridor, it was difficult to make eye contact and no one greeted her. When the liaison nurse asked about patients on the unit, staff would talk about some and not mention others. When questioned about the ones omitted, there were comments like, "Oh, I forgot about him." Or, "What would you want to know about her?"
>
> The nurse who brought the transferred patient to this unit attempted to explain to the head nurse about the patient's daily schedule during rehabilitation and to describe some of her preferences. "Oh, she's not going to be up that early here," said the head nurse. "None of our patients like to get up before breakfast. They all go slow in the morning."

The family on the midrange of the continuum allows for more autonomy on the part of the family members. However, an over-riding sense that people are essentially evil and therefore in need of strict control promotes the attitude towards child-rearing that makes it a battle. Definitions of good and evil exclude basic human qualities of anger, sexuality, and ambivalence. Since the expectation is always in absolutes, members of such families are constantly disappointed by the behavior of others. The rigidity of the system promotes sadness, depression, low-keyed bickering, and scapegoating. There is resistance to change, but hope is maintained through an "if-only" stance that things might be better if only some change occurred.

TABLE C–1 TYPES OF FAMILY SYSTEMS [3]

Seriously Disturbed	Midrange	Healthy
Lack of individual boundaries	Severely restricted autonomy	High degree of autonomy
Strong sense of timelessness	Human nature seen as evil	Human nature good or neutral
Poor parental coalition	Poor parental coalition or subjugation of one parent	Good parental coalition
Frequent speaking for others	Frequent scapegoating	Power shared, no domination
Unresponsive to one another	Feeling tones vary from polite to angry or depressed	Frequent real encounters and sharing
Individual choice impossible	Ubiquitous referee dominates	Feeling tone positive, frequent laughter
Poor task	Resistant to change, but hope for good change is alive.	High task efficiency
	Child-rearing seen as a battle for control	Extremely open and receptive

Table by W. Robert Beavers. Adapted from *The Minister As Crisis Counselor*, edited by David K. Switzer. Copyright 1974 by Abington Press. Used by permission.

On such a patient care unit it is difficult for staff to allow patients to express anger and for staff to express anger toward each other and toward patients. Patients are often put into "good" and "bad" categories, since ambivalent feelings of liking and disliking the same person are difficult to accept. "Good" patients are usually quiet and compliant. Patients are viewed as asexual, and behavior such as masturbation or talk of sexual fantasies is not permitted. Staff and patients alike often bicker about whether they get their fair share of attention. Staff may focus on patient assignments, days off, and coffee breaks. Patients may demand special diets and tasks that keep the nurses running to the bedside. Staff may think patients try to do as little for themselves as possible, while patients are heard to complain that staff spend too much time in the nurses' station.

> Nurses on one unit that exhibited some of these characteristics lamented that they had no time to take patients outdoors. When it was suggested that on warm spring days some patients might not have a total bedbath to allow time for them to go outdoors, the head nurse said that they could not do this since all patients had to have a complete bath daily. (There was no hospital policy for this.) No staff disagreed. They decided that excursions to the lawn would be possible *if only* more nurses were assigned to their unit.
>
> On another such unit when the suggestion was made that patients might participate in decisions regarding the daily schedule, one nurse said, "If you give them an inch, they'll take a yard." Staff agreed that allowing patients "too much" decision making would get out of control, since patients "try to get as much as they can." The child-rearing battle of the nursery is re-enacted daily on that ward.

The organized yet flexible family system is characterized by clearly defined roles and an openness to express thoughts and feelings. Ambivalence is accepted and true negotiation of differences takes place, resulting in problem solving and compromise. There is an unspoken affirmation that people are basically good and trustworthy. Interactions are punctuated with laughter, inside jokes, and easy give-and-take. Children are clearly less powerful than parents, but their ideas are listened to and incorporated into family decisions. This type of family is an open system, receiving input from outside and adapting to change.

> Nurses on one unit opened a discussion one day concerning the presence on their ward of half a dozen alert female patients mixed in with some twenty-five others who were either comatose or whose brain damage made them only partially aware of their surroundings and with whom communication was difficult. The nurses decided to rearrange patient room assignments, placing the alert patients together, even though they recognized that these patients would probably compete with each other for the nurses' attention and might argue with one another at times. The nurses drew up a timetable for the change and decided which nurse would present the idea to each patient to ask for voluntary participation in what would be a time-limited trial. After several weeks they evaluated the new arrangement, sharing their own feelings about working in a different environment and the reac-

tions gleaned from the patients. They decided to keep the alert patients together and begin planning for other ways to make the living environment more pleasant for these women.

Liaison nurses begin their intervention with the staff on an individual unit with organized knowledge about how that particular unit generally functions. When they receive a consultation or a request for assistance, it is important for them to assess what is currently occuring in the milieu.

Family therapy developed as clinicians realized that it was often more productive to deal with families than to react to a single troubled individual. These clinicians came to realize that a young person having trouble at school might be more a symptom of a family in trouble than of a sick adolescent. Since families strive to maintain a modicum of balance or homeostasis, the behavior of the troubled person may be in the service of maintaining the balance, and to change the behavior without dealing with the whole family is to throw the system out of kilter. It is also apparent that a call for help in dealing with a behavior problem exhibited by a patient may mean that the relationships on the patient care units are in trouble, rather than that the problem lies only with the individual patient. The liaison model provides a method for dealing with underlying problems.

Virginia Satir, using knowledge about family dynamics acquired in her years as a family therapist, provides a framework for assessing family function that is applicable to patient care units. In a troubled family Satir evaluates:

- *Self-worth:* The feelings and ideas each person has about himself or herself.
- *Communication:* The ways people work out to make meaning to one another.
- *Rules:* What people use for how they should feel and behave.
- *Link to society:* The way in which family relates to people and institutions outside the family [4].*

How each individual feels about himself or herself provides the basis for viewing and dealing with the rest of the world. If individuals appreciate their own worth, they can realize and value the worth of others. They can be honest, compassionate, trusting, and hopeful.

---

*Reprinted by permission of the author and publisher. *Peoplemaking* by Virginia Satir. Science & Behavior Books, Inc. Palo Alto, CA 94306.

Individuals with low self-esteem are distrustful, defensive, and isolated. If they cannot value themselves, they are not open to value others.

The relatively helpless state of being a patient is a setup for a sense of worthlessness. It takes hard work on the part of patient care providers to develop a living situation for patients in which they can feel some worth as individuals. If there are times when the self-worth of the staff is at a low ebb, they have little energy to devote to providing for the patient's sense of well-being. Liaison nurses need to evaluate the sense of self-worth evident in staff members and patients. They must be alert to situations that detract from positive feelings. As interested outsiders, they are in a position to contribute to staff members' sense of worth by expressions of appropriate encouragement.

Communication is a complex process between two people. Senders use not only the words spoken but the tone of their voices, the expressions on their faces, and the movement of their bodies. Receivers not only receive the sight and sound, but they involve the past experiences with the senders, and with other people like the senders, as well as other experiences like the present one. Clear communication must be congruent, that is, the voice tone and body movement must match the word content. This happens when each person voices his or her reactions rather than keeping them secret [5].

For example, the nurse, seeing that the patient has eaten little from the tray says, "Eat your supper before it gets cold." The nurse is thinking that the patient needs to eat and feels helpless that he or she cannot make the patient eat. Since the nurse said none of this, the patient is left to guess the reason for the remark and may misinterpret the nurse's voice tone as anger. If the patient does not ask the nurse if he or she is angry, the nurse will never know of the patient's assumption. Small mole hills of miscommunication grow into mountains of misunderstanding. The liaison nurse can be an important teacher and role model for congruent communication.

Patient units, like families, develop rules about how people should feel and act. Many times it is assumed that everyone knows and understands the rules, even though they are unspoken and unwritten. Rules may concern which tasks are assigned to which level of staff and who makes what kinds of decisions. Rules also concern which kinds of feelings can be expressed, who can disagree with whom, when it is all right to ask for clarification, and which subjects are taboo.

It takes observant liaison nurses to discover the unspoken rules of the "family" on a patient care unit. Sometimes the discovery is made only when the nurse blunders by talking about something that is taboo or by voicing a feeling that is not allowed. However, bringing unspoken rules out into the open to discuss their validity and usefulness can be an important function of liaison nurses.

The way in which the unit relates to the outside world—that is, to the rest of the hospital, the community, the patients' families—gives indication as to whether the unit operates as an open or closed system. Another way of describing a family at the low end of the health continuum discussed earlier is as a "closed system."

Crucial to the linkage of a patient care unit to the outside world is the nursing person to whom the head nurse is responsible, such as the clinical coordinator, supervisor, or director of nursing. These persons can communicate to the unit a vision of the world that is hostile or hospitable, underscore the value of the individuals on the unit or deny their worth, or facilitate keeping the unit an open system. An alliance with such supervisory persons is obviously critical for liaison nurses.

Case examples show how an assessment of current functioning in these areas help liaison nurses plan an intervention.

Mr. C had been a patient in a chronic disease hospital for seven years. He had a degenerative neuromuscular disease, which was slowly robbing him of the ability to sit upright or to control the use of his arms and legs. He was presented to the liaison nurse as a totally unmanageable patient. He threw full urinals, berated staff nurses for their ineptness, and refused food and medication apparently on whim.

An interview with the patient, which indicated a normal mental status, brought forth a litany of complaints. Many episodes of what he considered poor nursing care had occurred two, three, even four years in the past. The patient described the neurological condition that confined him to bed and the complications that could follow improper nursing care. He was able to cite individual nurses who over the years had given what he described as good care.

A meeting with the nursing staff produced a crescendo of grievances. The patient was arbitrary, critical, dictatorial, and dangerous. He told certain nurses he did not want them to care for him, complained about one nurse to another, and insisted on a schedule different from everyone else.

An assessment of the functioning of this particular unit indicated that it usually fell on the midrange of the continuum. Patients were perceived as trying to do as little for themselves as possible. Although staff were able to talk with one another about their anger towards patients, at least when there was general agreement that a patient was infuriating, there was no tolerance for a nurse who might say that he or she liked or was not angered by such a patient.

Assessment of what was currently happening indicated several reasons why the patient's behavior might be escalating and why staff were asking for help. Several nurses on the unit were in their first year of employment after graduation from nursing school. When the patient told them they did not know how to take care of him, their fragile sense of self-worth was unable to withstand the attack. Either they became angrily defensive, or they tearfully believed him. Intervention by the liaison nurse aided the more experienced nurses to validate for the novices that their procedures were indeed done correctly and skillfully. This enabled the less confident nurses to respond to the patient's complaints with humor instead of defensive anger.

Communication between staff and the patient on the unit was unclear. Staff behavior and facial expressions showed anger, but no one was comfortable telling the patient when he or she was angry. The staff needed help to learn that telling the patient when they felt attacked and angry made them feel better and permitted the patient to voice his own anger, instead of letting it build to an explosive point.

The unspoken rules on the unit included the idea that patients were to be subordinate and compliant, and that the physician was in charge of the unit. A relatively new staff physician had taken a hands-off attitude, considering the problem with this patient a nursing care issue. Staff included this doctor in discussions of the problem and asked him for a more take-charge approach. Discussion about the patient's need to have some decision-making power and control over his life, however, did not lead to any change in their idea about the compliant role of the patient.

The intervention of liaison nurses is based on a growth model. Each interaction with staff and patients can be used as a building block. Upon this foundation staff and patients can grow in their abilities to relate to each other and to solve problems. Liaison nurses are involved in the relationship system, since they are also part of the hospital staff. They are rarely total outsiders. They model communication skills they are recommending and share their own thoughts and feelings about the situation, while listening carefully and being receptive to others. Thus they demonstrate their concern about what happens on the unit.

Intervention of this kind with staff and patients on a long-term care unit occurs over a relatively long time span. The initial action of the nurse is to share with the staff the recognition that they have a truly difficult patient who is not likely to change drastically. They might wish that the patient would go away, but since that is unlikely, the liaison nurse's role is to help the staff find ways to make taking care of the patient more tolerable. The indirect outcomes, of course, are that life also becomes more tolerable for the patient and that behavior changes occur on both sides.

Many times liaison nurses are consulted about a patient whose record shows fairly consistent behavior. The question is what has disrupted the balance on the unit? Or why is the behavior a problem now?

Miss K was an unhappy 70-year-old single woman who felt cheated and punished because a stroke had left her wheelchair-bound —unable to walk except for a few halting steps with a walker. Although she had the staff on her unit run ragged by her constant demands for attention, they generally took care of her with relative good humor. Yet when one day three glasses of water appeared at her bedside within a five-minute period as a result of requests to three different nurses, the staff called for help.

This particular unit functioned on the lower midrange of the continuum. There were a lot of group think and some fighting among staff about "right" and "wrong" behavior with no allowance for differences. The patient role was perceived as unprotesting compliance with staff orders. There was a strong sense of caring and pride in "our patients."

A conference with staff disclosed that although Miss K's demands had recently escalated, the general content of them had remained constant. Usually staff had set some limits on their responses. What was different now?

Just as a family may go along on a fairly even keel until something disrupts the balance, so also with the patient care unit. In the family maybe the mother begins part-time work outside the home, or the father's job calls for him to travel out of town two or three nights a week when previously he had been home every evening. When a patient's behavior changes, or when the staff's ability to cope with certain behavior fails, liaison nurses must look for the factor(s) that may have thrown the system off balance.

On this particular unit their supervisor had recently been very busy with a committee assignment and had also taken some time off for vacation. A rotation of relief supervisors during the vacation and less frequent visits from their own supervisor during the committee work period had left the staff feeling isolated and unsupported.

The liaison nurse asked the supervisor to join in a discussion with staff about their difficulties caring for Miss K. Her participation re-established her support. She recalled for them their limit setting with the patient in the past and offered the possibility of a float nurse on days when they were short staffed, since they were able, with help, to recognize that the patient's demands increased when there were fewer nurses. As a result, staff reported that Miss K became "easier to take care of" and "doesn't make us so angry." The supervisor also resumed her usual number of visits to the unit each week after the staff were able to tell her how important they thought her visits were.

Consultation based on family systems theory can be consultee-centered as well as case-centered. Conferences regularly scheduled with staff on a unit facilitate growth and movement toward the healthy end of the continuum. These conferences are similar to parent groups, for in the same way that parents struggle to understand and develop patterns of discipline, communication, and family member roles, so do staff in such meetings. Since staff members come from a variety of family experiences, ethnic and social backgrounds, and even geographical locations, it is important to provide a setting in which points of view can be expressed without fear of censure or disparagement and in which negotiations and compromise take place.

Concrete examples drawn from family life can often be helpful for nurses trying to understand patient behavior. For example, nurses recalled that in situations where they had been frightened—a child wanders off and is lost at the beach, a boyfriend had driven carelessly and almost had an accident—their reaction had been to get angry—to yell at the driver or to spank the child. They were then able to understand that the angry outbursts of a patient indicated that he was frightened. On one unit discussion by staff nurses of ideas concerning child-rearing helped them clarify their ideas about permissive versus strict rules for patients. Issues of control were illustrated for nurses on another unit with the discussion of the differences between telling college students studying at a distance that they could come home only for winter and spring vacations, or giving them their transportation money and letting them figure out when and how to use it.

Liaison nurses, without becoming involved in the intrapsychic or personal relationship problems of the nursing staff, can use their observations of these factors to deal effectively with unit problems. The focus, however, is always on the patient and patient care issues. Regular unit meetings provide liaison nurses with an opportunity to build their alliance with the nursing staff and to teach congruent communication skills by modeling, having what they say and do accurately express their own perceptions, thoughts, and feelings.

An advanced level of consultee-centered consultation involves staff and patients holding community meetings with liaison nurses as facilitators. Such a forum provides the opportunity for growth in all areas and for increased communication. Nurses can tell patients how they feel when everyone wants attention at the change of shift. Patients can suggest ways in which their quality of life can be improved on the unit. An attempt to begin such meetings would be appropriate on units on the higher side of the health continuum.

The use of a family system theory base for working as liaison nurses in a long-term care facility is a useful adjunct to the skills and methods described elsewhere in this book. Although similar dynamics are evident on any patient care unit, the long-term relationships that develop in chronic care hospitals and nursing homes provide a time frame for evaluation, understanding, and intervention based on such a system.

references

1. Frank Moss and Val S. Halamandaris, *Too Old, Too Sick, Too Bad* (New York: Anthelion Press, 1979), p. 8.
2. David K. Switzer, "The Minister as Crisis Counselor," in *The Application of Family Systems Theory to Crisis Intervention*, edited by W. Robert Beavers (Nashville: Abingdon, 1974), p. 182.
3. ———, pp. 184–185.
4. Virginia Satir, *Peoplemaking* (Palo Alto: Science & Behavior Books, Inc., 1972), p. 3.
5. Virginia Satir, *Conjoint Family Therapy* (Palo Alto: Science and Behavior Books, Inc., 1967), pp. 63–72.

bibliography

books

BONNER, CHARLES D. *Medical Care and Rehabilitation of the Aged and Chronically Ill.* Boston: Little, Brown & Co., 1974.

ORLANDO, IDA JEAN. *The Discipline and Teaching of Nursing Process.* New York: G. P. Putnam's Sons, 1972.

———. *The Dynamic Nurse–Patient Relationship.* New York: G. P. Putnam's Sons, 1961.

SATIR, VIRGINIA; STACHOWIAK, JAMES; and TASCHMAN, HARVEY A. *Helping Families to Change.* New York: Jason Aronson, Inc., 1975.

articles

COVERT, A. B. "Community Mental Health Nursing: The Role of the Consultant in the Nursing Home," *Journal of Psychiatric Nursing and Mental Health Services* 17:7 (July 1979): 15–19.

FRANLIEL, F. H. and CLARK, E. "Mental Health Consultation in Nursing Homes," *Journal of the American Geriatric Society* 17:4 (April 1969): 360–365.

FREEDBERG, L. E. and ALTMAN, C. S. "Psychiatric Consultation in Nursing Homes: A Two Year Experience," *Gerontologist* 15:2 (April 1975): 125–128.

GOLDSTEIN, S. E. "Psychiatric Needs of Geriatric Patients," *Dimensions of Health Services* 51:1 (January 1974): 53–55.

appendix d
stress and the stereotyping of nurses: consultation issues in the intensive care unit

Mrs. Thomas suffered a cardiac arrest and died at 9:30 AM. It is now 11 AM, and Ms. Elliot is restocking the code cart as she keeps her eye on Mr. Belman who has been a patient in the ICU for five weeks. A 46-year-old lawyer and married father of three, he is critically ill with lupus erythematosus and congestive heart failure. Although intubated he is awake and alert and communicates his helplessness and anger to Ms. Elliot by writing poignant notes. Mr. George arrives in the ICU at 11:10 AM accompanied by two physicians, a nurse, and a respiratory therapist. He has IVs in place and an N/G tube, while meds and blood are being administered. Mr. George is agitated as he is quickly transferred to what was Mrs. Thomas' bed. Tension and stress are apparent as Ms. Elliot efficiently and mechanically prepares to care for the patient. An observer might experience Ms. Elliot and the staff as competent yet unfeeling stereotypic ICU nurses. Does the stress create the stereotype? Is the stereotype accurate?

There are many sources of stress for nurses who work in the ICU. According to Engel, there are three major categories of causes of psychological stress. Stress can be caused by: (1) the loss or threatened loss of an object or person viewed as valuable; (2) actual or threatened bodily injury; and (3) the frustration of basic drives [1]. Stress is present in a situation that places an adjustment demand on an individual, one that threatens equilibrium [2]. Psychological stress results from processes that may originate within the environment or within the individual. These processes place a requirement on the individual to make a cognitive and emotional assessment. This assessment occurs prior to the involvement of any other bodily system [3]. Obviously, there is a strong interrelationship between physiological stress and psychological stress.

In an examination of stress theory and its application to nursing practice, the correlations are fundamental. The arena of professional practice is flooded with actual and potential stressful stimuli, as well as a system of expectations and responsibilities. "The position of the nurse is paradoxical. On the one hand, she is expected to be objective and firm; on the other, she is expected to emanate warmth and feeling. Maintenance of an appropriate balance in these opposing attitudes is itself a stress [4]." The mere fact that nurses are faced with actual as well as possible illness, loss, bodily injury, is, by definition, inherently stressful. All too often, however, nurses acknowledge the experience of stress in terms of patients, peers, and colleagues, and not in terms of themselves. Although quite skilled in identifying and minimizing stress for others, nurses tend to recognize it in themselves and admit that they feel stressed, only when either someone else brings it to their attention or they are on the brink of burn-out, that is emotional exhaustion. The majority of the time, nurses do quite well in dealing with and adapting to the stressors that are so characteristic of professional practice. In some instances, nurses probably do not receive sufficient recognition from peers, colleagues, and/or supervisors regarding their emotional strength, endurance, and clinical sophistication. Yet there are times when coping is not successful, as there are also times when no coping strategy can be identified. At these times, nurses may experience immobilization, impotency, or hopelessness—that is, there is no alternative but to try and "live through" a particular situation.

That which is experienced or described as stressful by one individual may not be experienced or described similarly by another. For example, the significance of the stressful event to the individual, be it real or fantasy, influences the nature of the response. The actual or potential implications of the event on the individual's life and self-esteem are also considered in understanding reactions to and views of stress. Character structure, previous experience, and usual defensive style are also significant. Typically, the individual responds in a consistent fashion. Some people may become withdrawn under stress, others may feel angry, silly, or frightened. Personal expectations as to what constitutes appropriate behavior during stress, along with the real and/or imagined expectations of peers, colleagues, supervisors, friends, and family, are important factors as well.

Does tolerance for stress increase if one is exposed to unrelenting stress? Does the individual become tougher, stronger in character, or immune, so to speak, to stress? Can an individual "break" under constant stress? How common are anxiety attacks, and what do they symbolize? In an attempt to answer these questions, the personal experience of stress is considered. Depending on the nature and significance of a specific stress, an individual may learn to adapt to it by use of denial, sublimation, resolution, or mastery. The individual may become overwhelmed by the stress, which may escalate into crisis. It is important to note that certain situations, which initially may have been perceived as stressful, may no longer be viewed as such. The situation itself has not changed. The individual has cognitively and emotionally matured. The individual becomes desensitized to the particular stress. For example, when first crossing a street by themselves, children are somewhat excited and proud of their independence, but they also experience anxiety. As more streets are crossed and time passes, the anxiety lessens. When first suctioning a patient, nurses may experience fearfulness and stress. Once the technical skills necessary to safely suction a patient are mastered and the nurse has successfully suctioned many patients, this procedure becomes routine and not especially stressful.

Anxiety attacks are commonly experienced and are not a definitive indication that the individual is about to fall apart. Anxiety is "a state of tension and distress akin to fear; but produced by the threatened loss of inner control rather than external danger [5]." Uncomfortable and unpleasant, anxiety can make the work situation impossible, affect sleep, and take away appetite or increase it. Anxiety attacks may be precipitated by a stressor or threat that may or may not be consciously recognized. Nurses often experience anxiety attacks when in charge of the ward, when faced with carrying out a complex care procedure for a patient, when directly confronted by the pain, fear, suffering, and body mutilation often experienced by patients in intensive care units. In addition, all nurses have some degree of death anxiety, regardless of the clinical area in which they work. Perhaps critical care nurses have a higher rather than lower degree of death anxiety as compared to nurses working in other clinical areas. *Death anxiety* is defined as the symbolic meaning and emotional reactions experienced when an individual considers his or her death as a real possibility [6]. Perhaps critical care nurses are more proficient in defending against this anxiety. The environment of an intensive care unit is a breeding ground for stress. "Stimuli are present to mobilize literally every conflictual area at every psychological developmental level [7]." Anxiety attacks may indicate the necessity for a "time-out" to understand the anxiety and to identify supports and solutions.

Recently, the literature has contained more articles dealing with

the emotional reactions and stressful experiences of nurses in intensive care units. The quality and outcome of patient care is dependent
on the health care providers, whose effectiveness, in turn, is influenced by their psychological state and their technical expertise [8].
The atmosphere of the critical care unit has been overly acknowledged as crisis-provoking for patients and their families. The sensory
and bodily stresses on patients and the scope of their possible
psychological reactions, as well as possible interventions, are well
described [9]. The stresses on nurses in such a setting and the scope of
their possible psychological reactions are now being acknowledged.
The inherited reputations of critical care nurses should be understood
and placed in perspective. The nurses who staff intensive care units
should not be expected merely to work with the inherent stresses. Interventions for stress reduction are essential, and it is in this special
clinical area that psychiatric liaison nurses can illustrate their
effectiveness.

As professionals, nurses are usually quite skilled in the use of
denial as a defense against stress. Liaison nurses remain sensitive to
the use of denial by critical care nurses since it is an indication that
stress is being experienced. Although there are various types of
denial, neurotic denial, which is most commonly demonstrated by
nurse consultees, is usually quite adaptive. If nurses constantly considered what they are responsible for doing to people—the sights,
sounds, and smells that nurses are forever faced with, the suffering
and life-versus-death situations that surround them—they would, in
all probability, never be able to go to work.

Although their clinical work preference is to continue in intensive care units, the nursing staff in these areas frequently suffer from
"ICU-itis" and burn-out. Understanding the factors in these reactions
is necessary for the practice of liaison nurses. The intermissions and
escapes from the highly demanding, draining, and stimulating
patient population are few and far between. The critical care nurse
can rarely leave the bedside unless relieved by another nurse. The
reputation and professional status that accompanies the clinical
autonomy and sophistication is well deserved. It is clearly the nature
of the work, however, and not the needs of individual nurses, that
requires the suppression of personal feelings and reactions. All too
often, critical care nurses are given neither the permission nor the
time to feel, let alone to express emotions related to patient care
experience. Nurses are often fearful of: (1) rejection or betrayal by
peers or patients, (2) being regarded as weak, incompetent, irrespon-
sible, negative, or (3) being misunderstood [10]. In an environment in

which the tension is high and the pace unrelenting, such fears may be greater and the opportunities for insight even less.

Concerns regarding the comfort and dignity of patients may be in conflict with the realities of highly technical care. Legal constraints may also influence care. Frequently, patient modesty cannot be maintained. This results in tremendous exposure of the often muti-lated human body. The ramifications for nurses in terms of their sense of body integrity and boundaries are significant. As a result of severe illness, patients may lose their "humanness." Critical care nurses often experience their patients as merely a part of the machinery. For some nurses this may be comforting, for others it is terrifying. These nurses have "a repetitive contact with death and an on-going contact with dying [11]." What could possibly be more stressful for nurses than to participate in actively focusing on the laboratory values, when they are acutely aware that the patient's prognosis, at best, is grim. Or could it be that focusing on the laboratory values may be an attempt to defend against the stress of acknowledging the prognosis?

Critical care nurses may be confronted with alert patients who beg them not to proceed with suctioning or not to carry out a specific procedure. They may plead with the nurses to be allowed to die. They may become paranoid and frightened of the nurses, who may be faced with restraining patients in order to safely treat them. Nurses may have to participate in a resuscitation while knowing that the patient and/or the family never wanted the heroics. They may have to participate while, in their own hearts, they are in conflict about the resuscitation.

In addition, families and patients usually want information and progress reports. The ward nurses commonly have the advantage in this regard. They frequently have positive information to share and reassurance to offer. Critical care nurses, like physicians, may find it very difficult to translate signs of progress to the family and offer reassurance and hope. In addition, the anxiety level of most patients and families is so high, that they may not be able to hear reassurance. These nurses may also be caught in a type of silent conspiracy of not being allowed to share the patient's actual prognosis when asked, because the physician(s) is in the process of deciding whether or not treatment should continue.

Patients in intensive care units and their families are often unclear as to the role of nurses. They often view nurses as being too powerful, and many patients project their fear and helplessness on to them. In other instances, they may translate their anxiety into magical thinking regarding the critical care nurse. Patients and fami-

lies often wish to participate in care decisions, but due to their high
anxiety, the complexity of each decision, the rapidity at which decisions must be made, and the philosophy of various members of the
health care team, this is not always possible. Limit setting with families is also difficult. Due to their anxiety and fear, they may frequently call the unit to inquire about the patient or forget visiting
policies and enter the unit inappropriately. In both of these situations, nurses may feel pulled away from patients and increasingly
stressed themselves.

Stress also results from the nurse's clinical responsibility in
"distinguishing between an immediate-action emergency and a wait-
until-the-physician-comes emergency [12]." Prioritizing emergencies
can be an awesome and stressful responsibility. Nurses must be constantly alerted to subtle cues as they strive not to become distracted
by the constant traffic and noise. Time is of the essence. A "treadmill
phenomenon" exists wherein incessantly repetitive routines are
carried out over and over again [13]. Generally, nonprofessional
nursing staff members in an intensive care unit have very limited
responsibilities, although new programs to educate acute care technicians have emerged. The major work load falls to the professional
nurse. Staffing patterns, floating policies, visiting policies, the needs
of families, physician availability, patient care demands, and
psychological responses to being in an intensive care unit—all may
be problematic. Communication and coordination between multiple
services simultaneously treating a patient, the potential physical
danger to nurses from sepsis, assaultive patients, and other circumstances, as well as the nature of support from nursing leader-
ship/administration, may contribute to the nurses' stress.

Nursing practice in an intensive care unit is characterized by an
increased sense of responsibility, power, and accountability. Life-
versus-death struggles are constant, and nurses cannot afford to be
unfamiliar with procedures, treatments, the signs and symptoms of
medical complications, and other key information. The margin for
error grows slimmer as the ramifications of mistakes are truly life-
threatening. Complex, sophisticated, and dangerous procedures are
carried out on the human body, already physiologically stressed by
major illness.

Obviously, there is personal and professional gratification for
nurses working in intensive care units. They tend to find the required
clinical sophistication and technical skill challenging, stimulating,
and exciting. There are patients who do get better—even if they do
not remember the intensive care unit experience and their nurses—

and families who are grateful. There is a sense of fulfillment in being able to provide the quality nursing care characteristic of an intensive care unit without the frustrations of ward nursing. Critical care nurses enjoy the quick pace and the professional respect that they receive and deserve from peers and colleagues. It is interesting to note, however, that when floated to another intensive care unit or when faced with visiting a friend or family member in an intensive care unit, the critical care nurse may be not only frightened, but also quite threatened. Perhaps it is the "esprit de corps" and/or denial that aids in making critical care nursing gratifying. When among an unfamiliar group of nurses, or when not on duty, perhaps these defenses are no longer as available.

Patients are placed in intensive care units in an attempt to assist them in fighting off death. This situation is paradoxical in that non-viable patients are also admitted to intensive care units, as are ventilator-assisted, no-code patients. Critical care units are increasingly specialized. This specialization has influenced the critieria for admission. The major implication for the critical care nurse is that the goal of the battle is not always the same. The critical care nurse has been described as "a type of soldier within an elite combat group marked by a strong sense of mission, loyalty, and group interdependence [14]." Characteristically, "what is rarely discussed and left ambiguous is the scope of the battle and the strength of the enemy's forces that place limits on the size of the possible victory [15]."

Patients and families need support, information, time, attention, and tolerance from the nursing staff. But what about the needs of the nursing staff? One area to consider when attempting to identify interventions to reduce stress is peer support. How openly supportive, as opposed to competitive, are members of the nursing staff? Interpersonal problems among all members of the health care team, as well as among nurses, have been cited as sources of stress [16]. How burdened and isolated are members of the nursing staff in contrast to being members of a cohesive, professional group? How does the belief that "miracles can happen" with patients interfere with peer support? How powerful, responsible, and vulnerable to peer criticism do the nurses feel? Without peer support, an additional stress is placed on the critical care nurse, that is, peer-induced stress.

Everyday life stresses accompany each nurse into the intensive care unit. The balance between personal issues and professional responsibilities is more difficult to maintain in an intrinsically stressful environment. Psychological issues may stimulate a variety of responses. Anxiety, stress, and discouragement run high when only macabre cards from deceased patients' families are on the staff bulletin board. Some nurses find comfort in religion. Some focus on remembering the patients that were helped. Others concentrate on clinical skills. Some nurses project unrealistic qualities onto comatose patients only to be disappointed when the patient becomes alert [17]. Some nurses deny issues, and others become angry and depressed or devalue their work. They may refer to the intensive care unit as "a pit" or a "crazy circus." Humor is often utilized, as is isolation and scapegoating. Some nurses cannot remember the patients' names, as if their egos were overdosed with painful realities. A critically ill, comatose, 20-year-old, handsome college student with a poor prognosis was "brought painfully alive" for the nurses. His mother had clipped a recent photograph of him to his vital sign sheet. When the liaison nurse arrived, the nurse pointed to the picture and said, "This is Carl, the person." She then pointed to the bed and said, "This is Carl, the patient." It was adaptive in this case, to de-personalize the patient. Nevertheless, some reactions such as ex-cessive humor, sarcasm, and devaluation may be symptoms of brew-ing problems. An increase of sick calls, errors in care, apathy, and increased competitiveness may indicate stress overdose and impend-ing burn-out. Perhaps the stress described produces the stereotype of an ICU nurse.

Stereotyping is an attempt by peers and colleagues to characterize the professional nurse in certain clinical areas. Ex-perience has shown that sometimes these legacies are complimentary, critical, or accusatory. Sometimes the legacies are accurate, but fre-quently they are very inaccurate. The behavioral and affectual expectations of the stereotype are that nurses in specific clinical areas must behave and feel a certain way. The resulting reputation serves as a prophecy as to what constitutes a "true" clinician, or at least a successful one. One might wonder if nurses become prey to fulfilling the prophecy, even though it is not gratifying. The prophecy may also be in direct opposition to the nurses' personal and professional values and beliefs.

Like many other individuals, regardless of whether they are health care professionals, nurses tend to generalize when assessing each other's behaviors. Assumptions may be treated as facts based on a conclusive knowledge base, when this is not so. Perhaps some pediatric nurses are more motherly than are some adult pulmonary nurses. Perhaps some general medical nurses are more psychologi-cally minded than are some surgical nurses. However, this does not preclude that nurses caring for adult patients are not sometimes motherly. Also, it does not mean that the pediatric patient always needs a nurse/mother. Pediatric nurses sometimes foster regression rather than autonomy. Sometimes this is therapeutic, other times it is countertherapeutic. Some medical nurses could hardly be described as "psychologically minded." One such nurse—a bright, highly motivated, skilled clinician—after introduction to the liaison nurse, responded with: "You seem nice enough, and you're probably pretty good at what you do, but I hate psychiatry. I have no use for it and besides, my patients have medical problems." The inherited reputation and the nurse did not match.

Beginning practitioners of psychiatric liaison nursing may be encouraged by colleagues, peers, and/or supervisors to stay away from "hostile/difficult" areas unless they specifically request consultation. They may be encouraged to focus their initial time and energy in building consultation alliances with units that are clearly open and receptive to their services. In reality, this is probably very sound advice. Nevertheless, being cognizant of reputations and legacies can place that advice in another light. Three clinical examples will illustrate stereotyping:

1. A first consultation request was received from pediatric nurses. Consultation was requested regarding the problematic management of a 6-year-old boy who was behaving bizarrely on the ward. The nurses did not understand the child's behavior and were unsure how to approach him. The liaison nurse attended a nursing conference on the ward. Upon arriving at the conference room, the liaison nurse found that the nurse consultees were already seated. Interestingly, it was apparent that they had moved the conference table over to the side of the room and were sitting in a circle. This was not the usual arrangement for nursing conferences. Was this a reflection of the stereotypic image of a psychiatric nurse? That is, whenever possible, psychiatric nurses sit in a circle? What were the expectations and reputation of the liaison nurse? The nurses had probably arranged the room in that manner to make the liaison nurse comfortable. Perhaps it was a supportive gesture, but a variety of feelings and anxieties were experienced by the beginning liaison nurse.

2. What about the expectations/reputations of the consultees? Were they warm and motherly? Some of them were, but some of them were furious with the child for his disruptive, weird behavior. Their anger did not abate even though they observed the patient interview in which the child's psychosis was demonstrated and later discussed. Even if nurses can recognize that patients are not responsible for their behavior, they may remain angry with them. Warm and motherly? Clearly, it is impossible for any nurses or mothers to be that way all the time. They can forget the psychosis, so to speak, and reprimand the patient, or they can attempt to bargain with patients or experience their outbursts as personal attacks.

3. Nurses often react by stereotyping patients who "bring on" their own illnesses. The expectation may be to feel angry rather than empathic. When patients are uncooperative, the problem is intensified. In an adult medical intensive care unit, the nurses were frustrated and angry with a group of patients who were suffering from severe liver disease secondary to alcoholism. The nurses were tired of the "flapping and fighting" when attempting to provide nursing care. Intellectually, they understood that the patients' behaviors were organically based and that the patients were not responsible for the "verbal ragtime" and combativeness. Nevertheless, the nurses felt persecuted by these patients. The nurses sometimes found themselves trying to explain procedures to these patients as if they possessed the cognitive ability to comprehend the information. Obviously, attempting to reason with a psychotic/combative patient is not successful. Yet, it is both difficult and very threatening to think of a patient as being really psychotic. Nurses may find that they are trying to talk patients out of their psychoses by reminding them that they have been told before not to touch the tubes or to leave their restraints alone.

Intensive care units are frequently described as "hostile/difficult" areas in which to provide psychiatric nursing consultation. The nurses who work in these units are often described as tough, aggressive, and controlling. Stereotypically, they are described as devaluing of psychiatry in general and are not concerned with psychological care issues. Just as it is not true that all psychiatric nurses sit in a circle whenever possible and discuss feelings, the inherited legacy of intensive care nursing is not always accurate. The majority of nurses have clinical work preferences. Why some nurses enjoy working in critical care units, while others prefer well-baby clinics, is a personal and individualized matter that should not be subject to judgment.

It is useful to consider issues relevant to the etiology of stress on the critical care nurse and possible methods of psychological adaptation when providing consultation. Stress reduction is a definable process. The first step is the acknowledgement of exactly what is experienced as stressful. The second step includes the identification of supports and options. The third step deals with the development of strategies to quickly mobilize support and options. The fourth step reflects the operationalization of these strategies.

Reputations, when inherited, can be dangerous. When not considered, they may prove to be the very worst type of enemy and a primary source of stress. Nurses who are working in a certain clinical area may be regarded in a particular light, and members of the health care team may respond to them as if that view was founded in accuracy. When labeled as "tough," "aggressive," or "controlling," ICU nurses may be perceived as not needing support. They may be hesitant to ask for support, or they may neither receive nor expect it. Individual views and values may be at odds with group reputations. In considering the nature of the stress in intensive care units, along with the nurses' reactions to that stress, liaison nurses attempt to differentiate nurses from the reputation. Effective intervention includes recognition of this distinction.

If the etiology of stress is identified and the nursing staff is cohesive, some resolution can be achieved. Cohesion results in mutually agreed-upon expectations, peer respect, healthy competition, collaboration, and trust. Professional goals are agreed upon and shared. Individual group members feel valued by each other and are therefore able to agree and disagree in service of problem solving. Peer-to-peer teaching is valued, and the methods that each nurse uses in facing stress are acknowledged and respected unless they prove detrimental to the group. Personal and professional self-esteem is enhanced when expectations and goals of practice are realistic and nurses accept the unknown, uncontrollable factors that influence patient care outcomes [18]. Although applicable to all areas of nursing practice, these issues become more obvious in physically close quarters.

An effective modality for providing psychiatric nursing consultation, which is also of primary importance for other reasons, is a nurses' group. Through a nurses' group, critical care nurses may gain peer support, develop cohesion, improve their communication patterns, and share common sources of stress. Difficult patient/family situations can be discussed, and possibly interventions can be developed. Identifying realistic expectations of self, peers, and patients is a useful focus of discussion within the group. Helpful methods of reducing stress are dealing directly with the stereotyping or the "inherited reputation" by recognizing its existence, problem solving situations in which stress may be unwittingly promoted, and defining strategies for educating the health care team regarding the inherent difficulties of ICU nursing.

The consistent and flexible availability of liaison nurses is helpful given the nature of intensive care nursing. Useful consultations may emanate from the liaison nurse's willingness to respond to emergencies and to provide "on-the-spot" in-service conferences on pertinent topics—such as death and dying, principles of conflict resolution, communication skills, relaxation techniques for staff and for patients, or psychological responses of patients in intensive care units. Inherited reputations of critical care nurses may be not only dangerous, but also frightening. The nurse who is new to the critical care area may feel that he or she must become "one of them and lose herself" in order to survive the stresses. Liaison nurses can be helpful in working with nursing staff as they struggle to become more aware of the legacy and how they may unknowingly be promoting it. Supporting critical care nurses as they identify and communicate their needs is accomplished through a nurses' group, on an individual basis, and by role modeling. Critical care nurses may be worried that there is something inherently wrong with them psychologically because they choose to remain in such a high-stress environment. Acknowledging the combination of clinical expertise and motivation, as well as personal preference that nurses must have to work in this area, is invaluable.

In accord with nursing leadership, liaison nurses may also suggest and support some of the following interventions:

- Rotating assignments on particularly difficult and stressful patients.
- Rotations out of the intensive care unit when needed.
- Pre- and post-cardiac arrest conferences to aid nurses in preparing for such events, as well as for obtaining closure.
- Patient follow-up post-discharge from the intensive care unit.
- Nursing research.
- Direct or indirect psychiatric nursing consultation to assist in patient management.
- Regularly scheduled milieu meetings for the entire ICU health care team to discuss mutual concerns and to strengthen professional cohesion.
- Professional networking within the institution and/or city or outlying communities.
- Educational programming and the promotion of professional identity through an ICU consortium.

The nursing staff may be encouraged to share patient care

responsibility by utilizing not only the liaison nurse, but also the psychiatrist, the social worker, and pastoral counselor when appropriate. In some critical care areas, liaison nurses have been instrumental in starting or co-leading family support/education groups, which are conducted in conjunction with members of the nursing staff. The stress-reducing effects of these groups are impressive.

Described by some as "hostile/difficult" clinical areas, intensive care units are very much in need of psychiatric nursing consultation. Although without anxiety they would probably experience a brand of numbness and boredom, which brings its own sort of discomfort, critical care nurses are being asked constantly to face enormously painful stresses. Acknowledgement of the stressors present in the ICU environment is not supportive in and of itself. The implementation of realistic stress-reducing interventions are necessary, because they not only aid in creating a less stressful environment for the nurse but also potentiate those facets of critical care nursing that are gratifying.

The effectiveness of liaison nurses is directly related to the depth of their understanding of the etiology of these stresses, an awareness of stereotyping, the nature of intensive patient care, and the relationship between physiological and psychological responses to stress. Their identification with liaison nurses as professional nurses tends to enhance and validate the ICU nurses' sense of being not only supported but understood. Knowledge of the nursing care needs of patients/families and of the nursing experience itself is an adjunct to the provision of effective psychiatric consultation.

references

1. M. J. Reichle, "Psychologic Aspects of the Acutely Stressed in an Intensive Care Unit," in *Respiratory Intensive Care Nursing*, edited by Sharon Bushnell (Boston: Little, Brown & Co., 1973), p. 214.
2. C. K. Hofling, M. M. Leininger, and E. A. Gregg, *Basic Psychiatric Concepts in Nursing*, 2nd ed. (Philadelphia: J. B. Lippincott Co., 1967), p. 558.
3. J. N. Baker and K. Sovensen, "A Patient's Concern with Death," *American Journal of Nursing* 63 (1963): 90.
4. R. Vreeland and G. Ellis, "Stresses on the Nurse in an Intensive Care Unit," *Journal of the American Medical Association* 208 (1969): 333.
5. Hofling, Leininger, and Gregg, p. 546.
6. T. W. Campbell, "Death Anxiety on a CCU," *Psychosomatics* 21:2 (February 1980): 135.
7. D. Hay and D. Oken, "The Psychological Stresses of the Intensive Care Unit," *Psychosomatic Medicine* 34 (1972): 110.
8. Hay and Oken, p. 109.
9. M. Adams, R. Hanson, D. Norkool, A. Beaulieu, E. Bellville, and K. Morss,

"The Confused Patient, Psychological Responses in Critical Care Units," *American Journal of Nursing* (September 1978): 1504–1512.

10. D. Q. Michaels, "Too Much in Need of Support to Give Any?" *American Journal of Nursing* (October 1971): 1932.

11. Hay and Oken, p. 110.

12. Vreeland and Ellis, p. 333.

13. Hay and Oken, p. 111.

14. ———, p. 109.

15. T. Q. Price and B. J. Bergen, "The Relationship to Death as a Source of Stress for Nurses on a Coronary Care Unit," *Omega* 8:3 (1977): 236.

16. L. Huckabay and B. Jagla, "Nurses' Stress Factors in the Intensive Care Unit," *Journal of Nursing Administration* (February 1979): 21–26.

17. Hay and Oken, p. 114.

18. A. Lewis and S. Goldberg, "Mechanisms for Peer Communication," An unpublished paper presented at *The National Primary Nursing Symposium, 1980*, sponsored by New England Medical Center Hospital, Boston, Mass.

bibliography

books

AGUILERA, D.; MESSICK, J.; FARRELL, M. *Crisis Intervention: Theory and Methodology.* St. Louis: The C. V. Mosby Company, 1978.

CLAUS, K. E. and BAILEY, J. T., eds. *Living with Stress and Promoting Well-Being. A Handbook for Nurses.* St. Louis: The C. V. Mosby Company, 1980.

JANIS, I. *Psychological Stress.* New York: John Wiley & Sons, Inc., 1958.

KAHANA, R. and BIBRING, C. "Personality Types in Medical Management," in *Psychiatry and Medical Practice in a General Hospital*, edited by N. E. Zinberg, New York: International Universities Press, Inc., 1964.

LAZARUS, R. S. *Psychological Stress and the Coping Process.* New York: McGraw-Hill Book Company, 1966.

LEVINE, S. and SCOTCH, N. *Social Stress.* Chicago: Aldine Publishing Co., 1970.

MONAT, A. and LAZARUS, R. S. *Stress and Coping: An Anthology.* New York: Columbia University Press, 1977.

ROBERTS, S. *Behavioral Concepts and the Critically Ill Patient.* Englewood Cliffs, N.J.: Prentice-Hall, Inc., 1976.

SELYE, H. *The Stress of Life.* New York: McGraw-Hill Book Company, 1956.

SIMON, N. *The Psychological Aspects of Intensive Care Nursing.* Washington, D.C.: Robert J. Brady Co., 1980.

STRAIN, J. and GROSSMAN, S. *Psychological Care of the Medically Ill: A Primer in Liaison Psychiatry.* New York: Appleton-Century-Crofts, 1975.

articles

ANDERSON, CHERYL ANN and BESTEYNS, MARGARET. "Stress and the Critical Care Nurse Reaffirmed," *Journal of Nursing Administration* 11:1 (January 1981): 31–34.

BALDWIN, C. ANN. "Mental Health Consultation in the Intensive Care Unit: Toward a Greater Balance and Precision of Attribution," *Journal of Psychiatric Nursing and Mental Health Services* (February 1978): 17–21.

BALLARD, K. "Identification of Environmental Stressors for Patients in a Surgical Intensive Care Unit," *Issues in Mental Health Nursing* 3:1–2 (January–June 1981): 89–108.

BILODEAU, C. B. "The Nurse and Her Reactions to Critical-Care Nursing," *Heart and Lung* 2:3 (May–June 1973): 358–363.

CALDWELL, TROY and WEINER, MYRON. "Stresses and Coping in ICU Nursing: I. A Review," *General Hospital Psychiatry* 3:2 (June 1981): 119–127.

CASSEM, N. H. and HACKETT, T. P. "Sources of Tension for the CCU Nurse," *American Journal of Nursing* 72 (1972): 1426–1430.

————. "Stress on the Nurse and Therapist in the Intensive Care Unit and the Coronary Care Unit," *Heart and Lung* 4:2 (1975): 252–259.

CHECK, D. S. "Unconscious Perception of Meaningful Sounds During Surgical Anesthesia as Revealed Under Hypnosis," *American Journal of Clinical Hypnosis* 1:101 (1959): 101–113.

DEMEYER, J. "The Environment of the Intensive Care Unit," *Nursing Forum* 11:3 (1957): 262–272.

DUBOVSKY, S. L.; GETTO, C. J.; GROSS, S. A.; and PALEY, J. A. "Impact on Nursing Care and Mortality: Psychiatrists on the Coronary Care Unit," *Psychosomatics* (August 1977): 20–27.

EISENDRATH, S. J. and DUNKEL, J. "Psychological Issues in Intensive Care Unit Staff," *Heart and Lung* 8:4 (1979): 751–758.

FREUDENBERGER, H. J. "Staff Burn-Out," *Journal of Social Issues* 30 (1974): 159–165.

GIBSON, K. T. "The Type A Personality: Implications for Nursing Practice," *Cardio-Vascular Nursing* 16:5 (September–October 1980): 25–28.

GROUT, JAMES; STEFFEN, SUSAN; and BAILEY, JUNE. "The Stresses and the Satisfiers of the Intensive Care Unit: A Survey," *Critical Care Quarterly* 3:4 (March 1981): 35–45.

HACKETT, T. P. "The Psychiatrist's View of the ICU," *Psychiatric Annals* 6:10 (October 1976): 14–27.

HOLMES, T. H. and RAHE, R. H. "The Social Readjustment Rating Scale," *Journal of Psychosomatic Research* 2 (1967): 213–218.

KORNFELD, D. S. "Psychiatric View of the Intensive Care Unit," *British Medical Journal* (1969): 108–110.

KOUMANS, A. J. "Psychiatric Consultation in an Intensive Care Unit," *Journal of the American Medical Association* 194 (1965): 633–637.

MICHAELS, D. "Too Much in Need of Support To Give Any?" *American Journal of Nursing* 71 (1971): 1922–1935.

MINCKLY, B. "The Multiphasic Human-to-Human Monitor (The ICU Model) Nursing Observations in the Intensive Care Unit," *The Nursing Clinics of North America* 3 (1968): 29–39.

OSKINS, S. L. "Identification of Situational Stressors and Coping Methods by Intensive Care Nurses," *Heart and Lung* 8:5 (1979): 953–960.

ROBINSON, A. "Professional Conflicts in the ICU/CCU," *RN* 72 (1972): 40–45.

STILLMAN, S. M. and STRASSER, B. L. "Helping Critical Care Nurses with Work-Related Stress," *The Journal of Nursing Administration* (January 1980): 28–31.

WEINER, MYRON and CALDWELL, TROY. "Stresses and Coping in ICU Nursing: II. Nurse Support Groups on Intensive Care Units," *General Hospital Psychiatry* 3:2 (June 1981): 129–134.

appendix e
psychiatric nurse-psychiatrist liaison team: a collaborative model

KATHLEEN BLANDFORD

A full evaluation of a patient's psychosocial needs requires more than the traditional diagnostic interview. Family dynamics, the milieu of the hospital, and its effect on the patient, as well as the patient–staff relationships, all contribute to the patient's experience of illness and hospitalization. Appreciation of these factors is a prerequisite to understanding the patient's intrapsychic and interpersonal dynamics.

The nurses on a ward have long served as key observers of the milieu–patient and staff–patient interactions. Psychiatrists on consultation-liaison services have identified the importance of incorporating nursing observations and assessments into their own evaluations [4,13] and, over the years of developing liaison services, have begun to identify the importance of the role of psychiatric liaison nurses in the general hospital [1,7,9].

At the same time, psychiatric nurses began extending their role from working on in-patient units and in community mental health centers to providing psychiatric nursing skills to patients and nursing staff in general hospitals [14,15]. Psychiatric liaison nurses recognized the integral role nurses play in identifying and meeting the psychosocial needs of hospitalized patients; often nurses provide major input in helping patients adjust to illness and regain adaptive defensive patterns that allow them to recover optimal physical and mental health. Psychiatric nurses' knowledge of nursing theory, psychiatric theory, and unique familiarity with the ward social system are the key factors making their consultative skills particularly relevant to nurses.

In many instances, psychiatrists and psychiatric liaison nurses have worked together, either informally or formally, on liaison teams in order to broaden the focus of each discipline in addressing the needs of patients and staff in the medical setting. The "liaison team" is one in which psychiatric staff, who regardless of professional discipline share the common goal of assisting hospital staff to meet the psychosocial needs of patients, coordinate their efforts and collaborate in their practice. Crawshaw and Keys mention several factors that are essential for a team such as this to operate effectively [5]. First, there must be administrative support for a professional practice that involves a physician and nurse functioning in a collaborative rather than supervisor–subordinate relationship. The nursing administration, along with the chiefs of psychiatry, medicine, and surgery, must agree with this mode of functioning. Second, each of the team members must understand and respect the contributions of the other. They must understand that as each specialty or discipline works to identify its particular contribution to the team, anxiety or conflict may develop with regard to the other members' contributions. These conflicts could lead to issues of territoriality and sharing of responsibility. Finally, although status factors can play an important role in the struggle for identity, one discipline should not feel it is subservient to the other.

The following addresses only the psychiatrist–psychiatric liaison nurse team and the elements involved in its functioning. It explores areas of role differentiation and role negotiation, models for team organization, and potential problems and benefits of this kind of collaborative practice.

models of psychiatrist–psychiatric liaison nurse teams

Most models for psychiatric liaison teams are variations on three basic themes. The first is one in which the entire team operates out of the department of psychiatry, and usually it is headed by a psychiatrist. Such teams often employ social workers, psychologists, and psychiatric residents in addition to liaison nurses. Often the liaison nurse does the initial screening and the psychiatrist serves as "back-up" or countersigns all consultations. In this model the liaison nurse is administratively as well as clinically responsible to the psychiatrist and has no formal tie to the department of nursing. The second model is one in which formal psychiatric liaison-consultation service is based in the department of psychiatry while a parallel service for nursing consultation is based in the department of nursing. There is a clear distinction made between a formal psychiatric consultation, which is done only by a psychiatrist, and nurse-to-nurse consultation around psychosocial patient care issues provided by a psychiatric liaison nurse. In this model each discipline reports to its professional department, and there are no formal ties between the two services. Ideally in this system there is good communication between the two services with many cross-referrals as one service recognizes the need for input from the other. The third model is one in which the departments of psychiatry and nursing each hire their own psychiatric personnel for liaison work, but the psychiatrist and liaison nurse collaborate in providing a psychiatric liaison-consultation service. Each one may also have other responsibilities in his or her own department. In this model, each discipline is administratively accountable to its own professional department, but there is an officially sanctioned combined liaison service. They both may respond to requests for formal psychiatric consultations, but they attempt to divide clinical responsibilities according to their particular area of expertise. This model differs from the first primarily in that the relationship is collaborative and neither one is administratively accountable to the other. It differs from the second in that there is more visible interrelationship and working together than is afforded in the "separate service" model.

This author is most familiar with the third model of practice, and the following is based on her experience working as a liaison nurse in this kind of organizational structure.

For both the psychiatric liaison nurse and the psychiatrist to understand and respect the contributions of the other team member, it is necessary that they each have an understanding of their own roles and areas of expertise. There is tremendous overlapping of roles, as well as role diffusion, in the field of psychiatry since all the disciplines share a related body of theoretical knowledge. There is differentiation among disciplines in terms of medical and clinical training and the depth of knowledge acquired. However, it is the educational process unique to each discipline and the primary focus of professional attention that distinguishes the clinical focus of one discipline from the other.

role of the psychiatric liaison nurse

Psychiatric liaison nurses combine nursing theory with psychiatric theory using the nursing process as a vehicle for implementing their practice. They utilize a health or wellness model, which defines the

patient in terms of optimal functioning and views illness as a dis-
equilibrating force that compels the patient to make adjustments and
adaptations to regain both physical and psychological functioning.
Their major area of expertise lies in the realm of patient management,
since this has been the hallmark of psychiatric nursing in all in-
patient settings. In providing their consultative skills to others,
liaison nurses may gather history from the patient or indirectly from
the nursing staff. This information would include data about the
patient's social and familial environment outside of the hospital.
They also assess the social and therapeutic milieu the patient experiences in the hospital. With this kind of information available,
psychiatric liaison nurses formulate their assessment of the key
factors that may be affecting the patient's adjustment to illness and/
or progression towards health. The assessment most often includes a
psychiatric and psychosocial formulation that explains the dynamics
of the case and identifies major psychological problems. The major
focus of their consultation lies in formulating a care plan that can be
integrated into the overall plan of nursing care for that patient. This
plan addresses management of the behavioral and psychosocial
factors in the patient's current situation. It requires that psychiatric
liaison nurses assist the nurse consultees in identifying the
psychological needs of a patient and in planning interventions that
meet these needs in an ego-constructive way. The liaison nurse
recommends interventions that establish an interpersonal and
physical environment in the hospital bolstering the healthy defenses
and coping mechanisms of the patients. The following is a case
example illustrating the liaison nurse's intervention in a patient
management problem:

> The liaison nurse was called by a staff nurse to consult on a
> 78-year-old retired RN admitted for treatment of a cellulitis of the left
> leg. The patient was obese and inattentive to her appearance.
> Although the pain and edema caused by cellulitis had diminished after
> antibiotic treatment was administered. the patient was resistant to am-
> bulating or participating in any self-care. She had been living alone
> prior to admission but told staff she believed she would be safer in a
> nursing home. Having made that decision, she seemed to have settled
> back and claimed she didn't have to do anything if she was going to a
> nursing home. The nurse described the patient as "demanding,
> manipulative, and uncooperative" in efforts to mobilize her. The
> patient was interviewed by both the liaison nurse and the staff nurse.
> She was cordial and loquacious, and volunteered her impression that
> she and her nurse didn't see "eye-to-eye" on things. She described a
> lifestyle of becoming increasingly isolated over the last few years and

felt she had worsened after the death of her dog, saying, "Walking him got me outside and kept me in touch with the other people." In discussing the interview, the staff nurse identified the fact that many of the patient's demands, particularly when the nurse was caring for others in the room, might have reflected loneliness and her fear that she would be forgotten when attention was diverted elsewhere. She also recognized that she had been so adamant about the goals for increased independence and mobility she had formulated for the patient, she hadn't adequately listened to the patient's complaints that she felt too much was being expected of her all at one time. A care plan was formulated, which included scaling down the nurse's goals to small, concrete goals that were negotiated with the patient, letting the patient know when the nurse was available to her and when she would be attending to others, and having the patient ambulate to the solarium where there would be other people with whom she could talk.

In the course of the consultation the liaison nurse also evaluated the patient for evidence of depression or other psychiatric disorder, but her primary interest was in helping the nurse find alternative ways of meeting the patient's psychological needs and "managing" her behavior, all in the interest of promoting a healthier adjustment.

Although the major clinical goal of liaison nurses' interventions is better patient care, their target population for consultation is the nursing staff. They utilize patient care conferences organized by the nursing staff as their major mode of consultation. By utilizing their psychiatric skills and knowledge at these conferences, they develop the staff nurses' assessment skills and capacity to identify patients' psychosocial needs in planning care. Since the patient has needs twenty-four hours a day, liaison nurses rely on the staff nurses to meet those needs. They teach psychological principles and concepts, which the staff nurses then use to plan their own patient interventions. Although some cases require liaison nurses to be more actively involved with the patient, they always involve the staff nurse too. To be effective, the liaison nurse must be familiar with the nursing care system on each particular unit, recognizing its current strengths and deficits, all of which will dictate the kinds of interventions possible. For example, on a unit that has low staffing and that is not utilizing primary nursing, the liaison nurse may rely on the head nurse or assistant head nurse to communicate the care plan to all the shifts.

role of the psychiatrist

In contrast to liaison nurses' emphasis on psychosocial assessments and strategies for promoting adjustment or management of maladaptive behavior, psychiatrists, by virtue of the focus of their education and experience, contribute their expertise in psychiatric diagnosis and in the behavioral aspects of medical practice. Psychiatrists are often called upon to assist medical staff in their diagnostic appraisal of patients. Lipowski describes four major categories of diagnostic problems addressed by psychiatric consultants [11]. Often they are called upon to differentiate between an organic versus psychiatric disorder. Another common request is for assistance in diagnosing the etiology of a patient's uncharacteristic behaviors. This differential requires a familiarity with personality changes, which can be caused by cerebral or systemic disorders as well as by psychiatric illness. A third type of request for assistance arises when a patient presents an obvious psychiatric disorder that the primary physician is not always comfortably able to diagnose or treat. Finally, psychiatrists are called upon to identify and explain illness behavior that may interfere with medical treatment.

Psychiatrists provide expertise in planning guidelines for action based on the determined diagnosis. They may recommend further medical interventions, such as laboratory studies or even the delay of or cancellation of treatment such as postponing surgery, due to a patient's clinical depression. Psychiatrists may also make recommendations for any further psychiatric interventions, such as psychotropic medications, psychological testing, or psychotherapy. The following is an example of the way in which a psychiatrist applied his diagnostic expertise to a complicated case:

A 35-year-old separated mother of three was admitted for the second time with a provisional diagnosis of multiple sclerosis. The patient had been hospitalized several months prior to this with the workup yielding only "soft positive" neurological findings. On this admission, she was noted to be regressed with marked inattention to her appearance, and she was withdrawn. She reported that her first neurological symptoms occurred within days of being hit in the neck by her estranged husband. Her symptoms had remitted during her last admission but recurred quickly after she returned home from rehabilitation. On this admission, she had reported to the intern that she had been planning to file for divorce, but the recurrence of symptoms had prevented this. The psychiatric liaison nurse saw the patient in response to her request for "support." During the course of several interviews, the liaison nurse noted a confusing presentation of psychological phenomena. The illness developed in the context of severe familial stress, and the patient herself wondered if some of the symptoms could be "psychosomatic." She showed a pronounced indifference to her appearance and to certain problems such as urinary and fecal incontinence. She demonstrated a vagueness in her speech, some short-term memory problems, and a somewhat detached affect which at times seemed euphoric.

Due to the complexity of the patient's presentation, the liaison nurse asked the liaison psychiatrist to evaluate the patient. On the basis of his interview, he felt that the patient was displaying both regression in the face of overwhelming debilitating illness and neurologic dysfunction—whether it was from the ACTH she was receiving or some cerebral process was unclear. As a result of his recommendations, some studies, including CT SCAN, were repeated since they hadn't been done in several months. Neuropsychological testing was also done to determine a baseline personality and defensive style. CT SCAN showed probable demylenating processes in the cortex, and the neuropsychological testing also confirmed some organic impairment. The test results described areas of strength for this woman as well as outlined her less adaptive defenses. This information was shared with the rehabilitation unit to which the patient was transferred so that her program could be tailored to capitalize on her psychological strengths.

In this case, the psychiatrist and liaison nurse worked together in the ongoing follow-up. While the psychiatrist reviewed study results and worked with the house staff and attending physician, the liaison nurse worked with the patient's primary nurse to address the patient's regression and control issues. The liaison nurse also met with the patient to review treatment and allow her to explore her reactions to her illness. Both the psychiatrist and the liaison nurse reviewed the case together during ward visit rounds attended by house staff and a teaching physician. The liaison nurse then shared the results of the conference with the patient's primary nurse. Just as the psychiatric liaison nurse directs her expertise primarily to nursing staff and their relationships with patients, the psychiatrist's target population is the medical staff. The psychiatrist can serve as the mediator between physician and patient and can have input into structuring the physician–patient relationship so that it is interpersonally as well as medically therapeutic.

Because both the psychiatrist and psychiatric liaison nurse share a common body of psychiatric theory, they each share knowledge of psychiatric diagnoses and treatment modalities. There is often overlap in their roles, particularly in the sphere of providing psychotherapy to patients seen in consultation. As they both become familiar with the other's area of expertise, there may be overlap in the recommendations they make to their consultees. Liaison nurses may recommend laboratory studies when they assess a patient and suspect a toxic delirium. Psychiatrists may include recommendations for orienting devices (a clock or calendar) or a predictable, written treatment schedule for a confused patient they have evaluated. Other areas of potential overlap occur in teaching and research. The role differentiation falls in their areas of emphasis and target populations. Given this framework for role differentiation, it is clear that the two roles complement each other and have great potential for promoting the maximal physical and psychosocial recovery of the patient.

negotiating a collaborative practice

The necessary complementary relationship between the liaison nurse and psychiatrist evolves over time, and it is influenced by the demands and structure of the institution. However, certain issues must be negotiated between the two for them to work effectively as a team. As noted above, a foundation for good collaboration is a sound understanding of and respect for the contributions of the other. Particularly in a setting where both parties respond to requests for formal psychiatric consultations, it is important that they each understand which consultations are always to be within the province of the psychiatrist and which fall into the province of the nurse. Both the nurse and the psychiatrist must spell out which kinds of patient problems require the input or back-up of the psychiatrist after the nurse has already seen the patient and which require the psychiatrist to be available to the nurse. Does it mean the psychiatrist is available only by phone? Or will the psychiatrist be willing to interview a patient with the nurse and collaborate on recommendations? Will there be flexibility in the timing of the back-up response to allow for acute crises? Is the nurse able to identify areas of practice that are outside the realm of his/her expertise? And will the liaison nurse call the psychiatrist in a timely fashion without concerns about a "loss of face"?

Just as there is a need for flexibility in providing psychiatric back-up to the nurse, it is important that they each agree to ways in which the liaison nurse provides assistance to the psychiatrist. For example, the psychiatrist may see a patient to evaluate for the presence of a clinical depression, recommend the use of anti-depressants, and begin some interim psychotherapy while the patient is on the medical unit. However, the patient's apathy, psychomotor retardation, and withdrawal may be interfering with his or her ability to cooperate with the plans for ambulation, nutrition, or self-care. The psychiatrist may then negotiate with the liaison nurse to become involved with the nursing staff to develop a nursing care plan that attempts to structure care so that it meets the medical needs of the patient while taking into account the psychological symptoms that interfere with compliance.

The following case demonstrates the way in which both the psychiatrist and the liaison nurse provide "back-up" to each other:

> A 25-year-old divorced woman was admitted to the medical service after taking about 40 tablets of Triavil shortly after admitting herself to a psychiatric unit. She was known to the liaison service from a prior medical admission during which she had been diagnosed with diabetes mellitus. The patient's history included prior Nembutal abuse, a suicide "gesture" at age 15, and chronic feelings of low self-esteem. The patient was first evaluated by the liaison nurse while she was still in the ICU. At that time, the staff wanted to know if she was "psychologically safe" for transfer to one of the medical floors. The liaison nurse found the patient to be mildly delirious with impairments in orientation and memory and to have active delusions and ideas of reference regarding her safety. She verbalized ambivalent feelings about her wish to die. After determining that the patient felt protected by the presence of hospital staff, the liaison nurse recommended that she be transferred to an observation room on a medical floor and that she be given one-to-one supervision by staff. She also told staff she would have the psychiatrist return with her later in the day to re-evaluate the situation, particularly with regard to her active psychosis and her suicide potential. All the steps were in accordance with the hospital's protocol for suicidal patients.

> During the rest of her hospitalization, the psychiatrist and the liaison nurse were actively involved in her care. She was started on psychotropic medications and kept on close observation until her psychosis cleared. The liaison nurse met with the nursing staff to discuss her situation and to provide some teaching around assessing suicidal feelings and making appropriate interventions to allay the patient's fears and provide for her safety. The psychiatrist and liaison nurse saw the patient together so they could adjust the treatment provided by her physicians and nurses in a coordinated way. When the patient's mental status cleared, she stated that she no longer felt so desperate and depressed and wanted to go home. The psychiatrist evaluated her suicide potential and considered various dispositions. The patient explained that part of the desperation that had prompted her overdose was her admission to a psychiatric unit, which she

perceived as the final blow to her self-esteem. She expressed an interest in pursuing psychotherapy to explore her feelings of worthlessness, which were compounded by her conflicted relationship with her parents. The psychiatrist met with her family and then with her internist, and they agreed to discharge the patient home with her family with plans for close follow-up by an out-patient psychiatrist and her internist. He also arranged an appointment for a family evaluation by social service.

The psychiatrist and liaison nurse were in touch daily about this patient and shared their impressions and recommendations for treatment with each other. Although, at times, they focused on different aspects of her care (the psychiatrist addressed medication and disposition while the liaison nurse addressed her safety needs and her relationships with care givers), their efforts were closely coordinated and fostered a comprehensive approach to her treatment.

As the psychiatrist and liaison nurse discuss their interrelationship and identify their differences, they will begin to develop a relationship that is collegial rather than supervisor–subordinate, so that "Who's the boss?" struggles are avoided. It is important that communication relative to clinical responsibilities be thorough, open, and respectful so that there can be carry-over to constructive negotiations around more tedious issues like work schedules, alloting time for consultations, dividing less desirable tasks like reports, attending meetings, or avoiding duplication of efforts.

Although liaison psychiatry is gaining in momentum, and although both psychiatrists and psychiatric liaison nurses are becoming a more visible part of general hospitals, there still can be much resistance to and testing of both roles on the part of nonpsychiatric physicians and nursing staff. Therefore it is important for the psychiatrist and the liaison nurse to work together in addressing these resistances, which often have the potential to split the team and have them become angry with each other. Some common resistances include the following:

1. A physician listens politely to the report of an evaluation done by the liaison nurse and then ignores all recommendations and calls for the psychiatrist.
2. A physician approaches the psychiatrist to "chat" about a case that the liaison nurse has been involved in, never mentioning her involvement, so that the psychiatrist unwittingly gets pulled into the case.
3. A physician puts in consultation requests to the liaison nurse only as a

means of avoiding utilizing the psychiatrist, with whom he or she feels competitive.

4. The nurses pose all questions about the patient to the liaison nurse even when the psychiatrist is a central figure in the case.
5. The nurses look to the input of the psychiatrist as a means of avoiding dealing with the liaison nurse.
6. Consultations are put in to liaison nurses because there is no charge for their services whereas there is a psychiatrist consultant fee.
7. Liaison nurses are seen as pseudopsychiatrists by consultees expecting input that is beyond the scope of their practice.

This latter problem can also lead to the dilemma of liaison nurses' identity being so tied up in doing formal diagnostic consultations that they begin to have little time available for liaison nursing conferences and groups. It is essential, though, that the psychiatrist and liaison nurse openly discuss each problem and plan together the response they feel is most appropriate. Sometimes the liaison nurse bows out of a case rather than insisting on being involved as a matter of principle; at other times the best response is for the psychiatrist to refuse to become involved, just to assuage the anger of a physician or nurse. When the liaison nurse and psychiatrist maintain open communication and reinforce to others the value they place on each other's work, most resistances are worked through and staff learn to work with each of them appropriately.

The literature on psychiatric liaison work cites many examples of the benefits derived from combining the efforts of a psychiatric liaison nurse and a psychiatrist on a liaison service [1,7,9,16]. Of primary importance are the benefits to the patients when all aspects of their psychosocial care, both medical and nursing, are addressed. A second major benefit comes from the psychiatrist and liaison nurse collaborating together in teaching both nurses and physicians. There is a rich cross-fertilization of ideas as each psychiatric consultant provides his or her conceptual framework to both the medical and nursing staff. This same professional sharing affords the two consultants opportunities for professional growth as they learn from each other.

A final benefit derived from collaborative practice is the opportunity it provides for positive role modeling of the doctor–nurse relationship. The physician and nursing staff are primary care providers in the hospital setting, and they work toward collaborating with each other to provide quality patient care. Professional relationships between these two groups are often fraught with issues of competition, subordination, and devaluation of the efforts of the other.

When the psychiatrist and liaison nurse have gained the respect of each other and of their medical and nursing colleagues, they can be instrumental in demonstrating how the two disciplines can work with each other. Seemingly small things like asking for the staff nurse's impressions or suggestions during a conference with medical and nursing staff can go a long way towards emphasizing the value of all care providers' input in planning or implementing treatment. The following example demonstrates the process of modeling this kind of collegial relationship:

> Ward visit rounds are held for medical house staff three days a week and are led by one of the attending physicians affiliated with the hospital. One session a month is set aside for psychiatry rounds and is led by the liaison psychiatrist although the liaison nurse always attends. The house staff present a patient, who is often interviewed by the psychiatrist. The interview is then followed by a discussion. The liaison nurse actively participates in the discussion, often contributing the observations of the patient she has learned from the staff nurses.
>
> Over several years of attending these rounds, the psychiatrist and liaison nurse would openly turn to each other for comments or suggestions about the case. Initially, all questions were directed to the psychiatrist, even when the patient being discussed had been evaluated by the liaison nurse. At these times, the psychiatrist would always redirect the questions to the liaison nurse. As the house staff observed the way the psychiatrist and liaison nurse utilized each other's skills, they too began to direct their questions more appropriately to each. The acknowledgment of their recognition of the importance of various input occurred when the house staff began inviting the patient's primary nurse to the case discussions.

A sound understanding of one's own area of psychiatric expertise and a healthy respect for that of the other are the first steps in negotiating a team effort between the psychiatrist and liaison nurse on a consultation-liaison service. Psychiatrists' primary population for consultation is the medical staff although often they will gather input from the nurses, social workers, or other care providers involved with the patient. Their diagnostic skills, particularly in terms of providing differential diagnosis, are invaluable and will serve as the basis for recommendations for psychiatric and medical interventions. Psychiatric liaison nurses' target population is the nursing staff, even though they may often gather input from the physicians, social workers, occupational therapists, or others involved in patient care. Open communication about their own differences and a willingness to tackle together any problems that develop between the team and its consultees are essential for the development of a collegial relationship. The payoff for the effort put into effective role negotiation comes in more comprehensive, collaborative efforts being made in patient care and a richer professional experience for both the liaison nurse and the psychiatrist.

references

1. D. Barton and M. Kelso, "The Nurse as a Psychiatric Consultation Team Member," *International Journal of Psychiatry in Medicine* 2:1 (1971): 108–115.
2. C. Bilodeau and S. O. O'Connor, "Role of Nurse Clinicians in Liaison Psychiatry," *Massachusetts General Hospital Handbook of General Hospital Psychiatry,* edited by T. Hackett and N. Cassem (St. Louis: The C. V. Mosby Company, 1978), pp. 508–523.
3. B. L. Bloom and H. J. Parad, "Interdisciplinary Training and Interdisciplinary Functioning: A Survey of Attitudes and Practices in Community Mental Health," *American Journal of Orthopsychiatry* 46:4 (October 1976): 669–677.
4. B. Bursten, "The Psychiatric Consultant and the Nurse," *Nursing Forum* 2 (1963): 7–23.
5. R. Crawshaw and W. Key, "Psychiatric Teams," *Archives of General Psychiatry* 5:4 (October 1961): 397–405.
6. A. Froese, L. Kamin, and C. Levine, "Teamwork: A Multidisciplinary Pediatric-Liaison Service," *International Journal of Psychiatry in Medicine* 7:1 (1976–77): 42–56.
7. S. Holstein and J. Schwab, "A Coordinated Consultation Program for Nurses and Psychiatrists," *Journal of the American Medical Association* 194:5 (November 1, 1965): 491–493.
8. A. Issacharoff, J. Godduhn, and G. Nachman, "Psychiatric Consultation Teamwork in a General Hospital: A Study in Group Process," *Group Psychotherapy* 24:3 (July 1974): 300–307.
9. N. Kaltreider, W. Martens, S. Monterrasa, and L. Sachs, "The Integration of Psychosocial Care in a General Hospital: Development of an Interdisciplinary Consultation Program," *International Journal of Psychiatry in Medicine* 5:2 (1974): 125–134.
10. J. Ludden, R. Winickoff, and S. Steinberg, "Psychological Aspects of Medical Care: A Training Seminar for Primary Care Providers," *Journal of Medical Education* 54:9 (September 1979): 720–724.
11. Z. J. Lipowski, "Consultation-Liaison Psychiatry: Past, Present, and Future," *Consultation-Liaison Psychiatry,* edited by R. O. Pasnau (New York: Grune & Stratton, Inc., 1975), pp. 17–18.
12. B. J. Lowery and D. Jarwulis, "Community Mental Health and the Unanswered Questions," *Perspectives in Psychiatric Care* 11:1 (January 1973): 26–28.
13. E. Meyer and M. Mendelson, "Psychiatric Consultations with Patients on Medical and Surgical Wards: Patterns and Processes," *Psychiatry* 24:1 (1961): 197–220.

14. J. Nelson and D. Schilke, "The Evolution of Psychiatric Liaison Nursing," *Perspectives in Psychiatric Care* 14:2 (1976): 61–65.

15. L. Robinson, "Liaison Psychiatric Nursing," *Perspectives in Psychiatric Care* 6:2 (1968): 87–93.

16. T. Wise, "Utilization of a Nurse Consultant in Teaching Liaison Psychiatry," *Journal of Medical Education* 49:11 (November 1974): 1067–1068.

appendix f
standards of psychiatric-mental health nursing practice*

standard I

DATA ARE COLLECTED THROUGH PERTINENT CLINICAL OBSERVATIONS BASED ON KNOWLEDGE OF THE ARTS AND SCIENCES, WITH PARTICULAR EMPHASIS UPON PSYCHOSOCIAL AND BIOPHYSICAL SCIENCES.

standard II

CLIENTS ARE INVOLVED IN THE ASSESSMENT, PLANNING, IMPLEMENTATION AND EVALUATION OF THEIR NURSING CARE PROGRAM TO THE FULLEST EXTENT OF THEIR CAPABILITIES.

standard III

THE PROBLEM-SOLVING APPROACH IS UTILIZED IN DEVELOPING NURSING CARE PLANS.

standard IV

INDIVIDUALS, FAMILIES AND COMMUNITY GROUPS ARE ASSISTED TO ACHIEVE SATISFYING AND PRODUCTIVE PATTERNS OF LIVING THROUGH HEALTH TEACHING.

standard V

THE ACTIVITIES OF DAILY LIVING ARE UTILIZED IN A GOAL DIRECTED WAY IN WORK WITH CLIENTS.

standard VI

KNOWLEDGE OF SOMATIC THERAPIES AND RELATED CLINICAL SKILLS ARE UTILIZED IN WORKING WITH CLIENTS.

standard VII

THE ENVIRONMENT IS STRUCTURED TO ESTABLISH AND MAINTAIN A THERAPEUTIC MILIEU.

standard VIII

Nursing participates with interdisciplinary teams in assessing, planning, implementing and evaluating programs and other mental health activities.

standard IX

Psychotherapeutic interventions are used to assist clients to achieve their maximum development

standard X

The practice of individual, group or family psychotherapy requires appropriate preparation and recognition of accountability for the practice.

standard XI

Nursing participates with other members of the community in planning and implementing mental health services that include the broad continuum of promotion of mental health, prevention of mental illness, treatment and rehabilitation.

standard XII

Learning experiences are provided for other nursing care personnel through leadership, supervision and teaching.

standard XIII

Responsibility is assumed for continuing educational and professional development and contributions are made to the professional growth of others.

standard XIV

Contributions to nursing and the mental health field are made through innovations in theory and practice and participation in research.

appendix g
epilogue

In this text, the focus of psychiatric liaison nursing has been on the delivery of psychological health care in the general hospital. The theory and many of the principles of clinical practice can be adapted with relative ease to other health care settings, both in-patient and out-patient. Most health care providers struggle with issues of fear, anger, disappointment, and other emotions, as do patients in all health care settings. The psychological needs of patients/families, coupled with those of health care providers, is an indication of the enormous potential of the role for liaison nurses.

Psychiatric nurses who wish to specialize in consultation-liaison nursing are provided with a dynamic array of professional opportunities. The psychological needs of the elderly, who are increasing in numbers with improved medical technology, is one specialty that warrants increasing attention. The nursing staff responsible for the health of the elderly living in nursing homes is another aspect of this specialty area. As the institution becomes the home of elderly patients, their complex needs become more clearly identified and the care required more sophisticated.

As the deinstitutionalization process proceeds, there are more "psychiatric" patients living in the community. In the past these patients, for the most part, received their medical care within the walls of the state psychiatric facilities. Now these patients, with increased frequency, are being treated in the general hospital. The role for the psychiatric liaison nurse is obvious.

Health maintenance organizations (HMO), in their commitment to cost-effective health care, employ nurse practitioners from all specialties to deliver care. With the advent of primary nursing and federal grants for primary care, more attention has been focused on the psychological care of patients. This stimulates more interest in and recognition of the need for psychiatric liaison nursing. Also, these same liaison skills can be used in the treatment of somatic problems in the in-patient psychiatric unit [1]. As the number of masters-prepared nurses increase, the outlook is hopeful that with more autonomy, accountability, and creativity, psychiatric nurses will become more resourceful in developing new roles under the consultation-liaison umbrella.

Research, which is a vital component of other health care disciplines, has not enjoyed the prominence or attention in nursing that it deserves. Research provides a way to evaluate practice [2]. Suggestions for change have been made to encourage clinical nursing research, such as:

1. instituting new forms of training for nursing research in the undergraduate and graduate curriculum.
2. providing funding and institutional support,
3. hiring nurse researchers in clinical settings, and
4. encouraging nurses in practice to obtain support for research [3].

The research process applied to psychiatric liaison nursing encourages practitioners to examine their clinical practice, validate it, and apply knowledge gained to new situations. Areas for consideration for research might be:

- What psychosocial factors influence a patient's emotional recovery post-operatively?
- Are there predictable psychological responses to certain illnesses, just as there are predictable reactions to grief?
- Is the intervention of the psychiatric liaison nurse cost-effective by decreasing complications?
- Does psychiatric liaison nursing intervention decrease the potential for patient care crises?
- Does psychiatric liaison nursing intervention prior to mutilating surgery influence recovery?
- Does the involvement of a psychiatric liaison nurse on the ward affect the number of formal psychiatric consultations?
- Does the practice of psychiatric liaison nursing influence the retention of nursing staff?

The possibilities are endless. Clinical practice can become mechanical without continued efforts to increase professional skills. The research process offers more than practical solutions to individual problems. Research allows the practitioner not only to systematically analyze clinical problems, but also provides intellectual stimulation. Currently, the nurse clinician and the nurse researcher are rarely the same. To bridge the gap between research and clinical practice in nursing, research must be meaningful on the one hand, and respected and valued on the other. Certainly not all questions can be addressed by research, but clinically sound data that is gathered to promote further investigation is a professional responsibility.

Nurses have in the past decade become more aware of the possibilities for independent practice. The increased opportunities for advanced education has in part made this possible. For example, the specialist educated at the master's level may practice as a clinician, a manager, an educator, or a consultant. The ANA program for certification of psychiatric nurses as generalists or specialists has the potential to strengthen the position of the independent practitioner. The purpose of certification is to acknowledge excellence and to establish standards and regulations for nurses practicing psychotherapy. The general awareness of the professional competency of the advanced psychiatric nurse becomes the precursor to independent practice.

Other factors have affected the development of independent practice. These include:

1. the cost-effectiveness of nurses,
2. the development of the clincal specialist,
3. the increasing number of available skilled nurses,
4. the women's liberation movement,
5. emphasis in health care on prevention, and
6. the influence of the economy.

The possibilities for independent practice are vast. Clinical nurse specialists may practice either together, or in an interdisciplinary group practice, or alone. Within that framework, psychiatric liaison nurses may work within an agency providing consultation. They may provide consultation-liaison services to other disciplines, contracting with hospitals, extended care facilities, nursing homes, VNAs, and the like. They may also independently provide consultation liaison services to private physicians or agencies.

The independent practice of psychiatric liaison nursing may include teaching or consultation to special programs. The following are illustrations of independent practice by the authors:

1. A federal grant for the further training of nurse practitioners, in the delivery of care to hypertensive patients, included the provision of a psychiatric liaison nurse as educator. Through consultation, the

psychiatric liaison nurse addressed the crucial issue of noncompliance. Patient interviews, case conferences, and didactic teaching seminars comprised the methodology to implement the goals of the grant.

2. An innovative program for the training of acute care technicians in the intensive care unit included the involvement of a psychiatric liaison nurse. These technicians had minimal prior experience working with patients. The stress of both the ICU and the integration of a new role in the hospital system were also recognized. The liaison nurse was integrated into the program at the onset.

3. Private psychiatric supervision to liaison nursing colleagues has been provided on a regular basis. Issues presented in supervision included patient problems, nursing care management, and systems problems. Supervisees have indicated the enormous value of this relationship both personally and professionally.

4. Psychiatric nursing consultation has been provided to physicians in their private practices in several ways. First, the psychological needs of a patient assume the highest priority. Second, the physicians have requested assistance because the psychological issues are affecting medical care. Third, the psychological needs of a patient are of less immediate concern, but they warrant evaluation and intervention.

5. Formal presentations concerning the psychological care of the medically ill have been requested by and provided to physicians in private group practice, religious groups, parents' groups, and organizations associated with specific diseases.

The supervision by liaison nurses of medical students, interns, and residents about psychological care occurs within university settings. This illustrates another potential for the liaison nurse to provide further consultation, sometimes on a private basis.

Some type of national health insurance may become a reality in this decade. The changes that this would promote in the care of the elderly, the needy, and the ill-served will provide continuing challenges to liaison nurses. The escalation of medical costs will focus more attention on cost-effective medical care. Nurses, long the recipient of low wages, will be stimulated to find creative ways both to provide care and to improve their professional status.

The future of psychiatric liaison nursing includes the further integration of principles of organizational development to the delivery of nursing care. Organizational development is closely associated with the idea that organizations are complex social systems, and questions about human behavior within the organization are viewed from the perspective of the social system [4]. Throughout this text, the social system and subsequent behaviors of patients and health care providers have been integrated into the theory and practice of psychiatric liaison nursing. The behavioral science consultant assists the organization to gain insight into its own processes, develop coping resources, and improve internal relationships [5]. Nurses with advanced preparation in organizational psychology would add a richer dimension to general nursing practice. Psychiatric liaison nurses with such knowledge and expertise would not only refine their clinical practice but also expand the scope of this specialty.

Psychiatric liaison nursing is stimulating, challenging, and receptive to the creative efforts of its practitioners. The future requires continued creativity, perserverance, education, and clinical sophistication. The possibilities in terms of role development, patient care, and professional self-esteem for both liaison nurses and their consultees are impressive. This specialty area in psychiatric nursing has been carved out. To sustain itself, however—to be well recognized, to mature, and to progress—it will need further refinement and continued involvement of the nursing profession. As the setting or delivery of health care is altered, new avenues for psychiatric liaison nursing practice will continue to emerge.

references

1. Richard Bernstein, "Liaison Psychiatry: A Model for Medical Care on a General Hospital Psychiatric Unit," *General Hospital Psychiatry* 2 (1980): 141.
2. Judith Kraush, "Nursing Research," chapter 10 in *Comprehensive Psychiatric Nursing* by Judith Haber et al. (New York: McGraw-Hill Book Company, 1978), p. 675.
3. Donna Diers, "This I Believe About Nursing Research," *Nursing Outlook* 18:11 (November 1970): 54.
4. E. Schein, *Organizational Psychology* (Englewood Cliffs, N.J.: Prentice-Hall, Inc., 1970), p. 3.
5. ———, p. 125.

bibliography

books

ALEXANDER, EDYTHE. *Nursing Administration in the Hospital Health Care System.* St. Louis: The C. V. Mosby Company, 1978.
BECKHARD, R. *Organization Development: Strategies and Models.* Reading, Mass.: Addison-Wesley Publishing Co., Inc., 1967.
BRINK, P. J. and WOOD, M. J. *Basic Steps in Planning Nursing Research.* Duxbury, Mass.: Duxbury Press, 1978.
HABER, J.; SCHUDY, S. M.; LEACH, A. M.; and SIDELEAU, B. F. *Comprehensive Psychiatric Nursing.* New York: McGraw-Hill Book Company, 1978.
JONAS, STEVEN, ed. *Health Care Delivery in the United States.* New York: Springer Publishing Co., 1977.

KALLISCH, PHILIP and KALLISCH, BEATRICE. *The Advance of American Nursing*. Boston: Little, Brown & Company, 1978.

KJERVIK, D. and MARTINSON, I. *Women in Stress: A Nursing Perspective*. New York: Appleton-Century-Crofts, 1979.

MUNDINGER, MARY. *Autonomy in Nursing*. Germantown, Md.: Aspen Systems Corporation, 1980.

O'TOOLE, ANITA. "Psychiatric Nursing," chapter 50, in *Comprehensive Textbook of Psychiatry*, Vol. 3, edited by H. Kaplan, A. Freedman, and B. Sadock. Baltimore: Williams and Wilkins, 1980, pp. 3001–3004.

POLIT, D. F. and HUNGLER, B. P. *Nursing Research: Principles and Methods*. Philadelphia: J. B. Lippincott Company, 1978.

SCHEIN, E. *Organizational Psychology*. Englewood Cliffs, N.J.: Prentice-Hall, Inc., 1979.

STUART, GAIL and SUNDEEN, SANDRA. *Principle and Practice of Psychiatric Nursing*. St. Louis: The C. V. Mosby Company, 1979.

articles

BARSKY, A. "Hidden Reasons Some Patients Visit Doctors," *Annals of Internal Medicine* 94:4 (April 1981): 492–498.

BUTLER, ROBERT. "Psychiatry and the Elderly: An Overview," *American Journal of Psychiatry* 132:9 (September 1975): 893–900.

CETA AMENDMENTS OF 1978. P. L. 95-524, Vocational Education Projects Under Section 204, Acute Care Technicians Training.

HAMILTON, M. "Mentorhood: A Key to Nursing Leadership," *Nursing Leadership* 4:1 (March 1981): 4–13.

JACOX, ADA. "Nursing Research and the Clinician," *Nursing Outlook* 22:6 (1974): 382–385.

KJERVIK, DIANE. "Women, Nursing and Leadership," *Image* 11:2 (June 1979): 34–36.

KRANT, MELVIN; DOSTER, NANCY; and PLOOF, SUSAN. "Meeting the Needs of the Late-Stage Elderly Cancer Patient: A Clinical Model," *Journal of Geriatric Psychiatry* 13:1 (1980): 53–62.

PHILIPS, JOHN R. "Health Care Provider Relationships: A Matter of Reciprocity," *Nursing Outlook* (November 1979): 738–741.

ROCHE, GERARD. "Much Ado About Mentors," *Harvard Business Review* (January–February 1979): 14–28.

SALMON, J. WARREN and BERLINER, HOWARD S. "Health Policy Implications of the Holistic Health Movement," *Journal of Health Politics, Policy and Law* 5:3 (Fall 1980): 535–553.

SPAN, PAULA. "Where Have All the Nurses Gone?" *New York Times Magazine* (February 22, 1981): 70.

STACHYRA, MARCIA. "Self-Regulation Through Certification," *Perspectives in Psychiatric Care* 11:4 (October–November–December 1973): 148–154.

STICKNEY, S. and HALL, Q. "The Role of the Nurse on a Consultation Liaison Team," *Psychosomatics* 22:3 (March 1981): 224–235.

VANCE, CONNIE. "Women Leaders: Modern Day Heroines or Social Deviants," *Image* 11:2 (June 1979): 37–41.

ZISOOK, S. and GAMMON, E. "Medical Noncompliance," *International Journal of Psychiatry in Medicine* 10:4 (1980–81): 291–303.

index